New Insights into Epidemiology

New Insights into Epidemiology

Edited by **Tony Andrew**

hayle medical

New York

Published by Hayle Medical,
30 West, 37th Street, Suite 612,
New York, NY 10018, USA
www.haylemedical.com

New Insights into Epidemiology
Edited by Tony Andrew

International Standard Book Number: 978-1-63241-298-0 (Hardback)

Printed in the United States of America.

Contents

Preface

Epidemiology is the scientific discipline that focuses on the study of the patterns, causes, and effects of health and disease conditions in various sets of defined populations. Epidemiology studies also rate of occurrence of diseases in different groups of people and their reasons. Epidemiological data is used to plan and evaluate strategies and policies towards prevention of illnesses and as a manual to the management of disease stricken patients. There are various areas of epidemiological study that include outbreak investigation, disease etiology, bio-monitoring, disease surveillance and screening and comparisons of treatment effects such as in clinical trials. Epidemiology is also an interdisciplinary field that often relies on other scientific disciplines like biology to better understand and grasp disease processes, social sciences to better understand proximate and distal causes, engineering for exposure assessment and statistics to make efficient use of the data and draw appropriate conclusions. This field can be said to be one of the cornerstones of public health, and is a foundation in policy decisions as well as helping in identifying risk factors for disease and targets for preventive healthcare. Epidemiologists often facilitate study design, interpretation and dissemination of results as well as collection and statistical analysis of data. Epidemiological research has thus helped in developing methodologies used in public health studies, clinical research and basic research in the biological sciences.

This book is an attempt to compile and collate all available research on epidemiology under one umbrella. I am grateful to those who put their hard work, effort and expertise into these research projects as well as those who were supportive in this endeavor.

Editor

1

Epidemiology of Multi-Drug Resistant Organisms in a Teaching Hospital in Oman: A One-Year Hospital-Based Study

Abdullah Balkhair,[1] Yahya M. Al-Farsi,[2] Zakariya Al-Muharrmi,[1] Raiya Al-Rashdi,[1] Mansoor Al-Jabri,[1] Fatma Neilson,[1] Sara S. Al-Adawi,[3] Marah El-Beeli,[2] and Samir Al-Adawi[4]

[1] *Department of Infection Control, Sultan Qaboos University Hospital, Sultan Qaboos University, Muscat, Oman*
[2] *Department of Family Medicine and Public Health, College of Medicine and Health Sciences, Sultan Qaboos University, P.O. Box 35, P.C. 123 Al-Khoud, Muscat, Oman*
[3] *Oman Medical College, Sohar Campus, Al Tareef, Sohar, Oman*
[4] *Department of Behavioral Medicine, College of Medicine and Health Sciences, Sultan Qaboos University, Muscat, Oman*

Correspondence should be addressed to Yahya M. Al-Farsi; ymfarsi@squ.edu.om

Academic Editors: J. L. Fisher, G.-X. Jiang, H. K. T. Ng, and M. Schootman

Background. Antimicrobial resistance is increasingly recognized as a global challenge. A few studies have emerged on epidemiology of multidrug resistant organisms in tertiary care settings in the Arabian Gulf. *Aim.* To describe the epidemiology of multi-drug resistant organisms (MDRO) at Sultan Qaboos University Hospital, a tertiary hospital in Oman. *Methods.* A retrospective review of MDRO records has been conducted throughout the period from January 2012 till December 2012. Organisms were identified and tested by an automated identification and susceptibility system, and the antibiotic susceptibility testing was confirmed by the disk diffusion method. *Results.* Out of the total of 29,245 admissions, there have been 315 patients registered as MDRO patients giving an overall prevalence rate of 10.8 (95% CI 9.3, 12.4) MDRO cases per 1000 admissions. In addition, the prevalence rate of MDRO isolates was 11.2 (95% CI 9.7, 12.9) per 1000 admissions. Overall, increasing trends in prevalence rates of MDRO patients and MDRO isolates were observed throughout the study period. *Conclusion.* Antimicrobial resistance is an emerging challenge in Oman. Continuous monitoring of antimicrobial susceptibility and strict adherence to infection prevention guidelines are essential to prevent proliferation of MDRO. Along such quest, stringent antibiotic prescription guidelines are needed in the country.

1. Introduction

Data emerging from different parts of the world have suggested that strains of highly multidrug resistant organisms (MDRO) have quadrupled in the past decade [1, 2]. MDRO are increasingly being recognized to be impervious to available antibiotics. When MDRO afflict a vulnerable individual, the risk of morbidity and mortality is heightened. This has other insidious negative repercussions including lengthening of hospital stay and increase in social and medical costs due to the emergence of MDRO [3, 4]. Prior to the turn of the century, among the healthcare planners, there was enthusiasm that there will be "Health for all by the year 2000" [5]. In retrospect, this was a far-fetched aspiration. Barely two decades into a new century, there were proliferations of infectious diseases which render the standard of public health in many parts of the world equivalent to preantibiotic era [6].

There are likely to be myriads of factors that contribute to the rising tide of nosocomial infections. Firstly, the many attempts to find alternative means including bacteriophage [7] and immune-enhancing strategies [8] have not been found to be a practical adjunct antibiotic. Secondly, the development of "new generation of antibiotics" has been hampered with existing regulations that are not amenable for the development of new antibiotics such as the lack of scientific strategies to develop new class of antibiotics [9–11]. For these reasons, there has been a long lull on the development of new antibiotics. Some critics have also argued that pharmaceutical companies have little incentive to invest in what could be an enormously costly venture to develop new antibiotics, while the profit margin of the newly developed antibiotics is lower compared to "lifestyle" medications [12]. Thirdly, there is strong indication that the global proliferation of strains of multidrug resistant bacteria may partly stem from the fact that there is pervasive overuse and misuse of antimicrobial agents [13]. There has been a universal call of judicious use of antimicrobial agents, but such message appears to be unheeded, as emergence of various strains of intractable and antibiotic resistant organism appears to be proliferating in different parts of the world [6]. Fourthly, present proliferation of different strains of multidrug resistant organisms is limited to not only overuse in humans, but also the significant contribution of antibiotic resistant organism in food supply due to overuse/abuse of antibiotics for treatment, prevention, and growth promotion in animals [14]. As yet, there are no feasible strategies to reduce antibiotic-resistant organism from entering the food chain [15].

In the age of globalization, advances in transportation and telecommunications infrastructure have not only increased cross-cultural and technological interchange and aided in the diffusion of organisms from one region to another, but also created fertile ground for internationalization of multidrug resistant bacteria. Oman, a country in the southern tip of the Arabian Peninsula, overlooking the continent of Asia and Africa, represent the place where globalization and Arabia intertwine. According to the 2010 census [16], its population is estimated to be 2,773,479. The country is classified by the World Bank as a "high-income economy" among the emerging economies [17]. Recent affluence due to exploitation of hydrocarbon has turned Oman as a hub for international shipment and trade. The country has attracted a number of foreign workers from different parts of the world, with all the consequences this may entail in terms of human, animal, and material exchanges as testified by infections that were linked to zoonotic events [18]. Some preliminary studies have alluded to the existence of MDRO. In the year 2005, Al-Muharrmi et al. [19] evaluated extended-spectrum β-lactamase (ESBL) isolates in a pediatric population in Oman. For over 12-month period of observation, the authors found that 13.3% of *E. coli* and 6.6% of *Klebsiella pneumoniae* isolated were ESBL producers. The study concluded that ESBL-producing organisms are becoming a major problem in Omani children. In reference to the pediatric population, Al-Muharrmi and colleagues [20] also investigated the *in vitro* activity of carbapenems, piperacillin-tazobactam, and ciprofloxacin alone or in combination with aminoglycosides against ESBL-producing strains isolated from clinical samples. It was found that ESBLs have high resistance profiles against piperacillin/tazobactam and ciprofloxacin. The study concluded that the ESBLs from Oman have a similar resistance pattern to those reported from the UK and USA. Other studies in the regions have also pointed out the emergence of multidrug resistant organisms [21–23]. More recently, Aly and Balkhy [24] have synthesized the prevailing situation in the region by reviewing published articles on nosocomial infections. These authors identified a total of 45 articles published between 1990 and 2011. On the whole, the review indicates emergence of MDRO. Accordingly, *Escherichia coli, Klebsiella pneumoniae, Pseudomonas aeruginosa*, methicillin-resistant *Staphylococcus aureus, Acinetobacter C. difficile,* and *Enterococcus* do exist in the region with variable rates of such strains of MDRO. Most of the studies have focused on one particular subspecialty of clinical departments. Studies are needed to garner comprehensive view, for example, of tertiary care hospitals where attendees of such hospitals are likely to have advanced pathology of the disease and to be highly immunocompromised and, therefore, more prone to succumb to vagaries of MDRO. Therefore, exploring epidemiology and types of multidrug resistant organisms in a tertiary care is imperative. Oman represents a fertile ground for such undertaking. To our knowledge, there is no previous comprehensive document of MDRO in Oman.

In order to consolidate the available information of MDRO in a tertiary care setting in Oman, this study aims to address the monthly cumulative frequencies and prevalence rates of hospital-acquired multidrug resistant organisms during the year of 2012. It also aims to describe the distribution of hospital-acquired MDRO by site of infection and types of bacteria.

2. Methods

A retrospective review was conducted to all reports of Gram-negative and Gram-positive isolates from all units at SQUH which is a 570-bed tertiary care teaching hospital in Muscat, Oman. The study has been conducted for a period from January 2012 to December 2012.

Gram-negative and Gram-positive organisms were identified and tested. Definition of MDRO was based on the recently proposed joint definition by the European Center for Disease Prevention and Control (ECDC) and the Centers for Disease Prevention and Control (CDC) [25].

Two prevalence rates were calculated: (1) prevalence rate of MDRO patients and (2) prevalence rate of MDRO isolates. Both prevalence rates were calculated by dividing the number of cases with index by number of monthly inpatient admissions for the whole year. The prevalence rates were reported per 1,000 admissions. The 95% confidence intervals (95% CI) of prevalence rates were calculated using the Poisson distribution method of binomial variables. The 95% CI were calculated using the GraphPad Prism 6.0 software.

The trend in the prevalence rates over a 12-month period was calculated and analyzed to identify a statistically significant increasing or decreasing trend using the Cochran-Armitage test for trend, and a cutoff value for statistical significance was taken at P value of 0.05. Statistical Package for Social Sciences (SPSS) (version 20.0, IBM) was used for all statistical analyses. Ethical approval for this study was obtained from the Institutional Review Board of Sultan Qaboos University, Medical Research Ethics Committee at College of Medicine and Health Sciences.

3. Results

Table 1 shows the cumulative frequencies and rates of hospital-acquired MDRO among patients and isolates at

Table 1: Cumulative frequencies and rates of hospital-acquired multidrug resistant organisms (MDRO) among patients and isolates at SQUH, Oman, 2012.

Month	Total admissions	MDRO patients	MDRO isolates	Rate per patient *R* (95% CI)[a]	Rate per isolate *R* (95% CI)[a]
January	2699	25	21	9.3 (4.8, 11.9)	7.8 (5.9, 11.9)
February	2506	19	16	7.6 (3.6, 10.4)	6.4 (4.4, 12.0)
March	2506	31	28	12.4 (7.6, 16.4)	11.2 (8.4, 17.6)
April	2561	9	7	2.7 (16.0, 28.1)	2.7 (1.2, 5.5)
May	2523	19	21	7.5 (4.4, 11.9)	8.3 (5.2, 12.7)
June	2488	10	11	4.0 (2.0, 7.2)	4.4 (2.0, 8.0)
July	2405	15	16	6.2 (3.3, 10.0)	6.7 (3.7, 10.8)
August	2150	13	16	6.0 (3.3, 10.2)	7.4 (4.2, 12.1)
September	2347	36	51	15.3 (10.7, 21.3)	21.7 (16.2, 28.2)
October	2255	40	51	17.7 (12.9, 23.9)	22.6 (16.9, 29.7)
November	2374	29	39	12.2 (8.0, 17.7)	16.4 (11.8, 22.3)
December	2431	33	42	13.6 (9.5, 18.9)	17.3 (12.3, 23.4)
Total	29245	315	329	10.8 (9.3, 12.4)	11.2 (9.7, 12.9)

[a]Rate calculated per 1000 admissions.

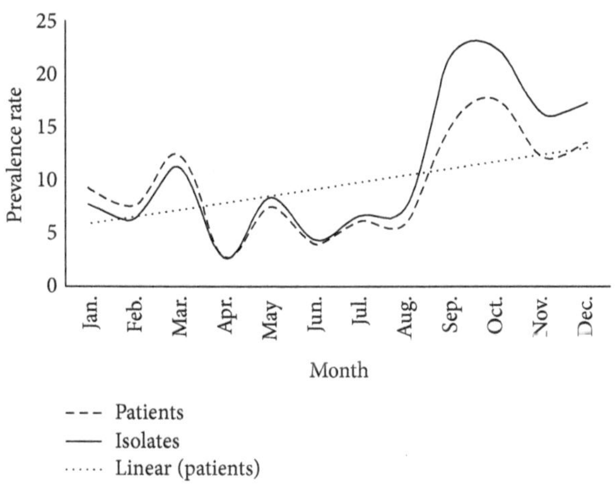

Figure 1: Prevalence rates of hospital-acquired multidrug resistant organisms (MDRO) at SQUH, Oman, 2012.

SQUH during the year of 2012. Overall and of the total of 29,245 admissions, there has been 315 patients who were registered as hosting MDRO, giving an overall prevalence rate of 10.8 (95% CI 9.3, 12.4) MDRO cases per 1000 admissions. In addition, there were 329 registered MDRO isolates giving a prevalence rate of 11.2 (95% CI 9.7, 12.9) MDRO isolates per 1000 admissions. The lowest prevalence rate was observed in June (4.0; 95% CI 2.0, 7.2), while the highest prevalence rate was observed in October (17.7; 95% CI 12.9, 23.9).

As shown in Figure 1, the prevalence rates of MDRO patients and isolates were relatively steady throughout the period from January to August 2012. In September, there was an abrupt increase in the prevalence rates which continuously elevated until the end of the year. Overall, the increasing trends for prevalence rates of MDRO patients and MDRO isolates were both found to be statistically significant (trend, $P = 0.04$, $P = 0.03$, resp.).

Table 2: Distribution of hospital-acquired multidrug resistant organisms by site of infection at tertiary care centre in Oman, 2012.

Site of infection	*N* (Total = 329)	%
Bloodstream infection	81	24.6
Pneumonia	80	24.3
Urinary tract infection	62	18.8
Surgical infection	32	9.7
Others	74	22.5

Table 2 depicts that bloodstream infection and pneumonia were the most frequently occurring infections caused by hospital-acquired MDRO (24.6% and 24.3%, resp.) followed by urinary tract infection (UTI) (18.8%). Surgical infections were encountered among 9.7% of all MDRO affected patients.

As illustrated in Table 3, the number of types of bacteria was nine, namely, *Acinetobacter baumannii*, methicillin-resistant *S. aureus* (MRSA), *Escherichia coli*, *Escherichia coli* (CRE), *Klebsiella pneuminae*, *Klebsiella pneumoniae* (ESBL), *Enterobacter*, *Pseudomonas*, *Enterococcus* (VRE), *Burkholderia*, and *Stenotrophomonas maltophilia*. *Acinetobacter baumannii* was the most prevalent MDRO among the isolates (32.4%). *E. coli* comes next with a percentage of 18.4% followed by methicillin-resistant *S. aureus* (MRSA) (10.6%) and *Klebsiella pneumoniae* (ESBL) (10.3%). The frequencies of *Pseudomonas aeruginosa*, *Klebsiella pneumoniae* (CRE), and *Stenotrophomonas maltophilia* were nearly equal (8.1%, 7.8%, and 7.5%, resp.). The rest were encountered at a frequency of less than 2%.

4. Discussion

It has been estimated that nosocomial infections annually contract around two million in North America with a significant number of them requiring critical care. The colonization of MDRO tends to have an unexpectedly high rate of

Table 3: Distribution of hospital-acquired multidrug resistant organisms (MDRO) by type of bacteria at a tertiary care hospital in Oman, 2012.

Type of bacteria	N (Total = 329)	%
Acinetobacter baumannii	107	32.4
Escherichia coli (ESBL)	60	18.4
Methicillin-resistant *Staphylococcus aureus*	35	10.6
Klebsiella pneumoniae (ESBL)	34	10.3
Pseudomonas aeruginosa	27	8.1
Klebsiella pneumoniae (CRE)	26	7.8
Stenotrophomonas maltophilia	25	7.5
Escherichia coli (CRE)	5	1.6
Burkholderia cepacia	5	1.6
Enterobacter cloacae	4	1.2
Enterococcus faecalis/faecium (VRE)	2	0.6

ESBL: extended spectrum β-lactamases; VRE: vancomycin-resistant *Enterococcus*; CRE: carbapenem-resistant *Enterobacteriaceae*.

morbidity and mortality. The social, economic, and medical cost of nosocomial infections mount to a huge financial cost [26]. Such situation is not limited to North America; there are preliminary studies indicating that healthcare-associated infections constitute a global challenge in the GCC countries [27]. Previous surveys of Omani healthcare-associated infections were limited to specific clinical populations [19, 20]. To our knowledge, this study is the first of its kind that comprehensively explores monthly variations, prevalence rates, sites of infection, and type of MDRO in a tertiary care hospital.

As for the first hypothesis regarding monthly variations, there was an average of 2437 admissions with approximately 22.4 patients with MDRO and approximately 27 isolates, suggesting that some afflicted individuals have had more than one organism. There is a strong indication that climatic factors tend to influence the rate of nosocomial infections [28]. This study indicates that the nosocomial infections are invariably affected by the weather. In this study, healthcare-associated infections were shown to tend to dwindle in summer. In support of this, the summer season which normally peaks from April to September appears to be associated with fewer incidents of healthcare-associated infections. If this finding would withstand further scrutiny, countermeasures to mitigate healthcare-associated infections should consider factors such as monthly variation and the climatic conditions under which infections are more likely to occur.

The second related aim of this study is to gauge prevalence rates of hospital-acquired multidrug resistant organisms. Overall, the prevalence rate of MDRO patients was found to be 10.8 per 1000 admissions. There has been considerable variation in reported prevalence estimates of MDRO worldwide that ranged from 6 and 31 per 1000 admissions [29]. Despite that, all reports documented an increasing trend over the last few years. The prevalence of MDRO reported in this study was 10.8 per 1000 admissions, which falls within the international range. Estimation of prevalence is of great importance as it provides the health authorities with reliable data to plan adequate health care measures. This study indicates an increasing trend throughout 12 months of observation. In addition to climatic conditions, the increased prevalence of MDRO has been linked to antimicrobial use, inadequate antimicrobial therapy, and long antimicrobial exposures that may trigger emergence of resistance in a bacterium that was previously amenable to antibiotics. There is strong evidence suggesting that contaminated healthcare workers' hands or environmental surfaces may play a role in exacerbating MDRO [30]. Other factors associated with MDRO include gender, underlying comorbidity as well as those who are exposed to medical gadgets that cross different anatomical sites and breach the body's natural physical barriers, such as mechanical ventilations and catheters [31, 32].

The third aim of this study is to quantify the distribution of sites of infection at this particular tertiary care. The commonest site of MDRO infection was bloodstream and pneumonia. El-Saed et al. [33] reported that the most common sites in their study in Saudi Intensive Care Unit at a tertiary hospital for MDRO were respiratory and blood. Similar pattern was observed in other countries including Italy [34] and Finland [35]. However, other studies have pointed out different distributions for sites of MDRO infection. For example, Jaggi [36] traced bacterial cultures over a period of 45 months in a tertiary care hospital in Haryana, India. It was found that MDRO was isolated mostly from urine cultures which constituted 38% of the total bacterial cultures. Although the emergence of MDRO is a global phenomenon, it is likely to be across populations and geographical variations. Therefore, it was not surprising that, in Oman, the rate of MDRO appears to have monthly variations.

The final related aim of this study was to survey the commonest types of MDRO. Decades of research have identified various common multidrug resistant organisms including Vancomycin-resistant *Enterococci*, MRSA, *Klebsiella pneumonia*, carbapenemase producing Gram-negatives, *Enterococcus faecium*, *Staphylococcus aureus*, *Acinetobacter baumannii*, as well as those that fall under the broad category of multidrug resistant gram-negative rods. The most common MDRO were those related to *Enterobacter* species, *Acinetobacter baumannii*. The reported array of organisms in this study has similarities with other studies conducted in theregion. In an attempt to review the prevalence of antibiotic resistance in the GCC countries and the reasons behind this phenomenon, Aly and Balkhy [24] reported that the most prevalent microorganism was *E. coli* (44%) followed by *K. pneumoniae* (20%) and *P. aeruginosa* (18.7%). MRSA and *Acinetobacter* were found to be less frequently observed by nearly equal percentages (5.4% and 5%, resp.). In a previous study done on patients admitted to ICU in Riyadh Military Hospital in Saudi Arabia, similar isolates were obtained among which *Acinetobacter baumannii* was the most common MDRO (40.9%). In Saudi Arabia also, El Tahawy and Khalaf [37] evaluated 100 isolates and found that *P. aeruginosa*, *K. pneumoniae*, *E. coli*, and *Enterobacter* were the most commonly isolated, with imipenem, ciprofloxacin, and amikacin showing greatest efficacy. Another study carried out at a tertiary care hospital in Riyadh [38] over a one-year period showed the most frequent pathogens to be *P. aeruginosa, E. coli, S. aureus, K. pneumoniae*, and *S. marcescens*.

Our study is not without limitations. This single center study data may not reflect the MDRO prevalence trend in Oman as a whole. Therefore, a multisite study would be essential in order to lay groundwork for comparison between different healthcare settings. Another limitation is lack of certainty that all clinical specimens represented active infection. Not all of the isolates may represent active infections from the patients. In addition, we did not correlate the samples to admission data for each patient/clinical specimen, so we were unable to provide a more accurate description of community versus nosocomial onset of infection. Studies with more robust methodology would be needed in order to generalize the present findings.

In conclusion, this study demonstrated an increasing trend of MDRO in Oman, with an array of organisms that was similar to those reported in neighboring countries. These findings call for the prompt necessity in developing nationwide antibiotic policy and guidelines, which is essential nowadays due to the increasing resistance patterns. In addition, it calls for developing a local antibiogram database which will improve the knowledge of antimicrobial resistance patterns in Oman and will also help to improve treatment strategies based on unit-specific data.

Conflict of Interests

The authors declare that there is no conflict of interests regarding the work and the content of this study.

References

[1] Centers for Disease Control and Prevention, "Vital signs: carbapenem-resistant enterobacteriaceae," Morbidity and Mortality Weekly Report (MMWR), 2013, http://www.cdc.gov/mmwr/preview/mmwrhtml/mm6209a3.

[2] M. L. Cohen, "Changing patterns of infectious disease," *Nature*, vol. 406, no. 6797, pp. 762–767, 2000.

[3] L. H. Rosenberger, T. Hranjec, A. D. Politano et al., "Effective cohorting and "superisolation" in a single intensive care unit in response to an outbreak of diverse multi-drug-resistant organisms," *Surgical Infections*, vol. 12, no. 5, pp. 345–350, 2011.

[4] E. Morales, F. Cots, M. Sala et al., "Hospital costs of nosocomial multi-drug resistant Pseudomonas aeruginosa acquisition," *BMC Health Services Research*, vol. 12, article 122, 2012.

[5] H. Mahler, "The meaning of "health for all by the year 2000""," *World Health Forum*, vol. 2, no. 1, pp. 5–22, 1981.

[6] C. A. Arias and B. E. Murray, "Antibiotic-resistant bugs in the 21st century: a clinical super-challenge," *The New England Journal of Medicine*, vol. 360, no. 5, pp. 439–443, 2009.

[7] S. Matsuzaki, M. Rashel, J. Uchiyama et al., "Bacteriophage therapy: a revitalized therapy against bacterial infectious diseases," *Journal of Infection and Chemotherapy*, vol. 11, no. 5, pp. 211–219, 2005.

[8] B. Spellberg, J. G. Bartlett, and D. N. Gilbert, "The future of antibiotics and resistance," *The New England Journal of Medicine*, vol. 368, no. 4, pp. 299–302, 2013.

[9] G. Devasahayam, W. M. Scheld, and P. S. Hoffman, "Newer antibacterial drugs for a new century," *Expert Opinion on Investigational Drugs*, vol. 19, no. 2, pp. 215–234, 2010.

[10] A. R. M. Coates and Y. Hu, "Novel approaches to developing new antibiotics for bacterial infections," *British Journal of Pharmacology*, vol. 152, no. 8, pp. 1147–1154, 2007.

[11] R. M. Echols, "A long and winding road, evolution of antimicrobial drug development: crisis management," *Expert Review of Anti-Infective Therapy*, vol. 10, no. 11, pp. 1311–1319, 2012.

[12] D. M. Shlaes and B. Spellberg, "Overcoming the challenges to developing new antibiotics," *Current Opinion in Pharmacology*, vol. 12, no. 5, pp. 522–526, 2012.

[13] A. Alumran and X. Y. Hou, "Hurst assessing the overuse of antibiotics in children in Saudi Arabia: validation of the parental perception on antibiotics scale (PAPA scale)," *Health and Quality of Life Outcomes*, vol. 11, article 39, 2013.

[14] C. Verraes, S. van Boxstael, E. van Meervenne et al., "Antimicrobial resistance in the food chain: a review," *International Journal of Environmental Research and Public Health*, vol. 10, no. 7, pp. 2643–2669, 2013.

[15] J. M. Rolain, "Food and human gut as reservoirs of transferable antibiotic resistance encoding genes," *Frontiers in Microbiology*, vol. 4, article 173, 2013.

[16] Central Intelligence Agency, *The World Factbook: Oman*, 2013, http://www.umsl.edu/services/govdocs/wofact2001/geos/mu.html.

[17] The World Bank. Oman, 2013, http://data.worldbank.org/country/oman.

[18] C. Reusken, B. L. Haagmans, M. üller MA et al., "Middle East respiratory syndrome coronavirus neutralising serum antibodies in dromedary camels: a comparative serological study," *The Lancet Infectious Diseases*, vol. 13, no. 10, pp. 859–866, 2013.

[19] Z. Al-Muharrmi, A. Rafay, A. Balkhair, and A. A. Jabri, "Antibiotic combination as empirical therapy for extended spectrum beta-lactamase," *Oman Medical Journal*, vol. 23, no. 2, pp. 78–81, 2008.

[20] Z. Al Muharrmi, A. M. Rafay, A. Balkhair, S. Al-Tamemi, A. Al Mawali, and H. Al Sadiri, "Extended-spectrum β-lactamase (ESBL) in Omani children: study of prevalence, risk factors and clinical outcomes at Sultan Qaboos University Hospital, Sultanate of Oman," *Sultan Qaboos University Medical Journal*, vol. 8, no. 2, pp. 171–177, 2008.

[21] N. K. Saeed, A. M. Kambal, and N. A. El-Khizzi, "Antimicrobial-resistant bacteria in a general intensive care unit in Saudi Arabia," *Saudi Medical Journal*, vol. 31, no. 12, pp. 1341–1349, 2010.

[22] A. M. Somily, "Comparison of E-test and disc diffusion methods for the in vitro evaluation of the antimicrobial activity of colistin in multi-drug resistant gram-negative bacilli," *Saudi Medical Journal*, vol. 31, no. 5, pp. 507–511, 2010.

[23] A. M. Somily, A. S. Al-Khattaf, and A. M. Kambal, "Antimicrobial activity of tigecycline against bacterial isolates from intensive care units in a teaching hospital in Central Saudi Arabia," *Saudi Medical Journal*, vol. 31, no. 1, pp. 18–24, 2010.

[24] M. Aly and H. H. Balkhy, "The prevalence of antimicrobial resistance in clinical isolates from Gulf Corporation Council countries," *Antimicrobial Resistance and Infection Control*, vol. 1, no. 1, article 26, 2012.

[25] A.-P. Magiorakos, A. Srinivasan, R. B. Carey et al., "Multidrug-resistant, extensively drug-resistant and pandrug-resistant bacteria: an international expert proposal for interim standard

definitions for acquired resistance," *Clinical Microbiology and Infection*, vol. 18, no. 3, pp. 268–281, 2012.

[26] D. R. Scott, *The Direct Medical Costs of Healthcare-Associated Infections in U.S.Hospitals and the Benefits of Prevention*, 2009, http://www.cdc.gov/hai/pdfs/hai/scott_costpaper.pdf.

[27] H. H. Balkhy, M. S. Bawazeer, R. F. Kattan et al., "Epidemiology of Acinetobacter spp.-associated healthcare infections and colonization among children at a tertiary-care hospital in Saudi Arabia: a 6-year retrospective cohort study," *European Journal of Clinical Microbiology and Infectious Diseases*, vol. 31, no. 10, pp. 2645–2651, 2012.

[28] Y. A. Al-Tonbary, O. E. Soliman, M. M. Sarhan et al., "Nosocomial infections and fever of unknown origin in pediatric hematology/oncology unit: a retrospective annual study," *World Journal of Pediatrics*, vol. 7, no. 1, pp. 60–64, 2011.

[29] M. Rodríguez-Créixems, L. Alcalá, P. Muñoz, E. Cercenado, and T. Vicente, "Bouza Bloodstream infections: evolution and trends in the microbiology workload, incidence, and etiology, 1985–2006," *Medicine*, vol. 87, no. 4, pp. 234–249, 2008.

[30] G. Bearman, A. E. Rosato, T. M. Duane et al., "Trial of universal gloving with emollient-impregnated gloves to promote skin health and prevent the transmission of multidrug-resistant organisms in a surgical intensive care unit," *Infection Control and Hospital Epidemiology*, vol. 31, no. 5, pp. 491–497, 2010.

[31] P.-R. Hsueh, L.-J. Teng, P.-C. Yang, S.-W. Ho, and K.-T. Luh, "Emergence of nosocomial candidemia at a teaching hospital in Taiwan from 1981 to 2000: increased susceptibility of Candida species to fluconazole," *Microbial Drug Resistance*, vol. 8, no. 4, pp. 311–319, 2002.

[32] Y. Fukuta, R. R. Muder, M. E. Agha et al., "Risk factors for acquisition of multidrug-resistant *Acinetobacter baumannii* among cancer patients," *American Journal of Infection Control*, vol. 41, no. 12, pp. 1249–1252, 2013.

[33] A. El-Saed, H. H. Balkhy, H. M. Al-Dorzi, R. Khan, A. H. Rishu, and Y. M. Arabi, "Acinetobacter is the most common pathogen associated with late-onset and recurrent ventilator-associated pneumonia in an adult intensive care unit in Saudi Arabia," *International Journal of Infectious Diseases*, vol. 17, no. 9, pp. e696–e701, 2013.

[34] S. Esposito and S. Leone, "Antimicrobial treatment for intensive care unit (ICU) infections including the role of the infectious disease specialist," *International Journal of Antimicrobial Agents*, vol. 29, no. 5, pp. 494–500, 2007.

[35] P. Ylipalosaari, T. I. Ala-Kokko, J. Laurila, P. Ohtonen, and H. Syrjälä, "Epidemiology of intensive care unit (ICU)-acquired infections in a 14-month prospective cohort study in a single mixed Scandinavian university hospital ICU," *Acta Anaesthesiologica Scandinavica*, vol. 50, no. 10, pp. 1192–1197, 2006.

[36] N. Jaggi, P. Sissodia, and L. Sharma, "Control of multidrug resistant bacteria in a tertiary care hospital in India," *Antimicrobial Resistance and Infection Control*, vol. 1, no. 1, article 23, 2012.

[37] A. T. A. E. El Tahawy and R. M. F. Khalaf, "Antibiotic resistance among gram-negative non-fermentative bacteria at a teaching hospital in Saudi Arabia," *Journal of Chemotherapy*, vol. 13, no. 3, pp. 260–264, 2001.

[38] S. M. H. Qadri, J. Akhter, and G. C. Lee, "Etiology of ICU infections and antibiogram of the isolates at a referral center in Riyadh," *Saudi Pharmaceutical Journal*, vol. 4, no. 3-4, pp. 174–178, 1996.

2

Risk of Coronary Heart Disease among HIV-Infected Patients: A Multicenter Study in Brazil

Sandra C. Fuchs,[1,2,3] Paulo R. Alencastro,[3] Maria Letícia R. Ikeda,[1] Nêmora T. Barcellos,[1,3] Fernando H. Wolff,[1,3] Ajácio B. M. Brandão,[3] Ricardo A. A. Ximenes,[3,4] Demócrito de B. Miranda-Filho,[3,4,5] Heloísa Ramos Lacerda,[5] Maria de Fátima P. M. de Albuquerque,[6] Ulisses Ramos Montarroyos,[7] Max W. Nery,[8] and Marilia D. Turchi[3,8]

[1] *Postgraduate Studies Program in Cardiology, School of Medicine, Clinical Research Center, No. 5 Andar, Hospital de Clinicas de Porto Alegre, Universidade Federal do Rio Grande do Sul, Rua Ramiro Barcelos 2350, 90035-903 Porto Alegre, RS, Brazil*

[2] *Postgraduate Studies Program in Epidemiology, School of Medicine, Universidade Federal do Rio Grande do Sul, 90035-003 Porto Alegre, RS, Brazil*

[3] *National Institute for Health Technology Assessment (IATS/CNPq), Hospital de Clinicas de Porto Alegre, 90035-903 Porto Alegre, RS, Brazil*

[4] *Department of Clinical Medicine, Universidade de Pernambuco, 50670-901 Recife, PE, Brazil*

[5] *Department of Tropical Medicine, Universidade Federal de Pernambuco, 50610-110 Recife, PE, Brazil*

[6] *Research Center Aggeu Magalhães, Fundação Oswaldo Cruz, 50.670-420 Recife, PE, Brazil*

[7] *Institute of Biological Sciences, Universidade de Pernambuco, 50670-901 Recife, PE, Brazil*

[8] *Institute of Tropical Pathology and Public Health, Universidade Federal de Goiás, 74605050 Goiania, GO, Brazil*

Correspondence should be addressed to Sandra C. Fuchs; scfuchs@terra.com.br

Academic Editors: A. Mosavi-Jarrahi, E. A. Okiro, and E. Paci

Cardiovascular disease has emerged as a crescent problem among HIV-infected population. This study aimed to determine the 10-year risk of coronary heart disease using the Framingham risk score among HIV-infected patients from three regions of Brazil. This is a pooled analysis of three cohort studies, which enrolled 3,829 individuals, 59% were men, 66% had white skin color, and mean age 39.0 ± 9.9 years. Comparisons among regions showed that there were marked differences in demographic, socioeconomic, clinical, and HIV-related characteristics. Prevalence of Framingham score ≥10 was 4.5% in the Southern, 4.2% in the Midwest, and 3.9% in the Northeast of Brazil. The Framingham score ≥10 was similar between regions for males, patients aged ≥60 years, with obesity, central obesity, hypertension, and diabetes mellitus. Women were three times more likely to have coronary heart disease in 10 years than men. Hypertension and diabetes increased more than four times the risk of coronary heart disease, followed by central obesity, obesity, and prehypertension. The use of antiretroviral agents and time since HIV diagnosis were not risk factors for coronary artery disease in 10 years. In conclusion, hypertension and diabetes are the strongest independent predictors of 10-year risk of coronary heart disease among HIV-infected population.

1. Introduction

Cardiovascular disease (CVD) has emerged as a growing problem among HIV-infected population. With the advent of highly active antiretroviral therapy (HAART), there was a reduction in AIDS-related mortality, increasing of life expectancy, and the exposure to traditional cardiovascular risk factors [1–3]. On the other hand, the infection itself, as well as HAART, seems to be involved in changing the profile of cardiovascular risk factors [4, 5]. Dyslipidemia and hyperglycemia are adverse effects of HAART, which were associated with metabolic syndrome and are intermediate steps in the development of cardiovascular events [6, 7].

In Brazil, the use of antiretroviral therapy (ART) is available to the public free of charge, as well as blood pressure-lowering agents, and other medications to control risk factors and prevent CVD. However, there are limited data on coronary heart disease (CHD) in the HIV-infected population [8, 9]. Cardiovascular risk can be evaluated by means of equations that combine several risk factors to provide a quantitative estimate of the risk [10]. The Framingham risk equation has been widely used to estimate the risk of development coronary heart disease over a fixed period of time, usually 10 years, in the general population [11], but the information in the HIV-infected population need to be further addressed [12].

Since the creation of the original equation [11], the Framingham risk score has been modified [13], and some concerns about its use were raised [14]. Although it has been suggested that a specific score needs to be used [15, 16], it is still uncertain the magnitude of CHD burden in the HIV-infected population. Moreover, the diversity of exposure to risk factors and socioeconomic conditions among patients from different clinical settings in Brazil may require the inclusion of different components in the score. Therefore, this study aimed to determine the 10-year risk of coronary heart disease using the Framingham risk score in HIV-infected patients from three regions of Brazil.

2. Methods

This is a cross-sectional with joint database analysis of baseline characteristics of three cohort studies, conducted in the Northeast, Midwest, and Southern Brazil, addressing characteristics associated with the Framingham risk score among HIV-infected individuals. In Recife, capital of the state of Pernambuco (Northeast), HIV-infected patients, aged 17 to 74 years, seen in two of the largest public outpatient centers (Hospital Universitario Oswaldo Cruz, from Universidade de Pernambuco, and Hospital Estadual Correia Picanço, from Health Secretariat of the state) for HIV/AIDS were enrolled. In Goiania, capital of the state of Goias (Midwest), HIV-infected patients, attending an outpatient public referral center for infectious diseases (Hospital das Clinicas da Universidade Federal de Goias), aged 20 to 75 years, with no clinical evidence of active opportunistic diseases at enrollment, were eligible to participate. In Porto Alegre, capital of the state of Rio Grande do Sul (Southern Brazil), HIV-infected patients aged 18 years or older, who have been seen in the outpatient clinic of the Hospital Sanatorio Partenon (SAT), of the Health State Department, were enrolled. In all studies, pregnant women, patients with mental retardation, and under restriction of freedom were excluded. The data collection was conducted in 2007–2009 (Recife), 2009–2011 (Goiania), and 2006–2008 (Porto Alegre). All research projects have been approved by the Institutional Review Board of the institutions, which are accredited by the Office of Human Research Protections, and all participants signed an informed consent.

Patients were interviewed using similar standardized questionnaires, anthropometric and blood pressure measurements, while HIV-related variables were obtained from medical records. Data collection was performed on routine visits, by certified physicians and research assistants, using similar questions pertaining demographic characteristics (age, categorized as <50, 50–59, or ≥60 years; self-reported skin color, categorized as white or nonwhite), socioeconomic level (number of years of formal education completed successfully, further categorized as ≥10 or <10), lifestyle (physical activity, categorized as yes or no; lifetime smoking, and binge drinking), clinical characteristics (self-reported previous morbidity, blood pressure lowering agents, antidiabetic agents, and drugs used in the dyslipidemia treatment), HIV-related characteristics (current or past cocaine or crack cocaine use, categorized as yes or no; reported use of antiretroviral medicine, also confirmed by medical records, and duration of HIV infection since the date of diagnosis, categorized as <8 or 8–29 years), and other risk factors for coronary heart disease (body mass index, waist circumference, diabetes mellitus, and hypertension status). In all studies, smoking was investigated by several questions: current status, number of cigarettes smoked per day, and smoking cessation, which allowed classifying individuals as never, former or current smokers. In two studies (in the Northeast and Southern Brazil), these questions were asked to those who reported having smoked at least 100 cigarettes during lifetime [17]. Alcohol consumption was investigated using a standardized questionnaire [18], including type, quantity, and frequency of each beverage consumed and binge drinking, defined by a consumption of five or more drinks on a single occasion [19].

Weight and height were obtained to calculate body mass index (kg/m^2), classified as <25, 25–29, or ≥30 kg/m^2. Central obesity was determined by waist circumference, which was measured in duplicate and classified as ≥102/88 cm for men and women, respectively. In Porto Alegre, there were four standardized measurements of blood pressure in two visits, using oscillometric monitor OMRON CP-705, and blood pressure was classified based on the average. In Recife and Goiania, there were two and three, respectively, measurements of blood pressure using calibrated aneroid sphygmomanometer (WelchAllyn/Tycos), and the average was used to classify blood pressure on <120/80, 80–89 and 120–139, or ≥140/90 mmHg, or use of antihypertensive medication. Laboratory tests were performed on fasting blood samples, with three months around the date of the interview. Diabetes mellitus was diagnosed based on fasting glucose ≥126 or use of antidiabetic agents.

Framingham scoring was calculated based on age, sex, total cholesterol, HDL cholesterol, LDL cholesterol, smoking status, diabetes mellitus, and blood pressure [11, 20], besides the reported use of using blood pressure, diabetes, or cholesterol lowering agents. Estimates of the Framingham score are more robust for total cholesterol than for LDL-cholesterol [21], and since LDL is the main treatment target [13], the lipid profile (total cholesterol, HDL, and LDL cholesterol) was maintained in the score calculation. The total score was calculated based on the original score sheets, which provide risk of CHD compared to people of the same age and sex [11]. The 10-year risk of CHD score was categorized as <10 (low) or ≥10 (intermediate or high risk, due to the expected low number of participants with high scores) to calculate prevalence and independent risk ratios with 95%CI (confidence intervals). This cutoff was based on the recommendations of the Adult Treatment Panel III (ATP III), which identified categories of cardiovascular risk to determine goals for lipid-lowering therapy [13].

Table 1: Characteristics of HIV-infected patients from regions of Brazil [n (% or mean ± SD)].

	Total (n = 3829)	Northeast (n = 2016)	Midwestern (n = 289)	Southern (n = 1224)	P value
Men	2086 (59.1)	1249 (62.0)	221 (76.5)	616 (50.3)	<0.001
Age (years)	39.0 ± 9.9	39.5 ± 9.6	37.3 ± 11.0	38.6 ± 10.1	<0.001
Nonwhite skin color	1194 (33.8)	529 (26.2)	145 (50.2)	520 (42.5)	<0.001
Years at school ≥10	1419 (40.2)	846 (42.0)	172 (59.5)	401 (32.8)	<0.001
Lifetime smoking	1424 (40.4)	480 (23.8)	137 (47.4)	807 (65.9)	<0.001
Physical activity	1171 (33.2)	389 (19.3)	74 (25.6)	708 (57.8)	<0.001
Binge drinking	747 (21.2)	475 (23.6)	66 (22.8)	206 (16.8)	<0.001
Current or past cocaine use	618 (17.5)	220 (10.9)	33 (11.6)	365 (29.8)	<0.001
Body mass index (kg/m^2)					<0.001
≤25.0	2240 (63.9)	1357 (67.3)	184 (68.9)	699 (57.1)	
25.0–29.9	961 (27.4)	517 (25.6)	69 (25.8)	375 (30.6)	
≥30.0	306 (8.7)	142 (7.0)	14 (5.2)	150 (12.3)	
Waist circumference ≥102/88 cm	666 (19.0)	379 (18.8)	31 (11.6)	256 (20.9)	0.002
Hypertension status					<0.001
Normal	1406 (39.8)	721 (35.8)	102 (35.3)	583 (47.6)	
Prehypertension	1107 (31.4)	574 (28.5)	129 (44.6)	404 (33.0)	
Hypertension	1016 (28.8)	721 (35.8)	58 (20.1)	237 (19.4)	
Diabetes mellitus	473 (13.4)	364 (18.1)	10 (3.5)	99 (8.1)	<0.001
Antiretroviral use	2544 (72.1)	1544 (76.6)	192 (66.4)	808 (66.0)	<0.001
Time >8 years since HIV diagnosis	864 (24.5)	553 (27.4)	39 (13.5)	272 (22.2)	<0.001

2.1. Statistical Analysis. A conceptual model through a hierarchical procedure was adopted in the data analysis in order to take confounding factors into account. The construction of the hierarchical model was based in two levels, and details are provided elsewhere [22]. Briefly, independent variables were grouped into socioeconomic (education), demographic factors (sex, age, and skin color), lifestyle (smoking, cocaine use, binge drinking, and physical activity), HIV characteristics (ARV use, length of HIV diagnosis) leading to direct determinants (obesity, hypertension, and diabetes mellitus) of cardiovascular disease [23]. Characteristics of the samples are expected to vary by regions, so an additional variable—the study site—was included in the multivariate analysis. At each hierarchical level, one regression equation was fitted including confounding factors which have been associated with Framingham score in the bivariate analysis (P level <0.2) or based on the literature. At the first level, the risk ratios (95% CI) were adjusted for the study site, sex, age, years at school, smoking, cocaine use, binge drinking, antiretroviral therapy, and years of the HIV diagnosis, and, at the second level, there was additional control for waist circumference, hypertension status, and diabetes mellitus. Multivariate analysis was performed using modified Poisson regression (robust variance estimates) [24], and analysis of prevalence of risk factors by regions was carried out using the chi-squared test, in the Statistical Package for Social Sciences (SPSS Inc., version 18, Chicago, IL, USA).

Statistical power was calculated to assess the size of odds ratios that could be detected in this joint analysis using the Epidata statistical software (version 3.1, Pan-American Health Organization, Washington D.C., USA). The association between Framingham risk score ≥10 among participants with prehypertension versus normal blood pressure, for instance, with a 1.27 ratio of unexposed to exposed, significance level of 0.05 (two tailed), and 80% of statistical power would require a sample size of 1284 unexposed and 1011 prehypertensive participants to detect a risk ratio of 2.5.

3. Results

Table 1 shows the characteristics of 3,829 men (59.1%) and women (40.9%) evaluated in this pooled analysis of patients infected with HIV. Most were white (66%) had, on average, 39.0 ± 9.9 years, ranging from 18 to 84 years, but only 1.8% were older than 60 years and 40% finished 10 years or more in school. Comparisons among regions showed that there were marked differences in demographic, socioeconomic, clinical, and HIV-related characteristics. Compared with smoking prevalence detected in Southern Brazil, in the Midwest was about twice and in the Northeast three times more prevalent. In the Midwest, the prevalence of central obesity was about half of the prevalence identified in the Northeast and Southern Brazil.

The prevalence of Framingham score ≥10 was 4.5% in the Southern, 4.2% in the Midwest, and 3.9% in the Northeast of Brazil. The prevalence of intermediate or high Framingham score was similar between regions for males, patients aged ≥60 years, with obesity, central obesity, hypertension, and diabetes mellitus (Table 2). The association between alcohol abuse and intermediate or high Framingham score was detected only in the Northeast, while cocaine use was not associated with risk of CHD in Midwestern.

Results of the multivariate analysis showed that age over 50 years was an independent risk factor for coronary heart disease in 10 years (Table 3). Women were three times more likely to have coronary heart disease than men, regardless

TABLE 2: Association of risk factors with intermediate and high Framingham risk score among HIV-infected patients by regions of Brazil (n (%)).

	Northeast (n = 2016)	Midwestern (n = 289)	Southern (n = 1224)
Sex			
Men	24 (1.9)	3 (1.4)	18 (2.9)
Women	55 (7.2)	9 (13.2)	37 (6.1)
P value	<0.001	<0.001	0.008
Age (years)			
<50	20 (1.2)	1 (0.4)	9 (0.9)
50–59	42 (16.9)	7 (26.9)	24 (17.9)
≥60	17 (35.4)	4 (40.0)	22 (55.0)
P value	<0.001	<0.001	<0.001
Skin color			
Nonwhite	28 (5.3)	4 (2.8)	18 (3.5)
White	51 (3.4)	8 (5.6)	37 (5.3)
P value	0.06	0.2	0.13
Years at school			
<10	53 (4.5)	8 (6.8)	38 (4.6)
≥10	26 (3.1)	4 (2.3)	17 (4.2)
P value	0.1	0.06	0.8
Lifetime smoking			
No	58 (3.8)	4 (2.6)	14 (3.4)
Yes	21 (4.4)	8 (5.8)	41 (5.1)
P value	0.6	0.17	0.17
Physical activity			
No	64 (3.9)	9 (4.2)	25 (4.8)
Yes	15 (3.9)	3 (4.1)	30 (4.2)
P value	0.9	0.9	0.6
Binge drinking			
No	72 (4.7)	7 (3.1)	50 (4.9)
Yes	7 (1.5)	5 (7.6)	5 (2.4)
P value	0.002	0.11	0.12
Current or past cocaine use			
No	77 (4.3)	10 (4.0)	50 (5.8)
Yes	2 (0.9)	1 (3.0)	5 (1.4)
P value	0.02	0.8	<0.001
Body mass index (kg/m^2)			
≤25.0	45 (3.3)	4 (2.2)	17 (2.4)
25.0–29.9	20 (3.9)	6 (8.7)	25 (6.7)
≥30.0	14 (9.9)	1 (7.1)	13 (8.7)
P value	0.001	0.06	<0.001
Waist circumference (cm)			
<102/88	46 (2.8)	5 (2.1)	27 (2.8)
≥102/88	33 (8.7)	6 (19.4)	28 (10.9)
P value	<0.001	<0.001	<0.001
Hypertension status			
Normal	12 (1.7)	0	3 (0.5)
Prehypertension	11 (1.9)	3 (2.3)	15 (3.7)
Hypertension	56 (7.8)	9 (15.5)	37 (15.6)
P value	<0.001	<0.001	<0.001
Diabetes mellitus			
No	25 (1.5)	6 (2.2)	32 (2.8)

TABLE 2: Continued.

	Northeast (n = 2016)	Midwestern (n = 289)	Southern (n = 1224)
Yes	54 (14.8)	6 (60.0)	23 (23.2)
P value	<0.001	<0.001	<0.001
Antiretroviral use			
No	22 (4.7)	2 (2.1)	14 (3.4)
Yes	57 (3.7)	10 (5.2)	41 (5.1)
P value	0.3	0.2	0.17
Time since HIV diagnosis (years)			
8–29	27 (34.2)	3 (25.0)	7 (12.7)
<8	52 (65.8)	9 (75.0)	48 (87.3)
P value	0.17	0.2	0.08

of age, socioeconomic status, lifestyle, and characteristics related to HIV. Age was the strongest predictor of CHD, even after the control for confounding factors. Binge drinking reduced CHD prevalence, independently of confounding factors, but there was a borderline significance. Hypertension and diabetes mellitus increased more than four times the risk of coronary heart disease, compared with the absence of these conditions, even after adjustment for confounding factors. Hypertension and diabetes were the strongest predictors of intermediate or high CHD risk, followed by central obesity, obesity, and prehypertension. The use of antiretroviral agents and time since HIV diagnosis were not independent risk factors for coronary artery disease in 10 years. Since most of risk factors are established at the age of 60 years, a subanalysis was carried out among participants younger than 50 years. Most of the associations between risk factors and intermediate or high Framingham score were also detected for those less than 50 years old, but some of the associations had even greater risk estimates, such as BMI, hypertension, and diabetes (data not shown). Independent of other confounding factors, an annual increase of age elevated by 30% a 10-year risk of an intermediate or high score (RR = 1.3, 95% CI: 1.2–1.4).

4. Discussion

The main objective of this study was to evaluate the association of risk factors and coronary heart disease in 10 years among HIV-infected patients from three regions of Brazil. Traditional risk factors such as age, hypertension, and diabetes mellitus were confirmed as independent risk factors, while HIV-related characteristics were not independently associated. Prehypertension was also independently associated with risk of CHD, which has been described in subjects not infected with HIV. Furthermore, the prevalence of risk factors by regions showed marked differences, suggesting that HIV-infected individuals living in several parts of Brazil did not share many characteristics besides infection.

These findings were not surprising, since age is a strong predictor of CHD risk and one of the main drivers of the Framingham score [20], while hypertension is prevalent and has accounted for almost half of ischemic heart disease cases worldwide [25]. Diabetes mellitus has been pointed out as an important risk factor for CHD [26] in HIV-infected individuals, but the risk detected in this pooled analysis was higher than previously described [27]. Among HIV-positive residents near Kampala, Uganda, in Africa, it was found that more than a quarter had hypertension, similar to the overall prevalence detected in this study, but it was assumed that no participant was smoker. Even so, there was an excessively high prevalence of Framingham score above 10% among men (42% versus 3.7% of women) [28]. In another study, conducted in Germany, about half of HIV-infected participants were smokers and a fifth had high blood pressure. However, approximately 22% and 18% of patients, respectively, were categorized as being at moderate or high 10-year risk for CHD [29]. Results of theoretical models [1, 30] and based on clinical data suggest an increased risk of myocardial infarction, due to the use of antiretroviral treatment. However, these results were found to be specific antiretroviral agents such as indinavir, lopinavir, ritonavir, didanosine, and abacavir [30–32]. In Brazil, most of these agents has been withdrawn or has not been employed in the public health system, and two non-NRTI agents, out of seven, were associated with risk of myocardial infarction.

In this study, prevalence of high 10-year CHD risk (>10%) was very low, as previously reported in Brazil [12, 33]. Among potential explanations, one is that the HIV-infected population was under 60 years old and had low prevalence of cardiovascular risk factors. Furthermore, the Framingham risk score may not be the best tool for assessing cardiovascular risk [34]. Furthermore, it was developed in a subsample of the American population—middle-aged, mostly Caucasians—free of CHD at baseline, whereas the HIV-infected population has a diverse ethnicity and is, on average, younger [15]. It also has been pointed out that the 10-year risk model may underestimate the lifetime risk [35]. However, Framingham risk score has been largely validated against risk detected in the individual data of cohort studies [36], and its simplicity matches the aims of prevention [37].

Besides that, other limitations should be taken into account when interpreting the results. The use of the Framingham score may not capture the true risk for the HIV-infected population, and a specific score, taking into account the use of specific antiretroviral agents, might work differently [16]. In addition, the number of possible combinations of ARV agents and the duration of treatment makes it difficult to isolate individual effects on the risk of coronary heart disease.

Table 3: Risk factors for intermediate and Framingham risk score among HIV-infected patients from Brazil.

	RR (95% CI)	*P* value
Study site in Brazil*		0.12
Northeast	1.0	
Midwestern	0.8 (0.4–1.4)	
Southern	0.7 (0.5–0.9)	
Sex*		<0.001
Men	1.0	
Women	3.0 (2.1–4.2)	
Age (years)*		<0.001
<50	1.0	
50–59	16.3 (10.8–24.7)	
≥60	43.4 (28.5–66.0)	
Skin color*		0.7
Nonwhite	1.0	
White	1.1 (0.8–1.4)	
Years at school*		0.9
<10	1.0	
≥10	1.0 (0.7–1.4)	
Lifetime smoking*		<0.001
No	1.0	
Yes	2.2 (1.6–3.0)	
Physical activity*		0.9
No	1.0	
Yes	1.0 (0.7–1.4)	
Binge drinking*		0.04
No	1.0	
Yes	0.6 (0.4–1.0)	
Current or past cocaine use*		0.13
No	1.0	
Yes	0.6 (0.3–1.2)	
Body mass index (kg/m^2)*		<0.001
≤25.0	1.0	
25.0–29.9	1.3 (0.9–1.8)	
≥30.0	2.3 (1.5–3.4)	
Waist circumference (cm)*		0.001
<102/88	1.0	
≥102/88	1.7 (1.3–2.4)	
Hypertension status**		<0.001
Normal	1.0	
Prehypertension	2.1 (1.2–3.6)	
Hypertension	4.6 (2.7–7.9)	
Diabetes mellitus**		<0.001
No	1.0	
Yes	4.7 (3.4–6.5)	
Antiretroviral use*		0.7
No	1.0	
Yes	0.9 (0.7–1.3)	
Time since HIV diagnosis (years)*		0.6
<8	1.0	
8–29	0.8 (0.4–1.4)	

*Risk ratio was adjusted for study site, sex, age, years at school, smoking, binge drinking, cocaine use, antiretroviral use, and length of the HIV diagnosis.
**Risk ratio additionally adjusted for waist circumference, hypertension, and diabetes mellitus.

In conclusion, this study showed that cardiovascular risk factors are present in the HIV-infected population and account for risk of coronary heart disease in 10 years. Even with the variation on risk factor prevalence among regions, the main risk factors—hypertension and diabetes mellitus—were identified in all settings as risk factors for coronary heart disease.

Conflict of Interests

The authors declare that there is no conflict of interests regarding the publication of this paper.

Acknowledgments

The financial support was provided by the CNPq (National Council for Scientific and Technological Development), Ministry of Health/Secretariat of Health Surveillance/National STD and AIDS Program (MOH/SHS/NAP), FIPE-HCPA (Fundo de Apoio a Pesquisa, Hospital de Clínicas de Porto Alegre), and the National Institute for Health Technology Assessment (IATS/CNPq), Porto Alegre, RS, Brazil. The sponsors did not take part in the design or conduct of the study, including data collection, management, analysis, and interpretation of the data and preparation, review, or approval of the paper.

References

[1] M. Law, N. Friis-Möller, R. Weber et al., "Modelling the 3-year risk of myocardial infarction among participants in the Data Collection of Adverse Events of Anti-HIV Drugs (DAD) study," *HIV Medicine*, vol. 4, no. 1, pp. 1–10, 2003.

[2] N. Friis-Möller, C. A. Sabin, R. Weber et al., "Combination antiretroviral therapy and the risk of myocardial infarction," *The New England Journal of Medicine*, vol. 349, no. 21, pp. 1993–2003, 2003.

[3] W. M. El-Sadr, J. D. Lundgren, J. D. Neaton et al., "CD4+ count-guided interruption of antiretroviral treatment," *The New England Journal of Medicine*, vol. 355, no. 22, pp. 2283–2296, 2006.

[4] B. M. Bergersen, L. Sandvik, J. N. Bruun, and S. Tonstad, "Elevated Framingham risk in HIV-positive on highly active antiretroviral therapy: results from a Norwegian study of 721 subjects," *European Journal of Clinical Microbiology and Infectious Diseases*, vol. 23, no. 8, pp. 625–630, 2004.

[5] K. Mondy, E. T. Overton, J. Grubb et al., "Metabolic syndrome in HIV-infected patients from an urban, midwestern US outpatient population," *Clinical Infectious Diseases*, vol. 44, no. 5, pp. 726–734, 2007.

[6] P. Vergara-Rodriguez, S. Vibhakar, and J. Watts, "Metabolic syndrome and associated cardiovascular risk factors in the treatment of persons with human immunodeficiency virus and severe mental illness," *Pharmacology and Therapeutics*, vol. 124, no. 3, pp. 269–278, 2009.

[7] K. Samaras, H. Wand, L. Matthew, S. Emery, D. Cooper, and A. Carr, "Prevalence of metabolic syndrome in HIV-infected patients receiving highly active antiretroviral therapy using International Diabetes Foundation and Adult Treatment Panel III criteria: associations with insulin resistance, disturbed body fat compartmentalization, elevated C-reactive protein, and

hypoadiponectinemia," *Diabetes Care*, vol. 30, no. 1, pp. 113–119, 2007.

[8] J. C. Z. Amaral, H. R. L. Melo, V. M. G. Albuquerque et al., "Angina pectoris in patients with HIV/AIDS: prevalence and risk factors," *Brazilian Journal of Infectious Diseases*, vol. 16, no. 1, pp. 1–8, 2012.

[9] P. Monteiro, D. B. Miranda-Filho, F. Bandeira et al., "Is arterial stiffness in HIV-infected individuals associated with HIV-related factors?" *Brazilian Journal of Medical and Biological Research*, vol. 45, no. 9, pp. 818–826, 2012.

[10] M. M. Moreira Guimarães, D. Bartolomeu Greco, Á. H. Ingles Garces, A. R. De Oliveira Jr., R. Bastos Fóscolo, and L. J. de Campos MacHado, "Coronary heart disease risk assessment in HIV-infected patients: a comparison of Framingham, PROCAM and SCORE risk assessment functions," *International Journal of Clinical Practice*, vol. 64, no. 6, pp. 739–745, 2010.

[11] P. W. F. Wilson, R. B. D'Agostino, D. Levy, A. M. Belanger, H. Silbershatz, and W. B. Kannel, "Prediction of coronary heart disease using risk factor categories," *Circulation*, vol. 97, no. 18, pp. 1837–1847, 1998.

[12] Z. M. Barros, R. A. de Alencar Ximenes, D. B. Miranda-Filho et al., "Comparison between the Framingham and Prospective Cardiovascular of Münster scores for risk assessment of coronary heart disease in human immunodeficiency virus-positive patients in Pernambuco, Brazil," *Metabolic Syndrome and Related Disorders*, vol. 8, no. 6, pp. 489–497, 2010.

[13] National Cholesterol Education Program (NCEP) Expert Panel on Detection, Evaluation, and Treatment of High Blood Cholesterol in Adults (Adult Treatment Panel III), "Third report of the National Cholesterol Education Program (NCEP) Expert Panel on detection, evaluation, and treatment of high blood cholesterol in adults (Adult Treatment Panel III) final report," *Circulation*, vol. 106, no. 25, pp. 3143–3421, 2002.

[14] M. Schambelan, P. W. F. Wilson, K. E. Yarasheski et al., "Development of appropriate coronary heart disease risk prediction models in HIV-infected patients," *Circulation*, vol. 118, no. 2, pp. e48–e53, 2008.

[15] R. B. D'Agostino Sr., "Cardiovascular risk estimation in 2012: lessons learned and applicability to the HIV population," *Brazilian Journal of Infectious Diseases*, vol. 205, supplement 3, pp. S362–S367, 2012.

[16] N. Friis-Möller, R. Thiébaut, P. Reiss et al., "Predicting the risk of cardiovascular disease in HIV-infected patients: the Data collection on Adverse Effects of Anti-HIV Drugs Study," *European Journal of Cardiovascular Prevention and Rehabilitation*, vol. 17, no. 5, pp. 491–501, 2010.

[17] H. Ryan, A. Trosclair, and J. Gfroerer, "Adult current smoking: differences in definitions and prevalence estimates. NHIS and NSDUH, 2008," *Journal of Environmental and Public Health*, vol. 2012, Article ID 918368, 11 pages, 2012.

[18] L. B. Moreira, F. D. Fuchs, R. S. Moraes, M. Bredemeier, and B. B. Duncan, "Alcohol intake and blood pressure: the importance of time elapsed since last drink," *Journal of Hypertension*, vol. 16, no. 2, pp. 175–180, 1998.

[19] A. A. Steffens, L. B. Moreira, S. C. Fuchs, M. Wiehe, M. Gus, and F. D. Fuchs, "Incidence of hypertension by alcohol consumption: is it modified by race?" *Journal of Hypertension*, vol. 24, no. 8, pp. 1489–1492, 2006.

[20] R. B. D'Agostino Sr., R. S. Vasan, M. J. Pencina et al., "General cardiovascular risk profile for use in primary care: the Framingham heart study," *Circulation*, vol. 117, no. 6, pp. 743–753, 2008.

[21] E. G. Burke, J. Nelson, J. Kwong, and P. F. Cook, "Cardiovascular risk assessment for persons living with HIV," *Journal of the Association of Nurses in AIDS Care*, vol. 23, no. 2, pp. 134–145, 2012.

[22] C. G. Victora, S. R. Huttly, S. C. Fuchs, and M. T. A. Olinto, "The role of conceptual frameworks in epidemiological analysis: a hierarchical approach," *International Journal of Epidemiology*, vol. 26, no. 1, pp. 224–227, 1997.

[23] S. C. Fuchs, L. B. Moreira, S. A. Camey, M. B. Moreira, and F. D. Fuchs, "Clustering of risk factors for cardiovascular disease among women in Southern Brazil: a population-based study," *Cadernos de Saude Publica*, vol. 24, supplement 2, pp. S285–S293, 2008.

[24] A. J. D. Barros and V. N. Hirakata, "Alternatives for logistic regression in cross-sectional studies: an empirical comparison of models that directly estimate the prevalence ratio," *BMC Medical Research Methodology*, vol. 3, article 1, pp. 1–13, 2003.

[25] World Health Organization, *The World Health Report 2002: Reducing Risks, Promoting Healthy Life*, World Health Organization, Geneva, Switzerland, 2002.

[26] S. R. Preis, M. J. Pencina, S.-J. Hwang et al., "Trends in cardiovascular disease risk factors in individuals with and without diabetes mellitus in the framingham heart study," *Circulation*, vol. 120, no. 3, pp. 212–220, 2009.

[27] S. W. Worm, S. de Wit, R. Weber et al., "Diabetes mellitus, preexisting coronary heart disease, and the risk of subsequent coronary heart disease events in patients infected with human immunodeficiency virus the data collection on adverse events of anti-HIV drugs (D:A:D Study)," *Circulation*, vol. 119, no. 6, pp. 805–811, 2009.

[28] F. J. Mateen, S. Kanters, R. Kalyesubula et al., "Hypertension prevalence and Framingham risk score stratification in a large HIV-positive cohort in Uganda," *Journal of Hypertension*, vol. 31, no. 7, pp. 1372–1378, 2013.

[29] N. Reinsch, K. Neuhaus, S. Esser et al., "Are HIV patients undertreated? Cardiovascular risk factors in HIV: results of the HIV-HEART study," *European Journal of Preventive Cardiology*, vol. 19, no. 2, pp. 267–274, 2012.

[30] S. W. Worm, C. Sabin, R. Weber et al., "Risk of myocardial infarction in patients with HIV infection exposed to specific individual antiretroviral drugs from the 3 major drug classes: the data collection on adverse events of anti-HIV drugs (D:A:D) study," *Journal of Infectious Diseases*, vol. 201, no. 3, pp. 318–330, 2010.

[31] S. Lang, M. Mary-Krause, L. Cotte et al., "Impact of individual antiretroviral drugs on the risk of myocardial infarction in human immunodeficiency virus-infected patients: a case-control study nested within the French hospital database on HIV ANRS cohort CO4," *Archives of Internal Medicine*, vol. 170, no. 14, pp. 1228–1238, 2010.

[32] C. A. Sabin, S. W. Worm, R. Weber et al., "Use of nucleoside reverse transcriptase inhibitors and risk of myocardial infarction in HIV-infected patients enrolled in the D:A:D study: a multi-cohort collaboration," *The Lancet*, vol. 371, no. 9622, pp. 1417–1426, 2008.

[33] P. Cahn, O. Leite, A. Rosales et al., "Metabolic profile and cardiovascular risk factors among Latin American HIV-infected patients receiving HAART," *Brazilian Journal of Infectious Diseases*, vol. 14, no. 2, pp. 158–166, 2010.

[34] G. C. Siontis, I. Tzoulaki, K. C. Siontis et al., "Comparisons of established risk prediction models for cardiovascular disease: systematic review," *British Medical Journal*, vol. 344, Article ID e3318, 2012.

[35] K. H. Schlendorf, K. Nasir, and R. S. Blumenthal, "Limitations of the Framingham risk score are now much clearer," *Preventive Medicine*, vol. 48, no. 2, pp. 115–116, 2009.

[36] R. B. D'Agostino Sr., S. Grundy, L. M. Sullivan, and P. Wilson, "Validation of the Framingham coronary heart disease prediction scores: results of a multiple ethnic groups investigation," *Journal of the American Medical Association*, vol. 286, no. 2, pp. 180–187, 2001.

[37] J. S. Berger, C. O. Jordan, D. Lloyd-Jones, and R. S. Blumenthal, "Screening for cardiovascular risk in asymptomatic patients," *Journal of the American College of Cardiology*, vol. 55, no. 12, pp. 1169–1177, 2010.

Association of Blood Pressure and Hypertension with Alcohol Consumption in HIV-Infected White and Nonwhite Patients

Maria Leticia R. Ikeda,[1,2] Nêmora T. Barcellos,[3,4] Paulo R. Alencastro,[2,4] Fernando H. Wolff,[3,4] Ajácio B. M. Brandão,[3] Flávio D. Fuchs,[1,4] and Sandra C. Fuchs[1,3,4]

[1] *Postgraduate Program in Cardiology, School of Medicine, Universidade Federal do Rio Grande do Sul, R. Ramiro Barcelos 2600, 90035-003 Porto Alegre, RS, Brazil*
[2] *Hospital Sanatório Partenon, Health State Department of Rio Grande do Sul 3722, Avenida Bento Gonçalves, 90650-001 Porto Alegre, RS, Brazil*
[3] *Postgraduate Program in Epidemiology, School of Medicine, Universidade Federal do Rio Grande do Sul, R. Ramiro Barcelos 2600, 90035-003 Porto Alegre, RS, Brazil*
[4] *National Institute for Health Technology Assessment (IATS/CNPq), Clinical Research Center, Hospital de Clinicas de Porto Alegre, R. Ramiro Barcelos 2350, 90035-003 Porto Alegre, RS, Brazil*

Correspondence should be addressed to Sandra C. Fuchs; scfuchs@terra.com.br

Academic Editors: H. A. Beydoun, G.-X. Jiang, and L. Kuller

Introduction. Although alcohol abuse is associated with hypertension in whites and nonwhites, it has been scarcely investigated in HIV-infected patients. *Objective.* To investigate whether the association of alcohol abuse with hypertension is influenced by skin color in HIV-infected individuals. *Methods.* Cross-sectional study in HIV-infected individuals aged 18 years or older. Demographic characteristics, lifestyle, and HIV infection were investigated. Alcohol abuse was defined as ≥15 (women) and ≥30 g/alcohol/day (men), and binge drinking by the intake of ≥5 drinks on a single occasion. Hypertension was defined by blood pressure ≥140/90 mmHg or use of blood pressure-lowering agents. *Results.* We studied 1,240 individuals, with 39.1 ± 10 years, 51% males and 57% whites. Age and body mass index were associated with blood pressure, and there was an independent association of alcohol abuse with hypertension in whites (RR = 1.9, 95% CI 1.1–3.3) and nonwhites (RR = 2.4, 95% CI 1.4 to 4.0). Among nonwhite individuals who were alcohol abusers, systolic (9.3 ± 3.2; $P = 0.001$) and diastolic blood pressures (6.4 ± 2.1; $P = 0.008$) were higher than in nonabusers. *Conclusion.* Alcohol abuse is a risk factor for hypertension in white and nonwhite HIV-infected individuals. The association of ethanol consumption with blood pressure is not explained by AIDS-related conditions.

1. Introduction

Hypertension is a major cardiovascular risk factor worldwide. Projections are that, by the year of 2025, 75.0% (or 1.17 billion people) of the people with hypertension in the world will be living in emerging nations [1]. In Brazil, about 29% of the Brazilian population has hypertension [2]. Alcohol abuse is associated with elevated blood pressure [3], regardless of other risk factors [4–6]. Different studies have shown prevalence rates of hypertension attributed to alcohol consumption ranging from 5 to 30% [7].

Risk factors for cardiovascular diseases, including hypertension and dyslipidemia, are determinants of reduced life expectancy in HIV-infected patients [8]. Hypertension prevalence in HIV-infected individuals ranges from 5.9 to 56.4% [9–12] and has been associated with alcohol abuse and other factors related to HIV infection [9, 10, 13]. In these individuals, the prevalence of alcohol abuse ranges from 8% [14, 15] to 50% [16–18], exceeding the rates in general populations of the United States [19], Europe [20], and Brazil [21], where the prevalence is between 2 and 41% in men and 0.1 and 21% in women [20].

The relationship between alcohol consumption and hypertension may be influenced by some characteristics, such as skin color [3, 22]. Skin color has been identified as a marker of lifestyle [3, 23, 24] and, in some countries, it may also be characterized as the socioeconomic status of the individuals [4]. In Brazil, the HIV-infected population tends to be more homogeneous in terms of socioeconomic status, affecting the less privileged ones. High blood pressure has been associated with low socioeconomic status [4] and skin color may also be a risk factor. Therefore, the objective of the present study was to investigate if the association between alcohol abuse, blood pressure, and hypertension in HIV-infected patients is influenced by skin color.

2. Materials and Methods

We conducted a cross-sectional study including HIV-infected individuals who were being followed up at the Outpatient Clinic of the Care and Therapy Service (SAT), Hospital Sanatório Partenon, State Department of Health of Rio Grande do Sul, Brazil. This clinic and all public health care centers provide medical care, antiretroviral therapy (ART), antihypertensives, and other medications free of charge for HIV-infected patients. We consecutively enrolled female and male patients, aged 18 or older, who were seen between June 2006 and December 2008. Pregnant women, individuals who were unable to provide written consent, or those incarcerated were excluded. Participants who were under the influence of alcohol or drugs at the time of the interview were asked to return for evaluation at another time.

Participants were interviewed on the day of the regular medical appointments. Since they had to consult every month, in order to get antiretroviral medication, they were seen often, which contributed to achieving high participation rate. Information was collected, using standardized questionnaires, for the following characteristics: demographic (age and skin color self-reported, classified as white or nonwhite), socioeconomic (educational attainment, number of school years), and lifestyle characteristics (alcohol consumption, physical activity, and smoking), as well as the use of antiretroviral therapy (ART), and time since diagnosis of HIV infection (in years, classified as ≥6 years, from 3.0 to 5.9 years, and <3 years). Data related to HIV infection as CD4 lymphocyte count (mm^3/mL), viral load (copies per mL of blood), and clinical information were confirmed by medical records. Alcohol consumption was investigated using a validated quantity-frequency questionnaire based on the kind of beverage consumed [21], administered by a physician or healthcare professional, containing questions about type, frequency, and amount of alcohol consumed in the last six months. Alcohol consumption was categorized into abstemious drinking, social drinking (>0 and <15 grams/day for women and >0 and <30 grams/day for men), or abusive drinking (≥15 grams/day for women and ≥30 grams/day for men) [21, 22, 25]. Binge drinking was characterized by a consumption of five or more drinks on a single occasion [22]. Frequency of consumption was classified as weekly (consumption on some days of the week, but not daily) or monthly (consumption on some days of the month but not every week), regardless of the amount. Physical activity was investigated using the IPAQ (International Physical Activity Questionnaire) [26], which investigates frequency and duration of physical activity. The intensity of exercise was classified as moderate or high versus low physical activity according to the IPAQ protocol [27]. Smoking was defined according to the information provided by the participants, classifying the amount of consumption in at least 100 cigarettes during their lifetimes.

Weight (Kg) and height (m) were measured twice with the participants being barefoot and wearing light clothes, using an anthropometric scale (Filizola, model 31 adult, Indústria Filizola S.A., São Paulo, SP, Brazil). Body mass index (BMI; kg/m^2) was calculated as the weight (kg) divided by the square of the height (m) and classified as normal (<25.0), overweight (25–29.9), and obesity (≥30.0). Standardized measurements of blood pressure were obtained in duplicate in two visits, using a validated oscillometric device (OMRON CP-705) [28]. The average of four BP measurements was used to detect hypertension if systolic blood pressure ≥140 mmHg or diastolic blood pressure ≥90 mmHg, or in use of blood pressure-lowering agents [25].

Certified researchers performed the interviews and measured anthropometric parameters and blood pressure. Approximately 5% of the interviews were repeated for quality control. Data were entered twice into the database of Epinfo, version 2000. The study was approved by the Research Ethics Committee of the Hospital de Clínicas de Porto Alegre, which is accredited by the Office of Human Research Protections. All participants signed an informed consent form.

Sample Size Calculation and Statistical Analysis. Sample size calculation was based on the estimated prevalence of hypertension between white and nonwhite participants with abusive alcohol consumption (30 and 35%, resp.) and abstemious drinking (18%), with 80% of power and a significance level of 0.05 (two-tailed). A sample size of 738 white and 398 nonwhite participants with a 1 : 5 ratio for exposed and unexposed participants to excessive alcohol consumption would be required to detect a hazard ratio of at least 1.7. The estimates were based on previous studies [22, 29].

Characteristics of the sample were expressed as mean and standard deviation. We used Pearson's chi-square test for the analysis of categorical variables and analysis of variance (continuous variables) to assess the association between these factors and the different outcomes. Confounding factors were controlled using the modified Poisson regression (robust variance estimates) [30] and analysis of covariance. Statistical analyses were performed using the Statistical Package for the Social Sciences (SPSS Inc., Chicago, Illinois, USA), version 18.0. Confounding factors were selected based on the literature [3, 31, 32] and P values lower than or equal to 0.2 in unadjusted analysis. Age, sex, educational attainment, smoking, physical activity, body mass index, time since HIV infection, and lifetime HAART use were considered confounding factors used in the multivariate models for whites and nonwhites. Partially adjusted models of alcohol consumption with systolic or diastolic blood pressure, including age, sex, and educational attainment, were run in order to better understand the associations and to interpret the risk ratios. A trend for association was determined by P values between 0.05 and 0.1.

TABLE 1: Characteristics of HIV-infected individuals according to skin color (n (%) or mean ± SD).

	Total (n = 1240)	Whites (n = 710)	Nonwhites (n = 530)	P value
Male	628 (50.6)	391 (55.1)	237 (44.7)	<0.001
Age (years)	39.1 ± 10.0	39.3 ± 10.3	38.9 ± 9.7	0.5
Educational attainment (years)	7.5 ± 4.1	8.3 ± 4.2	6.4 ± 3.7	<0.001
Smoking	525 (42.3)	298 (42.0)	227 (42.8)	0.4
Physical activity				0.049
Low	321 (25.9)	199 (28.0)	122 (23.0)	
Moderate	398 (32.1)	232 (32.7)	166 (31.3)	
High	521 (42.0)	279 (39.3)	242 (45.7)	
Alcohol consumption				0.7
Abstemious	414 (33.4)	233 (32.8)	181 (34.2)	
Social drinking	757 (61.0)	440 (62.0)	317 (59.8)	
Abusive drinking	69 (5.6)	37 (5.2)	32 (6.0)	
Frequency of alcohol consumption				0.7
Abstemious	414 (33.4)	233 (32.8)	181 (34.2)	
Monthly	440 (35.5)	249 (35.1)	191 (36.0)	
Weekly	386 (31.1)	228 (32.1)	158 (29.8)	
Binge drinking	211 (17.0)	117 (55.5)	94 (44.5)	0.7
Abstemious	414 (33.4)	233 (32.8)	181 (34.2)	
No	616 (49.7)	360 (50.7)	255 (48.1)	
Yes	210 (16.9)	117 (16.5)	94 (17.7)	
Body mass index (kg/m^2)	24.9 ± 4.4	24.8 ± 4.3	25.0 ± 4.7	0.4
Systolic blood pressure (mmHg)	121.8 ± 18.2	121.8 ± 17.7	121.8 ± 18.8	0.9
Diastolic blood pressure (mmHg)	76.6 ± 11.4	76.0 ± 10.7	77.3 ± 12.3	0.06
Hypertension	241 (19.4)	120 (16.9)	121 (22.8)	0.009
Time since HIV infection (years)				0.005
≥6.0	404 (32.6)	250 (35.3)	154 (29.1)	
3.0–5.9	350 (28.2)	176 (24.8)	174 (32.8)	
<3.0	485 (39.1)	283 (39.9)	202 (38.1)	
HIV/HCV coinfection	261 (22.2)	143 (21.2)	118 (23.5)	0.3
AIDS diagnosis	892 (72.2)	510 (72.0)	382 (72.3)	0.9
Lifetime HAART use	815 (65.7)	467 (65.8)	348 (65.7)	0.9
Lifetime protease inhibitor use	468 (37.7)	277 (39.0)	191 (36.0)	0.3
CD4 (cell/mm^3)				0.08
<350	476 (38.8)	258 (36.7)	218 (41.6)	
≥350	751 (61.2)	445 (63.3)	306 (58.4)	

HAART: highly active antiretroviral therapy; HCV: hepatitis C virus; HIV: human immunodeficiency virus; SD: standard deviation.

3. Results

Of the 1,295 HIV-infected patients screened, 1,255 were eligible and 1,240 were included. Thus, forty patients had not confirmed eligibility due to age under 18 years, incarceration, or pregnancy; fifteen refused to participate, and two patients were included in a second attempt due to alcohol intoxication at the first visit. Characteristics of the overall sample are presented in Table 1 by skin color. Participants were aged 39.1 ± 10, half of them were males, and 57% had white skin color. Overall, the distribution of most characteristics was similar among whites and nonwhites, but whites had higher education and time since HIV infection, and nonwhites had high physical activity and prevalence of hypertension.

Risk factors for hypertension among whites and nonwhites are shown in Table 2. The unadjusted analysis showed that only age and BMI were positively associated with hypertension for both categories of skin color. White smokers had lower prevalence of hypertension, whereas among nonwhites there was a trend for the association of alcohol abuse with hypertension. There was no association between variables related to HIV and hypertension.

Table 3 shows that association among the different patterns of alcoholic beverages consumption is roughly similar in whites and nonwhites; abusive consumption of alcohol was associated with hypertension in white and nonwhite HIV-infected individuals, independently of a large set of confounding variables. The frequency of alcohol consumption

Table 2: Risk factors for hypertension among HIV-infected individuals by skin color (n (%)).

	Whites (n = 710)		Nonwhites (n = 530)	
	Hypertension (%)	RR (95% CI)	Hypertension (%)	RR (95% CI)
Sex				
Female	48 (15.0)	1.0	65 (22.2)	1.0
Male	72 (18.4)	1.2 (0.9–1.7)	56 (23.6)	1.1 (0.8–1.5)
P value		0.2		0.7
Age (years)				
18–34	20 (7.4)	1.0	23 (11.4)	1.0
35–49	56 (16.9)	2.3 (1.4–3.7)	63 (24.3)	2.1 (1.4–3.3)
50–78	44 (40.4)	5.4 (3.4–8.8)	35 (50.7)	4.5 (2.8–7.0)
P value		<0.001		<0.001
Educational attainment (years)				
≥9	58 (17.8)	1.0	23 (17.8)	1.0
5–8	38 (16.2)	0.9 (0.6–1.3)	51 (22.2)	1.2 (0.8–1.9)
0–4	24 (16.0)	0.9 (0.6–1.4)	47 (27.5)	1.5 (1.0–2.4)
P value		0.8		0.14
Smoking				
No	85 (20.6)	1.0	76 (25.1)	1.0
Yes	35 (11.7)	0.6 (0.4–0.8)	45 (19.8)	0.8 (0.6–1.1)
P value		0.002		0.16
Physical activity				
High	39 (14.0)	1.0	48 (19.8)	1.0
Moderate	44 (19.0)	1.4 (0.9–2.0)	38 (22.9)	1.2 (0.8–1.7)
Low	37 (18.6)	1.3 (0.9–2.0)	35 (28.7)	1.4 (1.0–2.1)
P value		0.3		0.16
Alcohol consumption				
Abstemious	41 (17.6)	1.0	41 (22.7)	1.0
Social drinking	70 (15.9)	0.9 (0.6–1.3)	68 (21.5)	0.9 (0.7–1.3)
Abusive drinking	9 (24.3)	1.4 (0.7–2.6)	12 (37.5)	1.7 (1.0–2.8)
P value		0.4		0.08
Frequency of alcohol consumption				
Abstemious	41 (18.0)	1.0	41 (22.7)	1.0
Monthly	41 (17.6)	0.9 (0.6–1.3)	42 (26.6)	0.9 (0.6–1.3)
Weekly	38 (15.3)	1.1 (0.7–1.5)	79 (21.2)	1.2 (0.8–1.7)
P value		0.7		0.3
Binge drinking				
Abstemious	41 (17.6)	1.0	41 (22.7)	1.0
No	60 (16.7)	0.9 (0.7–1.4)	60 (23.4)	1.0
Yes	19 (16.2)	0.9 (0.6–1.5)	20 (21.5)	1.0 (0.6–1.5)
P value		0.9		0.8
Body mass index (kg/m^2)				
<25.0	36 (8.7)	1.0	45 (15.3)	1.0
25–29.9	58 (26.6)	3.1 (2.1–4.5)	40 (24.7)	1.6 (1.1–2.4)
≥30.0	26 (32.9)	3.8 (2.4–5.9)	36 (49.3)	3.2 (2.3–4.6)
P value		<0.001		<0.001
HIV/HCV coinfection				
No	96 (18.0)	1.0	85 (22.1)	1.0
Yes	22 (15.4)	0.9 (0.6–1.3)	29 (24.6)	1.1 (0.8–1.6)
P value		0.5		0.6

Table 2: Continued.

	Whites (n = 710)		Nonwhites (n = 530)	
	Hypertension (%)	RR (95% CI)	Hypertension (%)	RR (95% CI)
AIDS diagnosis				
No	29 (14.6)	1.0	36 (24.7)	1.0
Yes	90 (17.6)	0.8 (0.6–1.2)	84 (22.0)	1.1 (0.8–1.6)
P value		0.3		0.5
Time since HIV infection (years)				
<3.0	47 (16.6)	1.0	44 (21.8)	1.0
3.0–5.9	23 (13.1)	0.8 (0.5–1.2)	34 (19.5)	0.9 (0.6–1.3)
≥6.0	50 (20.0)	1.2 (0.8–1.7)	43 (27.9)	1.3 (0.9–1.8)
P value		0.18		0.17
Lifetime HAART use				
No	34 (14.0)	1.0	46 (25.3)	1.0
Yes	86 (18.4)	1.3 (0.9–1.9)	75 (21.6)	0.9 (0.6–1.2)
P value		0.14		0.3
Lifetime protease inhibitor use				
No	77 (22.7)	1.0	68 (15.7)	1.0
Yes	44 (23.0)	1.0 (0.7–1.4)	52 (18.8)	1.2 (0.9–1.7)
P value		0.9		0.3
CD4 (cell/mm^3)				
<350	39 (15.1)	1.0	50 (22.9)	1.0
≥350	80 (18.0)	0.8 (0.6–1.2)	69 (22.5)	1.0 (0.7–1.4)
P value		0.3		0.9

HAART: highly active antiretroviral therapy; HCV: hepatitis C virus; HIV: human immunodeficiency virus; RR: risk ratio.

Table 3: Association between alcohol consumption and hypertension according to skin color.

	Whites RR (95% CI)*	Nonwhites RR (95% CI)*
Alcohol consumption		
Abstemious	1.0	1.0
Social drinking	1.2 (0.8–1.7)	1.1 (0.8–1.5)
Abusive drinking	1.9 (1.1–3.3)	2.4 (1.4–4.0)
P value	0.09	0.004
Frequency of alcohol consumption		
Abstemious	1.0	1.0
Monthly	1.1 (0.7–1.6)	1.0 (0.7–1.5)
Weekly	1.4 (1.0–2.0)	1.3 (0.9–1.9)
P value	0.2	0.18
Binge drinking		
Abstemious	1.0	1.0
No	1.2 (0.8–1.7)	1.1 (0.6–1.8)
Yes	1.2 (0.8–1.9)	1.2 (0.8–1.6)
P value	0.6	0.7

*RR adjusted for age, sex, educational attainment, smoking, physical activity, BMI, time since diagnosis of HIV infection, and use of highly active antiretroviral therapy.

and acute intake of large amounts were not associated with hypertension.

Systolic and diastolic blood pressure was higher exclusively in nonwhite participants who abused alcohol, independently of confounding factors (Table 4). Systolic blood pressure was on average 9.3 ± 3.2 mmHg, and diastolic 6.4 ± 2.1 mmHg greater among abusers. These differences were independent of age, sex, and educational attainment (data not shown) and of full control for confounding factors. Among white participants, there were an association of diastolic blood pressure with weekly consumption of alcoholic beverages in comparison with nondrinkers and a borderline association versus monthly consumers.

4. Discussion

In this study, we found that the consumption of large amounts of alcohol was independently associated with hypertension in white and nonwhite HIV-infected individuals. Blood pressure, on the other hand, was higher exclusively in nonwhite abusers of ethanol, demonstrated after adjustment for confounding factors. However, even partially adjusted models showed the presence of negative confounding factors. Among, whites there was an association of blood pressure with the frequency of consumption. Taken together, these findings suggest that among nonwhite participants quantity is more important than the pattern of consumption, while for whites the frequency of drinking is more relevant.

The association between alcohol abuse and hypertension identified in our study is in agreement with findings from other populations [33]. The association of blood pressure with abusive consumption exclusively in nonwhites was similar to the observed one in the ARIC cohort study (Atherosclerosis Risk in Communities) [3] and in a cohort carried out in southern Brazil [22]. It is unlikely that this differential association of alcohol abuse and blood pressure by skin color is due

TABLE 4: Association of systolic and diastolic blood pressure with alcohol consumption by skin color.

Skin color	Alcohol consumption	BP ± SE (mmHg)	Delta of BP ± SE (mmHg)*†	P value*†	Delta of BP ± SE (mmHg)**†	P value**†
Systolic BP (mmHg)						
	Abstemious	120.5 ± 1.0	—		—	
Whites	Social drinking	122.5 ± 0.7	2.0 ± 1.3	0.3	—	
	Abusive drinking	123.3 ± 2.5	2.8 ± 2.8	0.7	0.9 ± 2.7	1.0
	Abstemious	120.8 ± 1.3	—		—	
Nonwhites	Social drinking	121.6 ± 0.9	0.8 ± 1.6	0.9	—	
	Abusive drinking	130.9 ± 3.0	10.1 ± 3.3	0.007	9.3 ± 3.2	0.01
Diastolic BP (mmHg)						
	Abstemious	74.9 ± 0.6	—		—	
Whites	Social drinking	76.6 ± 0.5	1.7 ± 0.8	0.1	—	
	Abusive drinking	77.4 ± 1.6	2.6 ± 1.7	0.4	0.9 ± 1.7	0.9
	Abstemious	76.6 ± 0.9	—		—	
Nonwhites	Social drinking	77.1 ± 0.6	0.5 ± 1.1	0.9	—	
	Abusive drinking	83.4 ± 2.0	6.9 ± 2.2	0.006	6.4 ± 2.1	0.008
	Frequency of alcohol consumption					
Systolic BP (mmHg)						
	Abstemious	120.5 ± 1.0	—			
Whites	Monthly	121.6 ± 1.0	1.1 ± 1.4	0.9	—	
	Weekly	123.5 ± 1.0	3.0 ± 1.5	0.4	2.3 ± 1.8	0.5
	Abstemious	120.8 ± 1.3	—			
Nonwhites	Monthly	121.3 ± 1.2	0.5 ± 1.8	0.8	—	
	Weekly	123.6 ± 1.4	2.8 ± 2.0	0.12	1.9 ± 1.4	0.5
Diastolic BP (mmHg)						
	Abstemious	74.9 ± 0.6				
Whites	Monthly	75.7 ± 0.6	0.8 ± 0.9	0.8		
	Weekly	77.6 ± 0.6	2.8 ± 0.9	0.008	2.0 ± 0.9	0.079
	Abstemious	76.7 ± 0.9				
Nonwhites	Monthly	77.5 ± 0.8	0.8 ± 1.2	0.9		
	Weekly	77.7 ± 0.9	1.0 ± 1.3	0.8	0.2 ± 1.2	0.9

SE: standard error; *delta in relation to abstemious drinking; **delta in relation to social drinking or monthly consumption; †analyses of covariance adjusted for age, sex, educational attainment, smoking, physical activity, body mass index, time since HIV infection, and lifetime HAART use.

to race or ethnicity, but probably relies on other behavioral characteristics of nonwhite individuals [34]. Anyway, blood pressure was higher exclusively in nonwhite abusers, suggesting that these individuals are at higher risk of the harmful effects of ethanol.

Our study adds a piece of mind in the investigation of the influence of HIV-related characteristics and higher incidence of cardiovascular disease. It has been suggested that the use of HAART may be associated with increasing blood pressure [9, 10, 35, 36]. In some studies, longer time of HAART was associated with hypertension [13, 37]. These associations were not identified in our study, since the use of antiretrovirals, time of HIV infection, AIDS, and CD4 count were not associated with hypertension.

Some limitations of our study deserve to be mentioned. The cross-sectional design does not allow inferring causality. Data on alcohol consumption were obtained from a standardized questionnaire containing detailed information, but it relies on memory, and because it was applied in the context of medical care, this might have led individuals to underreport consumption. Another aspect to be considered is the fact that blood pressure measurements were performed at the medical consultation, and therefore the possibility of a white coat effect cannot be discarded. Even underreporting alcohol consumption or the white coat effect, the association of alcohol abuse with hypertension has been confirmed by ambulatory monitoring of blood pressure [38]. The prospective planning, together with the extensive and detailed measurement of AIDS-related and nonrelated characteristics and adequate statistical power, is a strength of our investigation.

5. Conclusions

In conclusion, alcohol abuse is associated with increased risk of hypertension in white and nonwhite HIV-infected individuals. Blood pressure is higher only in nonwhite individuals who abuse alcoholic beverages and in whites who drink weekly. The association of ethanol consumption with blood pressure is not explained by AIDS-related conditions.

Conflict of Interests

The authors declare that they have no conflict of interests.

Acknowledgments

The financial support was provided by the National Council for Scientific and Technological Development (CNPq), Ministry of Health/Secretariat of Health Surveillance/National STD and AIDS Program (MOH/SHS/NAP), Research funding from Hospital de Clínicas de Porto Alegre (FIPE-HCPA), and National Institute for Science and Technology for Health Technology Assessment (IATS/CNPq), Porto Alegre, RS, Brazil. The sponsors did not take part in the design or conduct of the study, including data collection, management, analysis, and interpretation of the data, and preparation, review, or approval of the paper.

References

[1] P. M. Kearney, M. Whelton, K. Reynolds, P. Muntner, P. K. Whelton, and J. He, "Global burden of hypertension: analysis of worldwide data," *The Lancet*, vol. 365, no. 9455, pp. 217–223, 2005.

[2] R. V. Picon, F. D. Fuchs, L. B. Moreira, G. Riegel, and S.C. Fuchs, "Trends in prevalence of hypertension in Brazil: a systematic review with meta-analysis," *PloS ONE*, vol. 7, no. 10, Article ID e48255, 2012.

[3] F. D. Fuchs, L. E. Chambless, P. K. Whelton, F. J. Nieto, and G. Heiss, "Alcohol consumption and the incidence of hypertension. The Atherosclerosis Risk in Communities Study," *Hypertension*, vol. 37, no. 5, pp. 1242–1250, 2001.

[4] C. C. Gravlee, W. W. Dressier, and H. Russell Bernard, "Skin color, social classification, and blood pressure in Southeastern Puerto Rico," *American Journal of Public Health*, vol. 95, no. 12, pp. 2191–2197, 2005.

[5] S.-Y. Fu, W.-M. Li, Y.-J. Zhao et al., "Prevalence of hypertension and risk factors in Heilongjiang province in 2007," *Chinese Medical Journal*, vol. 123, no. 6, pp. 752–755, 2010.

[6] J. M. Núñez-Córdoba, M. A. Martínez-González, M. Bes-Rastrollo, E. Toledo, J. J. Beunza, and Á. Alonso, "Alcohol Consumption and the Incidence of Hypertension in a Mediterranean Cohort. The SUN Study," *Revista Espanola de Cardiologia*, vol. 62, no. 6, pp. 633–641, 2009.

[7] S. MacMahon, "Alcohol consumption and hypertension," *Hypertension*, vol. 9, no. 2, pp. 111–121, 1987.

[8] M. S. Freiberg and K. L. Kraemer, "Focus on the heart: alcohol consumption, HIV infection, and cardiovascular disease," *Alcohol Research and Health*, vol. 33, no. 3, pp. 237–246, 2010.

[9] M. Baekken, I. Os, L. Sandvik, and O. Oektedalen, "Hypertension in an urban HIV-positive population compared with the general population: influence of combination antiretroviral therapy," *Journal of Hypertension*, vol. 26, no. 11, pp. 2126–2133, 2008.

[10] C. Jericó, H. Knobel, M. Montero et al., "Hypertension in HIV-infected patients: prevalence and related factors," *American Journal of Hypertension*, vol. 18, no. 11, pp. 1396–1401, 2005.

[11] N. Friis-Møller, R. Weber, P. Reiss et al., "Cardiovascular disease risk factors in HIV patients—association with antiretroviral therapy. Results from the DAD study," *AIDS*, vol. 17, no. 8, pp. 1179–1193, 2003.

[12] S. Medina-Torne, A. Ganesan, I. Barahona, and N. F. Crum-Cianflone, "Hypertension is common among HIV-infected persons, but not associated with HAART," *Journal of the International Association of Physicians in AIDS Care*, vol. 11, no. 1, pp. 20–25, 2012.

[13] I. W. Manner, M. Baekken, O. Oektedalen, L. Sandvik, and I. Os, "Effect of HIV duration on ambulatory blood pressure in HIV-infected individuals with high office blood pressure," *Blood Pressure*, vol. 19, no. 3, pp. 188–195, 2010.

[14] M. Bonacini, "Alcohol use among patients with HIV infection," *Annals of Hepatology*, vol. 10, no. 4, pp. 502–507, 2011.

[15] M. S. Freiberg, K. A. McGinnis, K. Kraemer et al., "The association between alcohol consumption and prevalent cardiovascular diseases among HIV-infected and HIV-uninfected men," *Journal of Acquired Immune Deficiency Syndromes*, vol. 53, no. 2, pp. 247–253, 2010.

[16] S. J. Phillips, K. A. Freedberg, E. T. Traphagen, N. J. Horton, and J. H. Samet, "Screening for alcohol problems in HIV-infected primary care patients," *Journal of General Internal Medicine*, vol. 16, no. 1, p. S165, 2001.

[17] J. H. Samet, S. J. Phillips, N. J. Horton, E. T. Traphagen, and K. A. Freedberg, "Detecting alcohol problems in HIV-infected patients: use of the CAGE questionnaire," *AIDS Research and Human Retroviruses*, vol. 20, no. 2, pp. 151–155, 2004.

[18] J. Conigliaro, A. J. Gordon, K. A. McGinnis, L. Rabeneck, and A. C. Justice, "How harmful is hazardous alcohol use and abuse in HIV infection: do health care providers know who is at risk?" *Journal of Acquired Immune Deficiency Syndromes*, vol. 33, no. 4, pp. 521–525, 2003.

[19] B. F. Grant, D. A. Dawson, F. S. Stinson, S. P. Chou, M. C. Dufour, and R. P. Pickering, "The 12-month prevalence and trends in DSM-IV alcohol abuse and dependence: United States, 1991-1992 and 2001-2002," *Drug and Alcohol Dependence*, vol. 74, no. 3, pp. 223–234, 2004.

[20] N. Rehn, R. Room, and G. Edwards, *Alcohol in the European Region—Consumption, Harm and Policies*, Regional Office for Europe, World Health Organization, 2001.

[21] L. B. Moreira, F. D. Fuchs, R. S. Moraes, M. Bredemeier, and B. B. Duncan, "Alcohol intake and blood pressure: the importance of time elapsed since last drink," *Journal of Hypertension*, vol. 16, no. 2, pp. 175–180, 1998.

[22] A. A. Steffens, L. B. Moreira, S. C. Fuchs, M. Wiehe, M. Gus, and F. D. Fuchs, "Incidence of hypertension by alcohol consumption: is it modified by race?" *Journal of Hypertension*, vol. 24, no. 8, pp. 1489–1492, 2006.

[23] D. S. Minor, M. R. Wofford, and D. W. Jones, "Racial and ethnic differences in hypertension," *Current Atherosclerosis Reports*, vol. 10, no. 2, pp. 121–127, 2008.

[24] M. S. Mujahid, A. V. Diez Roux, R. C. Cooper, S. Shea, and D. R. Williams, "Neighborhood stressors and race/ethnic differences in hypertension prevalence (the Multi-Ethnic Study of atherosclerosis)," *American Journal of Hypertension*, vol. 24, no. 2, pp. 187–193, 2011.

[25] A. V. Chobanian, G. L. Bakris, H. R. Black et al., "The Seventh Report of the Joint National Committee on prevention, detection, evaluation, and treatment of high blood pressure," *Journal of the American Medical Association*, vol. 289, no. 19, pp. 2560–2572, 2003.

[26] C. L. Craig, A. L. Marshall, M. Sjöström et al., "International physical activity questionnaire: 12-country reliability and validity," *Medicine and Science in Sports and Exercise*, vol. 35, no. 8, pp. 1381–1395, 2003.

[27] https://sites.google.com/site/theipaq/scoring-protocol.

[28] E. O'Brien, F. Mee, N. Atkins, and M. Thomas, "Evaluation of three devices for self-measurement of blood pressure according to the revised British Hypertension Society Protocol. The Omron HEM-705CP, Philips HP5332, and Nissei DS-175," *Blood Pressure Monitoring*, vol. 1, no. 1, pp. 55–61, 1996.

[29] P. R. Alencastro, S. C. Fuchs, F. H. Wolff, M. L. Ikeda, A. B. M. Brandão, and N. T. Barcellos, "Independent predictors of metabolic syndrome in HIV-infected patients," *AIDS Patient Care and STDs*, vol. 25, no. 11, pp. 627–634, 2011.

[30] A. J. D. Barros and V. N. Hirakata, "Alternatives for logistic regression in cross-sectional studies: an empirical comparison of models that directly estimate the prevalence ratio," *BMC Medical Research Methodology*, vol. 3, article 1, 2003.

[31] N. T. Barcellos, S. C. Fuchs, and F. D. Fuchs, "Prevalence of and risk factors for HIV infection in individuals testing for HIV at counseling centers in Brazil," *Sexually Transmitted Diseases*, vol. 30, no. 2, pp. 166–173, 2003.

[32] C. G. Victora, S. R. Huttly, S. C. Fuchs, and M. T. A. Olinto, "The role of conceptual frameworks in epidemiological analysis: a hierarchical approach," *International Journal of Epidemiology*, vol. 26, no. 1, pp. 224–227, 1997.

[33] L. J. Beilin, I. B. Puddey, and V. Burke, "Alcohol and hypertension-kill or cure?" *Journal of Human Hypertension*, vol. 10, no. 2, supplement, pp. S1–S5, 1996.

[34] A. L. Klatsky, "Alcohol and cardiovascular health," *Physiology and Behavior*, vol. 100, no. 1, pp. 76–81, 2010.

[35] R. Thiébaut, W. M. El-Sadr, N. Friis-Møller et al., "Predictors of hypertension and changes of blood pressure in HIV-infected patients," *Antiviral Therapy*, vol. 10, no. 7, pp. 811–823, 2005.

[36] D. C. Chow, S. A. Souza, R. Chen et al., "Elevated blood pressure in HIV-infected individuals receiving highly active antiretroviral therapy," *HIV Clinical Trials*, vol. 4, no. 6, pp. 411–416, 2003.

[37] E. C. Seaberg, A. Muñoz, M. Lu et al., "Association between highly active antiretroviral therapy and hypertension in a large cohort of men followed from 1984 to 2003," *AIDS*, vol. 19, no. 9, pp. 953–960, 2005.

[38] J. L. Abramson, C. Lewis, and N. V. Murrah, "Relationship of self-reported alcohol consumption to ambulatory blood pressure in a sample of healthy adults," *American Journal of Hypertension*, vol. 23, no. 9, pp. 994–999, 2010.

4

HIV Infection and Cardiovascular Disease

Sandra C. Fuchs,[1,2,3] **Marina Beltrami-Moreira,**[1,4] **Bolanle Oyeledun,**[5,6] **Papa Salif Sow,**[7] **and Marco Vitoria**[8]

[1] *Postgraduate Studies Program in Cardiology, School of Medicine, Universidade Federal do Rio Grande do Sul, R. Ramiro Barcelos 2600, 90035-003 Porto Alegre, RS, Brazil*
[2] *National Institute for Health Technology Assessment (IATS/CNPq), Hospital de Clínicas de Porto Alegre, R. Ramiro Barcelos 2350, 90035-003 Porto Alegre, RS, Brazil*
[3] *Department of Nutrition, Harvard School of Public Health, 677 Huntington Avenue, Boston, MA 02115, USA*
[4] *Harvard Medical School, New Research Building, Avenue Louis Pasteur, Room 724, Boston, MA 02115, USA*
[5] *Centre for Integrated Health Programs (CIHP), Plot 1129 Kikuyu Close, Off Nariobi Street, Wuse II Abuja, FCT, Nigeria*
[6] *ICAP, Mailman School of Public Health Columbia University, 722 West 168th Street, New York, NY 10032, USA*
[7] *University of Dakar, Department of Infectious Diseases Fann Hospital, BP 5035, Dakar, Senegal*
[8] *HIV/AIDS Department, World Health Organization, 20, Avenue Appia, CH-1211 Geneva 27, Switzerland*

Correspondence should be addressed to Sandra C. Fuchs; scfuchs@terra.com.br

HIV infection has been considered as one of the major global public health threats of the last century, increasing several times the mortality rate in comparison to the cholera epidemic that swept London in the nineteenth century. Unlike the contamination caused by cholera bacillus, prevention of HIV infection requires other interventions than basic sanitation, and the antiretroviral agents currently remain the touchstone to transform the disease from subacute into a chronic condition. The introduction of highly active antiretroviral therapy (HAART) in the treatment of HIV-infected patients, in 1990s, has allowed better health status and greater longevity among people living with HIV, associated with a reduction in the viral transmission rate. For a while, it has been believed that universal access to HAART and the progressive increase in the efficiency of the prevention methods could save future generations [1]. However, it requires an enormous effort to expand HIV testing, maintenance of sustained treatment, and implementation of prevention programs. Nevertheless, HAART is not free of adverse effects.

With the significant reduction of the mortality and morbidity associated with HIV induced immunodeficiency in patients using HAART, the HIV infection is behaving as a long-term sickness [2]. HIV infection and its treatment have been associated with abnormal metabolic profile [3]; increased prevalence of noncommunicable diseases [4, 5] and mortality rate of AIDS-related have shifted to non-AIDS-related conditions [6, 7]. In the pre-HAART era, mortality from cardiovascular disease in infected persons occurred almost two decades earlier than in the general population. After the introduction of HAART, this difference went on to about nine years [8]. Even though the HIV-infected population is getting older, most still ar less than 50 years old and, in the United States, only half of the population will be 50 years in 2015 [9]. Therefore, the long-term management of patients with HIV infection has to be expanded to diagnosis, treatment, and prevention of cardiovascular risk factors and coronary heart disease. Even so, most current guidelines for the treatment of HIV infection are still focused only on antiretroviral treatment and do not take into account the treatment and prevention of comorbidities not related to AIDS [10–12]. However, bringing the paradigm of cardiovascular disease prevention for the scenario of HIV infection requires detection of the prevalence of cardiovascular risk factors and coronary heart disease in HIV-infected patients.

In this edition of this journal, a portrait of the Brazilian scenario of cardiovascular disease among HIV-infected patients was presented. Brazil is a country that has provided free access to HIV treatment for the entire population of infected people in the last two decades, and the use of HAART had a great impact on the costs of health care and the demand for the public health system. D. V. Araújo et al. showed that, in the last five years, the number of HIV/AIDS cases increased approximately by 40%, among patients under 50-years of age, yet the hospital admissions due to AIDS remained stable. Conversely, there was a marked increase in the hospitalizations due to acute myocardial infarction. R. K. Lazzaretti et al. provided data on genetic basis for understanding the complexity of the dyslipidemia in HIV infection. They detected that single nucleotide polymorphisms in six candidate genes (APO B, APO A5, APO E, APO C3, SCAP, and LDLR) were associated with dyslipidemia, showing that genetic factors contribute to determining the lipid profile in HIV-infected individuals on antiretroviral therapy.

Even so, there is a lack of robust evidence for prescribing agents to reduce dyslipidemia in HIV-infected patients. The new guidelines for cholesterol treatment highlighted the lack of randomized clinical trials on the potential benefits of statin therapy to reduce the risk of atherosclerotic cardiovascular disease in HIV-infected patients exceeding the risk of adverse events or drug interactions [13].

Another approach, previously described for the general population [14, 15], was to determine whether the association between consumption of alcoholic beverages and hypertension was modified by race in HIV-infected individuals. Among lifestyle characteristics, the consumption of large amounts of alcohol was independently associated with hypertension in white and nonwhite HIV-infected individuals. M. L. R. Ikeda et al. showed that there was an association of blood pressure with the frequency of consumption among the whites, while for nonwhite participants the amount of alcohol consumed was more important than the pattern of consumption in raising blood pressure. Although some of lifestyle characteristics are not modifiable, alcohol consumption is suitable for intervention.

In an attempt to compare some tools available to assess the overall cardiovascular risk profile of HIV-infected patients, M. W. Nery et al. calculated the traditional Framingham risk score, the Prospective Cardiovascular Münster (PROCAM) score; both originally developed for non-HIV-infected population; and the Data Collection on Adverse Effects on Anti-HIV Drugs (DAD) score, validated on HIV-infected patients. They found that the proportion of patients classified as being at moderate risk or higher was larger for the Framingham than for the PROCAM score. While these results have clinical follow-up and management implications, there was no comparison with data collected for the incidence of events. The use of Framingham score seems to have the advantage of allowing the comparison with other studies conducted in non-HIV-infected population [16]. Finally, a pooled analysis carried out in three cities of the Northeast, Midwest, and Southern Brazil showed that, irrespective of HIV status or treatment, classically risk-associated conditions, such as hypertension and diabetes, persist as the most relevant risk factors for cardiovascular disease. Moreover, these conditions were present at a younger age in the studied population. Of note is also the high prevalence of moderate and high risk according to the Framingham risk score among women. In this group, the diagnosis of cardiovascular disease and ischemic heart disease frequently occurs later than in men. This study reminds us that it is never too early to approach these problems and emphasize primary prevention of cardiovascular disease, even among populations with chronic conditions such as the HIV infection. We believe that the spectrum of cardiovascular manifestations among patients infected by HIV, pictured in this edition, allows the design and implementation of initiatives aimed at controlling and preventing the impact of cardiovascular disease.

Sandra C. Fuchs
Marina Beltrami-Moreira
Bolanle Oyeledun
Papa Salif Sow
Marco Vitoria

References

[1] A. S. Fauci and G. K. Folkers, "Toward an AIDS-free generation," *The Journal of the American Medical Association*, vol. 308, no. 4, pp. 343–344, 2012.

[2] S. G. Deeks, S. R. Lewin, and D. V. Havlir, "The end of AIDS: HIV infection as a chronic disease," *The Lancet*, vol. 382, no. 9903, pp. 1525–1533, 2013.

[3] P. R. Alencastro, F. H. Wolff, R. R. Oliveira et al., "Metabolic syndrome and population attributable risk among HIV/AIDS patients: comparison between NCEP-ATPIII, IDF and AHA/NHLBI definitions," *AIDS Research and Therapy*, vol. 9, no. 1, p. 29, 2012.

[4] J. E. Ho and P. Y. Hsue, "Cardiovascular manifestations of HIV infection," *Heart*, vol. 95, no. 14, pp. 1193–1202, 2009.

[5] F. Thienemann, K. Sliwa, and J. K. Rockstroh, "HIV and the heart: the impact of antiretroviral therapy: a global perspective," *European Heart Journal*, 2013.

[6] B. Grinsztejn, P. M. Luz, A. G. Pacheco et al., "Changing mortality profile among HIV-infected patients in Rio de Janeiro, Brazil: shifting from AIDS to non-AIDS related conditions in the HAART era," *PLoS ONE*, vol. 8, no. 4, Article ID e59768, 2013.

[7] J. E. Lake and J. S. Currier, "Metabolic disease in HIV infection," *The Lancet Infectious Diseases*, vol. 13, no. 11, pp. 964–975, 2013.

[8] N. Wada, L. P. Jacobson, M. Cohen, A. French, J. Phair, and A. Muñoz, "Cause-specific life expectancies after 35 years of age for human immunodeficiency syndrome-infected and human immunodeficiency syndrome-negative individuals followed simultaneously in long-term cohort studies, 1984–2008," *American Journal of Epidemiology*, vol. 177, no. 2, pp. 116–125, 2013.

[9] R. B. Effros, C. V. Fletcher, K. Gebo et al., "Workshop on HIV infection and aging: what is known and future research directions," *Clinical Infectious Diseases*, vol. 47, no. 4, pp. 542–553, 2008.

[10] S. Gupta, R. Granich, A. B. Suthar et al., "Global policy review of antiretroviral therapy eligibility criteria for treatment and prevention of HIV and tuberculosis in adults, pregnant women, and serodiscordant couples," *Journal of Acquired Immune Deficiency Syndromes*, vol. 62, no. 3, pp. e87–e97, 2013.

[11] G. Hirnschall, A. D. Harries, P. J. Easterbrook, M. C. Doherty, and A. Ball, "The next generation of the World Health Organization's global antiretroviral guidance," *Journal of the International AIDS Society*, vol. 30, no. 16, Article ID 18757, 2013.

[12] M. Doherty, N. Ford, M. Vitoria, G. Weiler, and G. Hirnschall, "The 2013 WHO guidelines for antiretroviral therapy: evidence-based recommendations to face new epidemic realities," *Current Opinion in HIV and AIDS*, vol. 8, no. 6, pp. 528–534, 2013.

[13] N. J. Stone, J. Robinson, A. H. Lichtenstein et al., "2013 ACC/AHA guideline on the treatment of blood cholesterol to reduce atherosclerotic cardiovascular risk in adults: a report of the American College of Cardiology/American Heart Association Task Force on Practice Guidelines," *Circulation*, 2013.

[14] F. D. Fuchs, L. E. Chambless, P. K. Whelton, F. J. Nieto, and G. Heiss, "Alcohol consumption and the incidence of hypertension: the Atherosclerosis Risk in Communities study," *Hypertension*, vol. 37, no. 5, pp. 1242–1250, 2001.

[15] A. A. Steffens, L. B. Moreira, S. C. Fuchs, M. Wiehe, M. Gus, and F. D. Fuchs, "Incidence of hypertension by alcohol consumption: is it modified by race?" *Journal of Hypertension*, vol. 24, no. 8, pp. 1489–1492, 2006.

[16] N. Friis-Møller, R. Thiébaut, P. Reiss et al., "Predicting the risk of cardiovascular disease in HIV-infected patients: the Data collection on Adverse Effects of Anti-HIV Drugs study," *European Journal of Cardiovascular Prevention and Rehabilitation*, vol. 17, no. 5, pp. 491–501, 2010.

5

Genetic Markers Associated to Dyslipidemia in HIV-Infected Individuals on HAART

Rosmeri K. Lazzaretti,[1] Aline S. Gasparotto,[2] Marina G. de M. Sassi,[2] Carísi A. Polanczyk,[1,3] Regina Kuhmmer,[1] Jussara M. Silveira,[4] Rossana P. Basso,[4] Cezar A. T. Pinheiro,[5] Mariângela F. Silveira,[5] Eduardo Sprinz,[6] and Vanessa S. Mattevi[2]

[1] *Serviço de Cardiologia, Hospital de Clínicas de Porto Alegre, Universidade Federal do Rio Grande do Sul, 90035-903 Porto Alegre, RS, Brazil*
[2] *Universidade Federal de Ciências da Saúde de Porto Alegre, Rua Sarmento Leite 245, Sala 309, 90050-170 Porto Alegre, RS, Brazil*
[3] *Serviço de Cardiologia, Hospital de Clínicas de Porto Alegre, Universidade Federal do Rio Grande do Sul, Instituto de Avaliação de Tecnologias em Saúde, 90035-903 Porto Alegre, RS, Brazil*
[4] *Hospital Universitário Dr. Miguel Riet Correa Jr., 96200-000 Rio Grande, RS, Brazil*
[5] *Serviço de Assistência Especializada em HIV/AIDS, Universidade Federal de Pelotas, 96030-001 Pelotas, RS, Brazil*
[6] *Serviço de Medicina Interna, Hospital de Clínicas de Porto Alegre, Universidade Federal do Rio Grande do Sul, 90035-903 Porto Alegre, RS, Brazil*

Correspondence should be addressed to Vanessa S. Mattevi; vmattevi@ufcspa.edu.br

Academic Editors: S. C. Fuchs, M. B. Moreira, and B. Oyeledun

This study evaluated the impact of 9 single nucleotide polymorphisms (SNPs) in 6 candidate genes (*APOB, APOA5, APOE, APOC3, SCAP*, and *LDLR*) over dyslipidemia in HIV-infected patients on stable antiretroviral therapy (ART) with undetectable viral loads. Blood samples were collected from 614 patients at reference services in the cities of Porto Alegre, Pelotas, and Rio Grande in Brazil. The SNPs were genotyped by conventional polymerase chain reaction (PCR) and real-time PCR. The prevalence of dyslipidemia was particularly high among the protease inhibitors-treated patients (79%). *APOE* (rs429358 and rs7412) genotypes and *APOA5* −1131T>C (rs662799) were associated with plasma triglycerides (TG) and low-density-lipoprotein cholesterol levels (LDL-C). The *APOA5* −1131T>C (rs662799) and *SCAP* 2386A>G (rs12487736) polymorphisms were significantly associated with high-density-lipoprotein cholesterol levels. The mean values of the total cholesterol and LDL-C levels were associated with both the *APOB* SP *Ins/Del* (rs17240441) and *APOB XbaI* (rs693) polymorphisms. In conclusion, our data support the importance of genetic factors in the determination of lipid levels in HIV-infected individuals. Due to the relatively high number of carriers of these risk variants, studies to verify treatment implications of genotyping before HAART initiation may be advisable to guide the selection of an appropriate antiretroviral therapy regimen.

1. Introduction

The use of antiretroviral therapy (ART) as a standard of care has changed the prognosis of human immunodeficiency virus (HIV) infection by decreasing mortality and improving quality of life [1, 2]. Despite the clinical benefits, long-term ART is associated with a complex spectrum of unwanted metabolic effects, including dyslipidemia that eventually might lead to increased risk of cardiovascular diseases [3].

Nevertheless, these side effects are not universal to all individuals on ART and even vary in individuals with comparable ART, demographic, immunologic, and virological characteristics. This variability suggests that host genetic factors and inherited predispositions may have a significant influence on the appearance of metabolic alterations [4].

The exact mechanism of dyslipidemia is not fully understood but is most likely multifactorial. In the general population, genetic variation accounts for approximately 43%–83% of the variability in lipid plasma levels [5]. Recent candidate gene studies [6–11] as well as genome-wide-based association studies have identified certain single nucleotide polymorphisms (SNPs) that could account for a significant portion of the variation in blood lipid levels [12–14].

In HIV infection, genetic predisposition may help to explain the variability among patients with respect to the effects of protease inhibitors (PIs) on lipid metabolism [10, 11]. We have hypothesized that this variation is attributable to the joint effect of HIV infection and ART together with the underlying genetic predisposition present in these individuals. The aim of this study was to investigate the frequencies of 9 SNPs in 6 candidate genes and to identify associations between these SNPs and the plasma lipid levels of patients on stable ART with undetectable viral loads.

2. Methods

2.1. Subjects. We conducted a cross-sectional study with 614 patients who were diagnosed with HIV-1 infection according to the criteria of the Centers for Disease Control and Prevention [15]. All subjects were more than 17 years old, had regularly used ART for at least 12 months, had a viral load below the detection limit of the test (50 copies/mL; Versant HIV-1 RNA 3.0 Assay (bDNA), Siemens, Germany), and were recruited from three referral centers in southern Brazil (HIV/AIDS Ambulatory Unit of Hospital de Clínicas from Porto Alegre/RS, HIV Ambulatory Care of Hospital Universitário Dr. Miguel Riet Correa Jr. from Rio Grande/RS, and HIV/AIDS Specialized Assistance Service from Pelotas/RS) from March 2006 to November 2008. Pregnant women and those with neurological disease that prevented understanding and proper consent were not included in the study. The study protocol was approved by the Research Ethics Committees of the three centers and of the Universidade Federal de Ciências da Saúde de Porto Alegre, and all participants signed an informed consent statement before they were included in the study (protocol numbers: 05/295, 718/08, 154/07, and 141/06, resp.).

2.2. Study Protocol. The routine evaluation consisted of visits every 4 months in each center for an evaluation by the patients' attending physicians as well as laboratory evaluations that included measurements of CD4 cell counts, viral load, and lipid levels. The patients were invited to participate in the study and had their information and a blood sample for DNA extraction collected during one of these visits.

An interview was performed at enrollment to obtain demographic and lifestyle information. Details of HIV infection (time from diagnosis as well as current and prior antiretroviral medications), lipid-lowering intervention, and relevant clinical variables were obtained from medical records. The interviewer phenotypically defined the patients' ethnicities because there might be a strong cultural tendency to claim European ancestry in Brazil [16]. Patients were classified as Euro- or Afro-descendants because the Amerindian contribution is very low in the Brazilian South Region [17].

2.3. Laboratory Analysis. Blood samples were collected and sent to the Molecular Biology Laboratory for DNA extraction. Lipid profiles included determinations of total cholesterol (TC), high-density lipoprotein (HDL-C), triglycerides (TG), and, when possible, low-density lipoprotein (LDL-C) after fasting for 12 hours. LDL-C was calculated using the Friedewald formula, LDL-C = TC − HDL-C − TG/5, if triglyceride levels were below 400 mg/dL.

Dyslipidemia was defined by fasting triglycerides plasma levels ≥150 mg/dL and/or fasting total cholesterol ≥200 mg/dL and/or LDL-C ≥130 mg/dL and/or HDL-C <40 mg/dL. Participants were instructed not to perform any vigorous physical activity or ingest alcohol in the 24 hours prior to the blood collection [18].

Genomic DNA was obtained from peripheral leukocytes by a standard salting-out technique [19]. The genotypes of apolipoprotein B gene (*APOB*) polymorphisms were determined using polymerase chain reaction (PCR) based procedures in 410 individuals from the outpatient clinic of the Hospital de Clínicas de Porto Alegre. The polymorphism of insertion/deletion of signal peptide SP *Ins/Del* (rs17240441) was amplified by PCR using primers as previously described [20] and directly analyzed by electrophoresis in 8% polyacrylamide gels. The *Xba*I, 7673C>T (rs693) polymorphism was amplified by PCR using the primers described by Pan et al. [21], and genotypes were determined by digestion with *Xba*I restriction endonuclease and electrophoresis in 2% agarose gels.

The SNPs of apolipoprotein A-V (*APOA5*) −1131T>C (rs662799) and S19W (56C>G; rs3135506), apolipoproteinE (*APOE*) 334T>C (E4; rs429358) and 472C>T (E2; rs7412), apolipoprotein C-III (*APOC3*) 3238C>G (rs5128), sterol regulatory element-binding factor cleavage-activating protein (*SCAP*) 2386A>G (rs12487736), and low-density lipoprotein receptor (*LDLR*) intron 19G>T (rs6511720) were genotyped by real-time PCR using the TaqMan methodology and are listed in Table 1. Candidate SNPs were selected via review of PubMed reports of SNP associations with dyslipidemia in the general population or among HIV-infected individuals [6–11].

2.4. Statistical Analyses. The results are expressed as the mean ± standard deviation (SD) for continuous variables and as proportions for categorical variables. Variables that did not have a normal distribution (triglycerides) were transformed into natural logarithms before the statistical tests were applied. Allele frequencies were estimated by gene counting. χ^2 analysis that was used to test for deviations in genotype frequencies from the Hardy-Weinberg equilibrium (HWE).

For the *APOC3* 3238C>G (rs5128), *APOA5* −1131T>C (rs662799) and S19W (56C>G) (rs3135506), *SCAP* 2386A>G (rs12487736), and *LDLR* intron 19G>T (rs6511720) polymorphisms, the association analyses were performed according

TABLE 1: Genotypic and allelic frequencies of polymorphisms analyzed.

Polymorphisms	Genotypic frequency	Allelic frequency		
APOA5 −1131T>C (rs662799)[a]		T	C	
T/T	515 (84.7)	0.92	0.08	
T/C	90 (14.8)			
C/C	3 (0.5)			
Total	**608**			
APOA5 S19W (56C>G; rs3135506)[a]		C	G	
C/C	500 (82)	0.90	0.10	
C/G	103 (16.9)			
G/G	7 (1.1)			
Total	**610**			
APOB SP *Ins/Del* (rs17240441)[a]		*Ins*	*Del*	
Ins/ins	193 (47.3)	0.70	0.30	
Ins/del	176 (43.1)			
Del/del	39 (9.6)			
Total	**408**			
APOB XbaI, 7673C>T (rs693)[a]		C	T	
C/C	122 (30)	0.55	0.45	
C/T	203 (49.9)			
T/T	82 (20.1)			
Total	**407**			
APOC3 3238C>G (rs5128)[b]		C	G	
C/C	478 (78.8)	0.89	0.11	
C/G	127 (20.9)			
G/G	2 (0.3)			
Total	**607**			
APOE[a]		E2	E3	E4
E2/E2	5 (0.8)	0.07	0.79	0.14
E2/E3	67 (11.2)			
E2/E4	9 (1.5)			
E3/E3	379 (63.6)			
E3/E4	120 (20.1)			
E4/E4	16 (2.7)			
Total	**596**			
LDLR intron 19G>T (rs6511720)[a]		G	T	
G/G	487 (80.2)	0.90	0.10	
G/T	113 (18.6)			
T/T	7 (1.2)			
Total	**607**			
SCAP 2386A>G (rs12487736)[a]		A	G	
A/A	168 (27.7)	0.52	0.48	
A/G	296 (48.9)			
G/G	142 (23.4)			
Total	**606**			

The difference in the number of individuals among single nucleotide polymorphisms (SNPs) is due to failure in genotyping some SNPs in the whole sample.
Genotypic frequencies presented as number of patients (%).
[a]χ^2 test for Hardy-Weinberg equilibrium; $P > 0.05$.
[b]χ^2 test for Hardy-Weinberg equilibrium; $P = 0.032$.

Table 2: Characteristics of the study participants.

	All study participants $n = 614$	PI-sparing ART $n = 311$	PI-based ART $n = 303$	P value
Demographic				
Age, years	43.0 ± 10	42 ± 10	43 ± 9	0.114[§]
Male sex, n (%)	341 (55.5)	179 (58)	162 (54)	0.348[*]
Ethnicity, n (%)				
Euro-Brazilians	349 (57)	166 (48)	183 (60)	0.094[*]
Afro-Brazilians	265 (43)	145 (47)	120 (40)	
Physical activity, n (%)	156 (25)	74 (24)	82 (27)	0.389[*]
Cigarette smoking, n (%)	186 (30)	103 (33)	83 (28)	0.153[*]
Clinical				
CD4, cells/uL	533 ± 266	516 ± 255	552 ± 277	0.095[§]
Therapy time (months)	68 ± 41	57 ± 38	76 ± 41	<0.001[§¥]
Lipid-lowering drugs, n (%)	105 (17)	42 (14)	63 (21)	0.021[*]
Metabolic				
Triglycerides, mg/dL	196 ± 171	170 ± 131	223 ± 202	<0.001[¶¥]
Total cholesterol, mg/dL	192 ± 48	189 ± 44	196 ± 52	0.056[§]
HDL-C, mg/dL	48 ± 16	51 ± 17	46 ± 14	<0.001[§]
LDL-C, mg/dL	107 ± 37	105 ± 34	109 ± 40	0.175[§]
Dyslipidemia, n (%)	455 (74)	215 (69)	240 (79)	0.006[*]
Hypertriglyceridemia	293 (49)	122 (40)	171 (59)	<0.001[*]
Hypercholesterolemia	245 (41)	118 (39)	127 (44)	0.267[*]
Low HDL-C	185 (31)	74 (24)	111 (38)	<0.001[*]

Data presented as mean ± SD or number of patients (%).
PI: protease inhibitors; ART: antiretroviral therapy; HDL-C: high-density lipoprotein; LDL-C: low-density lipoprotein.
[¥] P value expressed with tests performed with ln-transformed variable.
[§] Student t-test for independent samples.
[*] χ^2-Test with Yates correction.
[¶] Student t-test for independent samples with ln-transformed variable.

to the dominant model due to the low number of individuals who were homozygous for the minor allele and were pooled with subjects with the heterozygous genotype. As for *APOE* SNPs 334T>C (rs429358) and 472C>T (rs7412), which together define the *APOE* E2, E3, and E4 alleles, the subjects were analyzed in 3 genotype categories: E2/E3, homozygotes for the E3 allele and E3/E4. Subjects with the rare genotypes E2/E2 ($n = 5$), E2/E4 ($n = 9$), and E4/E4 ($n = 16$) were excluded from the statistical analyses.

The Testing Haplotype Effects in Association Studies Program (version 3.1, THESIAS, Paris, France) was used for the analysis of linkage disequilibrium between polymorphisms within the same gene [22].

General linear model analyses were used to test for the interaction between SNPs and variables and to adjust the lipid profile for covariables. The following variables were included in the models and underwent stepwise removal according to the greatest P values: ethnic group, gender, age, physical activity, cigarette smoking, use of lipid-lowering agents, PI use, body mass index (BMI), and the presence of polymorphism. Only those variables that were significant predictors were included in the final model. Correction for multiple testing was performed using the Bonferroni method. The data were analyzed with the Statistical Package for Social Sciences (version 20.0, SPSS, Chicago, Illinois). The value indicating statistical significance was $P < 0.05$.

3. Results

3.1. Study Participants. The main demographic, clinical, and metabolic characteristics of the individuals enrolled in the study are shown in Table 2. Of the 614 patients, 55.5% were males, 57% were characterized as Euro-descendants, and the mean patient age was 43 ± 10 years. The mean duration of ART was 68 ± 41 months. Regarding metabolic parameters, 245 (41%) patients had hypercholesterolemia, 293 (49%) had hypertriglyceridemia, and 185 (31%) had low HDL-C levels.

The total patient population was stratified according to current PI use or nonuse. The prevalence of dyslipidemia was particularly high among the PI-treated patients (79% versus 69% in nonusers; $P = 0.006$). Although the mean levels of TC and LDL-C did not differ significantly between the PI-treated and non-PI-treated subjects, the latter had higher

Table 3: Mean metabolic variables according to polymorphisms analyzed.

Polymorphisms	Total cholesterol (mg/dL)		LDL-C (mg/dL)		HDL-C (mg/dL)		Triglycerides (mg/dL)	
	N	M ± SD	*N*	M ± SD	*N*	M ± SD	*N*	M ± SD
APOA5 −1131T>C (rs662799)								
T/T	499	191 ± 80	458	106 ± 72	498	48 ± 88	499	187 ± 157
T/C + C/C	92	196 ± 78	83	107 ± 12	92	45 ± 16	92	243 ± 230
P value		0.549		0.953		0.047[$]		0.003[*£]
P value *corrected*[**]		1.000		1.000		0.376		0.024
APOA5 S19W (56C>G; rs3135506)								
C/C	486	192 ± 49	443	106 ± 37	485	48 ± 15	486	199 ± 177
C/G + G/G	106	197 ± 43	99	112 ± 35	107	50 ± 17	107	183 ± 144
P value		0.330		0.047[#]		0.130		0.398[*]
P value *corrected*[**]		1.000		0.376		1.000		1.000
APOB SP *Ins/Del* (rs17240441)								
Ins/ins	192	189 ± 42[a]	176	99 ± 31[c]	192	52 ± 15	193	195 ± 167
Ins/del	175	193 ± 51[ab]	158	106 ± 36[cd]	175	50 ± 14	176	195 ± 193
Del/del	39	210 ± 45[b]	37	120 ± 41[d]	39	54 ± 13	39	187 ± 103
P value		0.036[$]		0.006[$]		0.245		0.996[*]
P value *corrected*[**]		0.288		0.048		1.000		1.000
APOB XbaI, 7673C>T (rs693)								
C/C	122	183 ± 42[e]	112	95 ± 35[g]	122	52 ± 15	122	187 ± 126
C/T	202	194 ± 42[ef]	185	107 ± 31[h]	201	50 ± 14	203	193 ± 163
T/T	81	203 ± 59[f]	73	110 ± 41[ih]	82	51 ± 12	82	212 ± 248
P value		0.007[$]		0.002[$]		0.705		0.791[*]
P value *corrected*[**]		0.056		0.016		1.000		1.000
APOC3 3238C>G (rs5128)								
C/C	464	193 ± 48	424	107 ± 37	465	49 ± 16	440	191 ± 162
C/G + G/G	125	192 ± 49	115	108 ± 39	124	47 ± 15	124	210 ± 214
P value		0.718		0.833		0.295		0.905[*]
P value *corrected*[**]		1.000		1.000		1.000		1.000
APOE genotype								
E2/E3	64	188 ± 60	56	93 ± 34[j]	63	46 ± 14	64	263 ± 350[l]
E3/E3	365	193 ± 47	333	109 ± 37[k]	366	49 ± 16	366	186 ± 128[m]
E3/E4	119	198 ± 47	112	112 ± 38[k]	119	48 ± 17	119	195 ± 153[m]
P value		0.209		0.002[¶]		0.371		0.033[*§]
P value *corrected*[**]		0.836		0.008		1.000		0.132
LDLR intron 19G>T (rs6511720)								
G/G	475	193 ± 48	430	107 ± 36	476	48 ± 16	473	198 ± 184
G/T + T/T	114	191 ± 51	107	105 ± 41	113	50 ± 16	114	183 ± 109
P value		0.612		0.427		0.120		0.971[*]
P value *corrected*[**]		1.000		1.000		1.000		1.000

TABLE 3: Continued.

Polymorphisms	Total cholesterol (mg/dL)		LDL-C (mg/dL)		HDL-C (mg/dL)		Triglycerides (mg/dL)	
	N	M ± SD	*N*	M ± SD	*N*	M ± SD	*N*	M ± SD
SCAP 2386A>G (rs12487736)								
A/A	164	195 ± 49	146	107 ± 39	164	50 ± 17^{n}	164	201 ± 162
A/G	287	194 ± 48	263	107 ± 35	287	49 ± 15no	287	197 ± 197
G/G	137	188 ± 47	129	107 ± 41	137	45 ± 14°	138	188 ± 124
P value		0.443		0.970		0.032[¥]		0.971[*]
P value *corrected*[**]		1.000		1.000		0.128		1.000

HDL-C: high-density lipoprotein; LDL-C: low density lipoprotein.
[*] *P* value expressed with tests performed with logn-transformed variable.
[**] *P* value after Bonferroni correction for multiple testing.
[§] Adjusted for gender, age, and lipid-lowering agents use.
[¶] Adjusted for age, and lipid-lowering agents use.
[$] Adjusted for gender, cigarette smoking, and PI use.
[£] Adjusted for gender, age, lipid-lowering agents use, and PI.
[#] Adjusted for gender, age, ethnic group, BMI, and lipid-lowering agents use.
[¥] Adjusted for gender, cigarette smoking, ethnic group, and lipid-lowering agents use.
[ab] Tukey test, *Ins/Ins* versus *Ins/Del*, $P = 0.619$; *Ins/Ins* versus *Del/Del*, $P = 0.027$; *Ins/Del* versus *Del/Del*, $P = 0.145$.
[cd] Tukey test, *Ins/Ins* versus *Ins/Del*, $P = 0.231$; *Ins/Ins* versus *Del/Del*, $P = 0.006$; *Ins/Del* versus *Del/Del*, $P = 0.071$.
[ef] Tukey test, C/C versus C/T, $P = 0.053$; C/C versus T/T, $P = 0.007$; C/T versus T/T, $P = 0.598$.
[ghi] Tukey test, C/C versus C/T, $P = 0.006$; C/C versus T/T, $P = 0.008$; C/T versus T/T, $P = 0.830$.
[jk] Tukey test, E2/E3 versus E3/E3, $P = 0.011$; E2/E3 versus E3/E4, $P = 0.005$; E3/E3 versus E3/E4, $P = 0.628$.
[lm] Tukey test, E2/E3 versus E3/E3, $P = 0.003$; E2/E3 versus E3/E4, $P = 0.029$; E3/E3 versus E3/E4, $P = 0.875$.
[no] Tukey test, A/A versus A/G, $P = 0.594$; A/A versus G/G, $P = 0.014$; A/G versus G/G, $P = 0.071$.

plasma HDL-C levels (51 ± 17 mg/dL versus 46 ± 14 mg/dL; $P < 0.001$) and lower triglycerides levels (170 ± 131 mg/dL versus 223 ± 202 mg/dL, $P < 0.001$) than the PI-treated subjects. Therefore, PI use was tested as a covariate in all statistical analyses and was included when significant.

The genotype and allele frequencies of the analyzed SNPs are shown in Table 1. For all studied polymorphisms, there was no departure from Hardy-Weinberg equilibrium, except for *APOC3* 3238C>G (rs5128). Table 3 summarizes the association analysis of the SNPs with serum lipid concentrations.

3.2. Triglycerides. Two SNPs contributed significantly to the modification of TG levels. The plasma TG levels were different among *APOE* genotypes ($P = 0.033$), the E2 allele being associated with increased TG levels (Tukey test, E2/E3 versus E3/E3, $P = 0.003$; E2/E3 versus E3/E4, $P = 0.029$). However, this result was no longer significant after correction for multiple testing ($P_{corrected} = 0.132$).

The effect of the *APOA5* −1131T>C (rs662799) polymorphism on plasma lipids was observed in C-allele carriers, who presented higher triglyceride levels than those with the TT genotype (243 ± 230 mg/dL and 187 ± 157 mg/dL, respectively; $P = 0.003$). This nominal *P*-value remained statistically significant after Bonferroni correction for multiple comparisons ($P_{corrected} = 0.024$).

3.3. HDL Cholesterol. The *APOA5* −1131T>C (rs662799) polymorphism was also significantly associated with HDL-C levels. The TT homozygotes presented higher HDL-C concentrations than C-carriers ($P = 0.047$) after the same statistical approach and adjustment for covariates. Furthermore, a statistically significant association of the *SCAP* 2386A>G (rs12487736) variant was observed with HDL-C levels ($P = 0.032$). As shown in Table 3, the 2386GG homozygotes had lower HDL-C levels, while the 2386AA homozygotes showed an increase of 5 ± 2 mg/dL when compared to GG homozygotes (Tukey test, AA versus GG, $P = 0.014$). However, both associations were no longer significant after the Bonferroni correction for multiple comparisons.

3.4. Total Cholesterol and LDL Cholesterol. Initially, the average TC levels were associated with both the *APOB* SP *Ins/Del* (rs17240441; Table 3, $P = 0.036$) and *APOB XbaI*, 7673C>T (rs693; $P = 0.007$) polymorphisms. The *post hoc* test showed that there were differences between the homozygotes for both polymorphisms (Tukey test, *Ins/Ins* versus *Del/Del*, $P = 0.027$ and C/C versus T/T, $P = 0.007$, resp.). Neither results were significant after Bonferroni correction was applied ($P_{corrected} = 0.320$ and $P_{corrected} = 0.056$, resp.).

The mean LDL-C levels were also different between the genotypes ($P = 0.007$ and $P = 0.002$, resp.) for both polymorphisms and were statistically significant after Bonferroni correction was applied ($P_{corrected} = 0.048$ and $P_{corrected} = 0.016$, resp.). The Tukey test showed that, in the polymorphism of the signal peptide, differences were found between the homozygotes (*Ins/Ins* versus *Del/Del*, $P = 0.006$) and in the polymorphism in exon 26 of the gene the homozygous group with regard to the C allele differed from

TABLE 4: Effect of *APOB* Del T haplotype in total cholesterol and LDL-C.

Risk haplotype	TC (mg/dL)			LDL-C (mg/dL)		
	N	Mean ± SD	*P* value	*N*	Mean ± SD	*P*-value
Noncarriers	213	188 ± 42[a]	0.036	196	100 ± 32[b]	0.011
Heterozygous *Del* T	163	195 ± 51		147	108 ± 36	
Homozygotes *Del* T	27	212 ± 48[a]		25	118 ± 43[b]	

TC: total cholesterol; LDL-C: low density lipoprotein.
Results from analysis of variance.
[a]Tukey test noncarriers versus homozygous for *Del* T, $P = 0.036$.
[b]Tukey test noncarriers versus homozygous for *Del* T, $P = 0.038$.

the other groups (C/C versus C/T, $P = 0.006$; C/C versus T/T, $P = 0.008$).

A significant linkage disequilibrium ($D' = 0.72$, $P < 0.001$) was detected between polymorphisms associating alleles *Del* and T, as well as *Ins* and C. Based on these results, we analyzed the effect of the haplotype combining alleles *Del* and T on the levels of these lipid parameters. The haplotype analysis showed that homozygotes for the risk haplotype showed significantly higher mean levels of TC and LDL-C (Table 4). The *post hoc* test showed that the differences were found between noncarriers and homozygotes for the *Del* T haplotype (Tukey test, $P = 0.036$ and $P = 0.038$, resp.).

The *APOE* genotype was associated with elevated plasma LDL-C levels ($P = 0.002$; $P_{\text{corrected}} = 0.008$; Table 3). In contrast to what was observed regarding the TG levels, the E2 allele was associated with a decrease in the LDL-C levels, while the E4 allele was associated with an increase, as the differences were found between the E2 and E4 allele carriers (Tukey test, E2/E3 versus E3/E3, $P = 0.011$; E2/E3 versus E3/E4, $P = 0.005$).

Regarding *APOA5* S19W (56C>G) (rs3135506), there was a marginal association with LDL-C levels. Carriers of the G allele and C/C genotype showed a mean and an SD of 112 ± 35 mg/dL and 106 ± 37 mg/dL, respectively ($P = 0.047$), that was adjusted for gender, age, BMI, and use of lipid-lowering agents. However, it did not remain significant after Bonferroni correction.

No significant contribution to plasma TC, TG, HDL-C, or LDL-C was identified in the present dataset with regard to *APOC3* 3238C>G (rs5128) and *LDLR* intron 19G>T (rs6511720).

Analyses were also performed separately for users and nonusers of IPs (data not shown), and similar effects were observed in both groups, although in some cases these effects were not significant.

4. Discussion

The contributions of several polymorphisms to dyslipidemia in 614 HIV-1-infected patients on HAART were addressed in the present multicenter study. Nine polymorphisms in 6 candidate genes were analyzed for their association with dyslipidemia. As expected according to the literature, this adverse effect was more prevalent in patients receiving PIs ([23] and references therein). However, we found no statistically significant difference in TC and LDL-C levels between PI-treated and non-PI-treated patients, probably associated with the more prevalent use of lipid-lowering agents by the PI group (21 versus 14%, $P = 0.021$).

The allelic frequencies of the *APOB*, *APOA5*, *APOE*, *SCAP*, and *LDLR* genotypes were similar to those previously described in populations from the same geographical region or ethnicity [8–11]. The *APOC3* 3238C>G (rs5128) genotypic frequencies were not distributed according to what was expected under Hardy-Weinberg equilibrium ($P = 0.032$; Table 1). This small deviation was most likely due to the lower number of homozygotes (2 patients, 0.3%) for the rare allele observed in our study; 7 were expected according to Hardy-Weinberg's proportions. Nevertheless, the allele frequencies ($G = 0.11$) were very close to those found in previous studies of individuals not infected with HIV who live in Southern Brazil ($G = 0.10$), as shown by Fiegenbaum et al. [8], and to participants in the Swiss HIV Cohort Study (SHCS), which were $G = 0.10$ and $G = 0.09$, as shown by Rotger et al. [11] and Tarr et al. [24], respectively.

Our study demonstrated a strong association between the E3/E4 genotype and elevated plasma LDL-C, which is in agreement with the results of previous studies [25, 26]. The E4 variant is typically associated with increased levels of LDL-C and low plasma TG levels, whereas the E2 variant is associated with lower LDL-C levels in the general population [25, 26]. In a large meta-analysis, the E4 variant was associated with a 42% increase in cardiovascular disease risk [27]. Although E2 isoforms bind to LDL receptors much more weakly than E3 or E4 isoforms, the catabolism of the particle containing isoform E2 is slower; this may result in a lower rate of LDL-C formation. Moreover, according to the conclusion of the meta analysis of Bennet et al. [28], there is an approximately linear relationship between the *APOE* genotypes and both LDL-C levels and to the risk of cardiovascular disease.

Carriers of non-E3/E3 genotypes of *APOE* appear to be at risk of ritonavir-associated hypertriglyceridemia, and this risk appears to be enhanced by the association with *APOC3* variants [29]. According to the SHCS, the interaction between *APOE* and *APOC3* is associated with an extreme risk of developing hypertriglyceridemia in individuals treated with ritonavir [24]. Our data did not allow us to perform the same analyses, as the vast majority of our PI-users were on ritonavir. Nevertheless, our findings are in agreement with these data reinforcing the association of E2 allele and increased TG levels. With respect to the E3/E3 genotype, according to our data as well as to those of [30], HIV-positive patients have a lower risk of developing high triglyceride levels after starting HAART than non-E3/E3 genotypes.

APOA5 also plays an important role in the modulation of blood lipid metabolism; it is predominantly synthesized in the liver and is secreted into the plasma, where it plays a central role in regulating TG metabolism [31, 32]. Two polymorphisms in the *APOA5* gene, −1131T>C and S19W (56C>G), have been shown to be associated with elevated triglyceride levels in different populations [31, 33]. In our study, for *APOA5* −1131T>C, individuals with at least one C allele had higher TG levels and lower levels of HDL-C. However, only the association with TG levels remained significant after the Bonferroni correction was applied. These results are consistent with previous study in HIV-infected patients, indicated that −1131C carriers experienced marked increases in triglyceride levels during a 3-year follow-up, while no change was recorded in patients carrying the −1131T normal allele [34]. A similar effect, but of lesser magnitude, was demonstrated regarding changes in cholesterol [34].

To our knowledge, this is the first study conducted in an HIV-positive setting to assess the association of *SCAP* 2386A>G rs12487736 with dyslipidemia. The SCAP pathway controls cellular cholesterol homeostasis. Initially, in our analysis, we found that AA homozygous patients showed higher HDL-C levels; however, this result was no longer significant after Bonferroni correction was applied. Carriers of the 2386G allele from non-HIV-infected Brazilians treated with simvastatin exhibit reduced TC and TG levels, as shown by Fiegenbaum et al. [7], but no association was found with HDL-C levels.

The mean TC and LDL-C levels showed statistically significant differences for genotypes of both polymorphisms in the *APOB* gene: SP *Ins/Del* (rs17240441) and *Xba*I, 7673C>T (rs693). The homozygotes for the alleles T and *Del* had higher levels of these lipids than individuals heterozygous for both alleles, who had intermediate levels; this result is compatible with a co-dominant effect of these polymorphisms. These results are in agreement with published data showing that the *Del* and T alleles are associated with increased levels of TC and/or LDL-C in different populations with distinct diseases [9, 35–37]. However, Xu et al. and Ye et al. found no association of the polymorphism in the signal peptide of the gene with TC and LDL-C levels in the Finnish and Chinese populations, respectively [38, 39].

The significant linkage disequilibrium observed between polymorphisms, as reported in other studies [20, 39], led to an analysis of risk haplotype (patients with a combination of alleles *Del* and T). The patients who were homozygous for the risk haplotype showed higher total cholesterol and LDL-C, while an intermediate effect was observed in patients with the heterozygous haplotype. Rios et al. [9] also observed the association of the haplotype with LDL-C levels in a Brazilian population in a comparison of patients with and without coronary artery disease.

There are two possible causes for these changes in lipid metabolism related to both polymorphisms in the *APOB* gene. The first cause is that three amino acids, leu-ala-leu, that are included in the allele *Ins* and deleted in the allele *Del* could alter the hydrophobicity of the signal peptide of the protein and, thereby, alter the rate of translocation of new *APOB* peptides synthesized in the cytoplasm to the endoplasmic reticulum [38]. The second hypothesis is based on the fact that there is no amino acid change in the functional protein in both polymorphisms. These could then be in linkage disequilibrium with an unknown change in the DNA that may cause lipid abnormalities [20].

Two further SNPs that were proposed in the literature (*APOC3* 3238C>G (rs5128) and *LDLR* intron 19G>T (rs6511720) did not contribute to the plasma lipid levels in the present dataset, which may reflect a limited effect of these SNPs in HIV-infected patients.

All analyses were also performed by stratifying the patients according to PI use (data not shown); however, similar effects were observed in both groups. Furthermore, the variables were not statistically significant in some analyses, and this was most likely attributable to the reduction in the number of individuals when they are analyzed separately. This finding suggests that in our sample, the lipid-gene interaction is independent of the type of HAART used and that the variation observed is similar to that found in the general population.

We acknowledge some limitations of the present study. The cross-sectional design and the inclusion of patients receiving several different antiretroviral regimens, which is a difficulty inherent to any study involving current HAART, as by definition should include at least three different drugs. This fact might hinder the accomplishment of any pharmacogenomics study regarding this therapy. Furthermore, we found a deviation from the HWE observed in the current population for the *APOC3* 3238C>G (rs5128) SNP. Although this deviation may indicate genotyping error, laboratory procedures were in place to detect errors, including blinded, no-template controls and DNA sample replicates. Another limitation that we might acknowledge is the restricted number of SNPs analyzed. We cannot rule out the possibility that other SNPs in the genes investigated here are associated with the phenotypes studied.

In conclusion, our data support the importance of genetic factors on of lipid levels in HIV-infected individuals from a previously uninvestigated region of the world. We found no evidence of interaction of these genetic variants with the use of non-nucleoside transcriptase reverse inhibitors or protease inhibitors. Due to the relatively high number of carriers of these risk variants (e.g., *APOA5* −1131T>C = 15%, *APOB* risk haplotype = 47%, *APOE* = 20.1%), studies to verify treatment implications of genotyping are desirable.

Authors' Contribution

Eduardo Sprinz and Vanessa S. Mattevi were joint senior authors on this work. Aline S. Gasparotto and Marina G. de M. Sassi genotyped the patients and performed the experiments. Rosmeri K. Lazzaretti, Eduardo Sprinz, Regina Kuhmmer, Jussara M. Silveira, Rossana P. Basso, Cezar

A. T. Pinheiro, and Mariângela F. Silveira were responsible for recruiting and clinical evaluation of patients. Vanessa S. Mattevi conceived and designed the experiments. Carísi A. Polanczyk reviewed the paper. Rosmeri K. Lazzaretti and Vanessa S. Mattevi performed the statistical analyses. Rosmeri K. Lazzaretti, Vanessa S. Mattevi, and Eduardo Sprinz wrote the paper.

Disclosure

The number of contributors is justified by the performance of sample collections and patients' evaluations in three different reference centers.

Conflict of Interests

The authors declare that there is no conflict of interests.

Acknowledgments

A special acknowledgement *in memoriam* of Prof. Jorge Pinto Ribeiro, an example of scientist and educator. He will be sadly missed, but his enduring and substantial legacy will be intensely alive. The authors thank Grasiela Agnes for helping with qPCR experiments. This work was supported by Departamento de DST, AIDS e Hepatites Virais, Ministério da Saúde, Brazil; Conselho Nacional de Desenvolvimento Científico e Tecnológico (CNPq); Fundação de Amparo à Pesquisa do Estado do Rio Grande do Sul (FAPERGS); and PRONEX-FAPERGS/CNPq.

References

[1] B. O. Taiwo, X. Li, F. Palella et al., "Higher risk of AIDS or death in patients with lower CD4 cell counts after virally suppressive HAART," *HIV Medicine*, vol. 10, no. 10, pp. 657–660, 2009.

[2] J. R. P. Marins, L. F. Jamal, S. Y. Chen et al., "Dramatic improvement in survival among adult Brazilian AIDS patients," *AIDS*, vol. 17, no. 11, pp. 1675–1682, 2003.

[3] M. P. Dubé, J. H. Stein, J. A. Aberg et al., "Guidelines for the evaluation and management of dyslipidemia in human immunodeficiency virus (HIV)-infected adults receiving antiretroviral therapy: recommendations of the HIV Medicine Association of the Infectious Disease Society of America and the Adult AIDS Clinical Trials Group," *Clinical Infectious Diseases*, vol. 37, no. 5, pp. 613–627, 2003.

[4] J. Fox, M. Boffito, and A. Winston, "The clinical implications of antiretroviral pharmacogenomics," *Pharmacogenomics*, vol. 7, no. 4, pp. 587–596, 2006.

[5] M.-H. Chang, A. Yesupriya, R. M. Ned, P. W. Mueller, and N. F. Dowling, "Genetic variants associated with fasting blood lipids in the U.S. population: third National Health and Nutrition Examination Survey," *BMC Medical Genetics*, vol. 11, no. 1, article 62, 2010.

[6] F. M. de Andrade, S. W. Maluf, J. B. Schuch et al., "The influence of the S19W SNP of the APOA5 gene on triglyceride levels in southern Brazil: interactions with the APOE gene, sex and menopause status," *Nutrition, Metabolism and Cardiovascular Diseases*, vol. 21, no. 8, pp. 584–590, 2011.

[7] M. Fiegenbaum, F. R. Silveira, C. R. van der Sand et al., "Determinants of variable response to simvastatin treatment: the role of common variants of SCAP, SREBF-1a and SREBF-2 genes," *Pharmacogenomics Journal*, vol. 5, no. 6, pp. 359–364, 2005.

[8] M. Fiegenbaum, F. M. de Andrade, and M. H. Hutz, "Association between plasma lipid parameters and APOC3 genotypes in Brazilian subjects: effect of gender, smoking and APOE genotypes," *Clinica Chimica Acta*, vol. 380, no. 1-2, pp. 175–181, 2007.

[9] D. L. S. Rios, A. F. Vargas, M. R. Torres, A. J. Zago, S. M. Callegari-Jacques, and M. H. Hutz, "Interaction between SREBP-1a and APOB polymorphisms influences total and low-density lipoprotein cholesterol levels in patients with coronary artery disease," *Clinical Genetics*, vol. 63, no. 5, pp. 380–385, 2003.

[10] M. Arnedo, P. Taffé, R. Sahli et al., "Contribution of 20 single nucleotide polymorphisms of 13 genes to dyslipidemia associated with antiretroviral therapy," *Pharmacogenetics and Genomics*, vol. 17, no. 9, pp. 755–764, 2007.

[11] M. Rotger, C. Bayard, P. Taffé et al., "Contribution of genome-wide significant single-nucleotide polymorphisms and antiretroviral therapy to dyslipidemia in HIV-infected individuals: a longitudinal study," *Circulation*, vol. 2, no. 6, pp. 621–628, 2009.

[12] S. Kathiresan, C. J. Willer, G. M. Peloso et al., "Common variants at 30 loci contribute to polygenic dyslipidemia," *Nature Genetics*, vol. 41, no. 1, pp. 56–65, 2009.

[13] M. S. Sandhu, D. M. Waterworth, S. L. Debenham et al., "LDL-cholesterol concentrations: a genome-wide association study," *The Lancet*, vol. 371, no. 9611, pp. 483–491, 2008.

[14] C. Wallace, S. J. Newhouse, P. Braund et al., "Genome-wide association study identifies genes for biomarkers of cardiovascular disease: serum urate and dyslipidemia," *American Journal of Human Genetics*, vol. 82, no. 1, pp. 139–149, 2008.

[15] E. Schneider, S. Whitmore, K. M. Glynn, K. Dominguez, A. Mitsch, and M. T. McKenna, "Revised surveillance case definitions for HIV infection among adults, adolescents, and children aged <18 months and for HIV infection and AIDS among children aged 18 months to <13 years–United States, 2008," *Morbidity and Mortality Weekly Report*, vol. 57, no. 10, pp. 1–12, 2008.

[16] V. M. Zembrzuski, S. M. Callegari-Jacques, and M. H. Hutz, "Application of an African ancestry index as a genomic control approach in a Brazilian population," *Annals of Human Genetics*, vol. 70, no. 6, pp. 822–828, 2006.

[17] N. P. C. Santos, E. M. Ribeiro-Rodrigues, Â. K. C. Ribeiro-dos-Santos et al., "Assessing individual interethnic admixture and population substructure using a 48-insertion-deletion (INSEL) ancestry-informative marker (AIM) panel," *Human Mutation*, vol. 31, no. 2, pp. 184–190, 2010.

[18] Expert Panel on Detection, Evaluation, and Treatment of High Blood Cholesterol in Adults, "Executive summary of the third report of the National Cholesterol Education Program (NCEP) expert panel on detection, evaluation, and treatment of high blood cholesterol in adults (adult treatment panel III)," *Journal of the American Medical Association*, vol. 285, no. 19, pp. 2486–2497, 2001.

[19] D. K. Lahiri and J. L. Nurnberger Jr., "A rapid non-enzymatic method for the preparation of HMW DNA from blood for RFLP studies," *Nucleic Acids Research*, vol. 19, no. 19, p. 5444, 1991.

[20] P. E. Pajukanta, L. M. Valsta, A. Aro, P. Pietinen, T. Heliö, and M. J. Tikkanen, "The effects of the apolipoprotein B signal peptide

(ins/del) and XbaI polymorphisms on plasma lipid responses to dietary change," *Atherosclerosis*, vol. 122, no. 1, pp. 1–10, 1996.

[21] J.-P. Pan, A.-N. Chiang, J. J. Tai, S.-P. Wang, and M.-S. Chang, "Restriction fragment length polymorphisms of apolipoprotein B gene in Chinese population with coronary heart disease," *Clinical Chemistry*, vol. 41, no. 3, pp. 424–429, 1995.

[22] D. A. Tregouet and V. Garelle, "A new JAVA interface implementation of THESIAS: testing haplotype effects in association studies," *Bioinformatics*, vol. 23, no. 8, pp. 1038–1039, 2007.

[23] E. R. Feeney and P. W. G. Mallon, "HIV and HAART-associated dyslipidemia," *The Open Cardiovascular Medicine Journal*, vol. 5, pp. 49–63, 2011.

[24] P. E. Tarr, P. Taffe, G. Bleiber et al., "Modeling the influence of APOC3, APOE, and TNF polymorphisms on the risk of antiretroviral therapy—associated lipid disorders," *Journal of Infectious Diseases*, vol. 191, pp. 1419–1426, 2005.

[25] J. M. Ordovas, J. Lopez-Miranda, F. Perez-Jimenez et al., "Effect of apolipoprotein E and A-IV phenotypes on the low density lipoprotein response to HMG CoA reductase inhibitor therapy," *Atherosclerosis*, vol. 113, no. 2, pp. 157–166, 1995.

[26] J. Pedro-Botet, E. J. Schaefer, R. G. Bakker-Arkema et al., "Apolipoprotein E genotype affects plasma lipid response to atorvastatin in a gender specific manner," *Atherosclerosis*, vol. 158, no. 1, pp. 183–193, 2001.

[27] R. W. Mahley and S. C. Rall Jr., "Apolipoprotein E: far more than a lipid transport protein," *Annual Review of Genomics and Human Genetics*, vol. 1, no. 2000, pp. 507–537, 2000.

[28] A. M. Bennet, E. di Angelantonio, Z. Ye et al., "Association of apolipoprotein e genotypes with lipid levels and coronary risk," *Journal of the American Medical Association*, vol. 298, no. 11, pp. 1300–1311, 2007.

[29] J. Fauvel, E. Bonnet, J.-B. Ruidavets et al., "An interaction between apo C-III variants and protease inhibitors contributes to high triglyceride/low HDL levels in treated HIV patients," *AIDS*, vol. 15, no. 18, pp. 2397–2406, 2001.

[30] A. Marzocchetti, J. Schwarz, S. di Giambenedetto et al., "The effect of polymorphisms in candidate genes on the long-term risk of lipodystrophy and dyslipidemia in HIV-infected white patients starting antiretroviral therapy," *AIDS Research and Human Retroviruses*, vol. 27, no. 12, pp. 1299–1309, 2011.

[31] O. Seda and L. Sedova, "New Apolipoprotein A-V: comparative genomics meets metabolism," *Physiological Research*, vol. 52, pp. 141–146, 2003.

[32] E. S. Tai and J. M. Ordovas, "Clinical significance of apolipoprotein A5," *Current Opinion in Lipidology*, vol. 19, no. 4, pp. 349–354, 2008.

[33] C.-Q. Lai, E.-S. Tai, C. E. Tan et al., "The APOA5 locus is a strong determinant of plasma triglyceride concentrations across ethnic groups in Singapore," *Journal of Lipid Research*, vol. 44, no. 12, pp. 2365–2373, 2003.

[34] M. Guardiola, R. Ferré, J. Salazar et al., "Protease inhibitor-associated dyslipidemia in HIV-infected patients is strongly influenced by the APOA5-1131T → C gene variation," *Clinical Chemistry*, vol. 52, no. 10, pp. 1914–1919, 2006.

[35] A. Kay, W. März, M. M. Hoffmann et al., "Coronary artery disease and dyslipidemia within Europe: genetic variants in lipid transport gene loci in German subjects with premature coronary artery disease," *Atherosclerosis Supplements*, vol. 3, no. 1, pp. 27–33, 2002.

[36] P. R. Turner, P. J. Talmud, S. Visvikis, C. Ehnholm, and L. Tiret, "DNA polymorphisms of the apoprotein B gene are associated with altered plasma lipoprotein concentrations but not with perceived risk of cardiovascular disease: european Atherosclerosis Research Study," *Atherosclerosis*, vol. 116, no. 2, pp. 221–234, 1995.

[37] M. Benn, B. G. Nordestgaard, J. S. Jensen, P. Grande, H. Sillesen, and A. Tybjærg-Hansen, "Polymorphism in APOB associated with increased low-density lipoprotein levels in both genders in the general population," *Journal of Clinical Endocrinology and Metabolism*, vol. 90, no. 10, pp. 5797–5803, 2005.

[38] C.-F. Xu, M. J. Tikkanen, J. K. Huttunen et al., "Apolipoprotein B signal peptide insertion/deletion polymorphism is associated with Ag epitopes and involved in the determination of serum triglyceride levels," *Journal of Lipid Research*, vol. 31, no. 7, pp. 1255–1261, 1990.

[39] P. Ye, B. Chen, and S. Wang, "Association of polymorphisms of the apolipoprotein B gene with coronary heart disease in Han Chinese," *Atherosclerosis*, vol. 117, no. 1, pp. 43–50, 1995.

The Economic Burden of HIV/AIDS and Myocardial Infarction Treatment in Brazil

Denizar Vianna Araújo,[1,2] Luciana Bahia,[1,2] and Steffan Frosi Stella[2]

[1] *Department of Internal Medicine, State University of Rio de Janeiro, Boulevard 28 de Setembro, No. 77, Room 329, 20551-030 Rio de Janeiro, RJ, Brazil*

[2] *National Institute of Science and Technology for Health Technology Assessment (IATS), CNPq, Rua Ramiro Barcelos, No. 2359, 90035-903 Porto Alegre, RS, Brazil*

Correspondence should be addressed to Denizar Vianna Araújo; denizarvianna@gmail.com

Academic Editors: S. C. Fuchs and M. B. Moreira

Objective. To analyze the expenses of HIV/AIDS and acute myocardial infarction (AMI) treatment in Brazil. *Methods.* A search in the Brazilian epidemiological database (DATASUS) on AMI and AIDS hospitalizations and their costs was done from January 1998 to December 2011. The number of HIV/AIDS cases and antiretroviral treatment (ART) costs was obtained from public Brazilian databases. *Results.* In 5 years, HIV/AIDS cases increased 38.5%, mainly in patients aged 25–49. There were 180,640 patients in ART in 2007 at a cost of R$ 3,920 per patient/year. The hospitalizations due to AIDS were stable over the last 13 years; however, the hospitalizations due to AMI have increased 78%. In 2007, the expenses with hospitalizations for HIV/AIDS and AMI (25–49 years) were approximately 0.12 and 1.52% of the Ministry of Health budget allocated to reimburse inpatient costs. The expenses on ART totaled 1.5% of the total budget (all age groups). *Conclusion.* The prevalence of HIV/AIDS is still increasing in Brazil. There are scientific evidences suggesting an increased incidence of AIM in this population. Considering the high costs for the treatment of both diseases, an economic analysis is important to alert health managers to strengthen the preventive measures to guarantee the financial sustainability of such treatment.

1. Introduction

The Brazilian HIV/AIDS Program was established in May 1985 [1]. In 1996, the Brazilian Unified Health System (SUS) ensured the coverage of antiretroviral drugs (ART) to all those living with HIV/AIDS in Brazil, resulting in AIDS mortality reduction [2].

Following the development of drug resistance in HIV patients, the Brazilian Ministry of Health had to provide new drugs at higher costs, investing up to R$ 551 million in antiretroviral treatment in 2003. There was an increase in the investment in subsequent years due to the acquisition of patented drugs (up to R$ 960 million in 2006). The introduction of the first fusion inhibitor, enfuvirtide, in the therapeutic regimen of multidrug-resistant patients had a strong impact on total costs. It was provided to 1,030 patients at a daily cost of US$ 22.19, the accounting for 4.4% of antiretroviral expenditure in 2006 [3].

It remains controversial whether the exposure to combination antiretroviral (ART) treatment increases the risk of acute myocardial infarction (AMI). Friis-Møller et al. conducted a prospective observational study with 23,468 patients with HIV from 11 previously established cohorts to evaluate the risk factors and the incidence of myocardial infarction. The authors concluded that ART therapy was independently associated with a 26-percent relative increase in the rate of myocardial infarction per year of exposure during the first four to six years of use [4]. The Data Collection on Adverse Events of Anti-HIV Drugs (D:A:D) study assessed the risk of AMI in 13 anti-HIV drugs in an observational study. Over 178,835 person-years, 580 patients developed AMI. Of the drugs considered, only indinavir, lopinavir ritonavir,

Table 1: Number of patients covered in the HIV/AIDS Program (antiretroviral drugs) and their related costs in the Brazilian Unified Health System (SUS).

Year	Number of patients	Cost (reais)	Cost per patient (reais)
2002	125,175	R$668,783,673	R$5,342
2003	139,868	R$495,900,996	R$3,545
2004	156,670	R$596,016,153	R$3,804
2005	164,547	R$567,045,691	R$3,446
2006	174,270	R$1,002,732,562	R$5,753
2007	180,640	R$708,178,407	R$3,920

Source: Vieira 2009 [8], monthly report for Assessment and Use of HIV Drugs, and STD/AIDS Program Care and Treatment Unit.

didanosine, and abacavir were associated with a significantly increased risk of AMI (12 to 13%) [5]. Islam et al. estimated the relative risk of cardiovascular disease (CVD) among people living with HIV (PLHIV) compared with the HIV-uninfected population. The authors conducted a systematic review and meta-analysis of studies and showed that the relative risk of CVD was 1.61 (95% CI 1.43–1.81) among PLHIV without ART compared with HIV-uninfected people. The relative risk of CVD was 2.00 (95%CI 1.70–2.37) among PLHIV on ART compared with HIV-uninfected people and 1.52 (95% CI 1.35–1.70) compared with treatment-naïve PLHIV [6].

Given the importance and the high costs of treating both conditions in Brazil, this analysis aimed to estimate and analyze the costs of HIV/AIDS and AMI treatment and their impact on the public budget of the Brazilian Unified Health System.

2. Methods

A search in the Brazilian epidemiological database (DATA-SUS) on AMI and AIDS hospitalizations and their costs was done from January 1998 to December 2011. The survey was restricted to patients aged 25–49 (group with the highest prevalence of HIV/AIDS in the Brazil). Data were registered as the number of hospitalizations and reimbursed expenditures in Reais (R$). The annual number of HIV/AIDS reported cases was obtained from the TABNET database of the Brazilian Ministry of Health [7].

Data from a previously published study about the antiretroviral treatment costs were analyzed. The authors analyzed the Ministry of Health's total spending on drugs and its programs between 2002 and 2007 [8]. The Federal Government antiretroviral drug acquisitions were analyzed separately, obtained from a federal purchase website (ComprasNet) [9].

The Brazilian Public Health System perspective, which considers only direct costs that are reimbursed to health care providers was adopted. In this scenario, indirect costs are not computed in the database.

3. Results

From 1980 to June 2007, 474,273 HIV/AIDS cases were reported. In June 2012, this number increased to 656,701 registered cases (Figure 1). Data on the number of patients on antiretroviral therapy between 2002 and 2007 and the annual total and per patient costs of HIV/AIDS treatment are described in Table 1, comprising almost 100% HIV of the reported cases (Brazilian Ministry of Health, 2008).

The number of hospitalizations for AMI and AIDS and their costs (patients aged 25–49; 1998–2011) is shown in Figures 2 and 3, respectively.

4. Discussion

In Brazil, the age-standardized mortality from cardiovascular diseases decreased by 26% in the last decade, and this decrease was partially due to the successful implementation of health policies that led to the reduction of smoking and the expansion of access to basic health care [10]. However, the prevalence of diabetes, arterial hypertension, and HIV/AIDS is increasing parallel with the prevalence of overweight and aging population, which may be reflected in unfavorable trends in mortality from cardiovascular diseases in the next decade.

Cardiovascular diseases represented the third leading cause of hospitalizations in the Brazilian Unified Health System, having been responsible for the greater spending on hospitalization, accounting for a total of R$ 1.9 billion or 19% of the total cost of hospitalizations. Acute coronary syndrome (unstable angina and acute myocardial infarction) accounted for 7% of all deaths in Brazil, associated with substantial direct and indirect costs to healthcare systems and society [11].

In the last 5 years, the number of HIV/AIDS registered cases increased 38.5% [12]. The age group where AIDS is more prevalent in both sexes is the one with 25–49 year olds, reflecting an early age group with an increased risk of developing cardiovascular events. The indirect costs, such as productivity loss in this age group, are a major concern to health policy makers and the whole society.

The number of hospitalizations due to AIDS related conditions was stable over the last 13 years; however, the number of hospitalizations due to AMI in patients aged 25 to 49 has increased approximately 78% in the same period. This age group has a low risk of cardiovascular events, but the combination of HIV exposure and HIV/AIDS treatment could be a possible reason for this increase in the incidence of AIM.

The total costs with hospitalization have increased in both conditions, but with a more substantial growth in the AMI

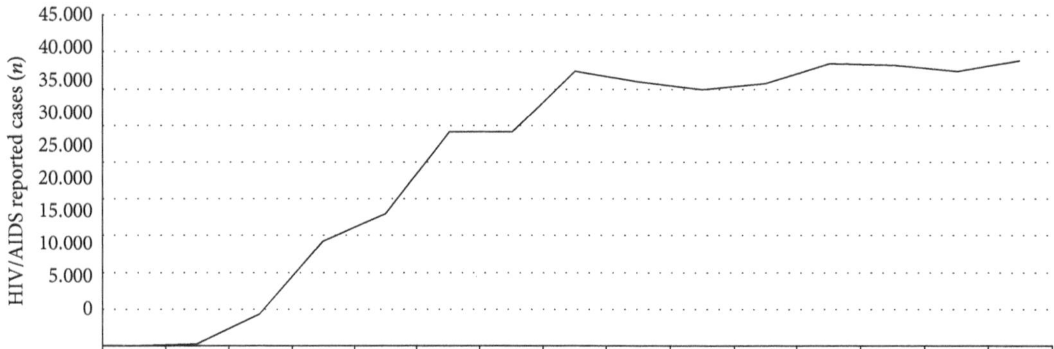

	1980	1984	1988	1992	1994	1998	2000	2002	2004	2006	2007	2008	2009	2010	2011
Patients	1	130	4.323	14.258	18.040	29.109	29.233	37.379	35.947	34.931	35.718	38.529	38.188	37.359	38.776

FIGURE 1: Annual HIV/AIDS reported cases in Brazil, 1980–2011.

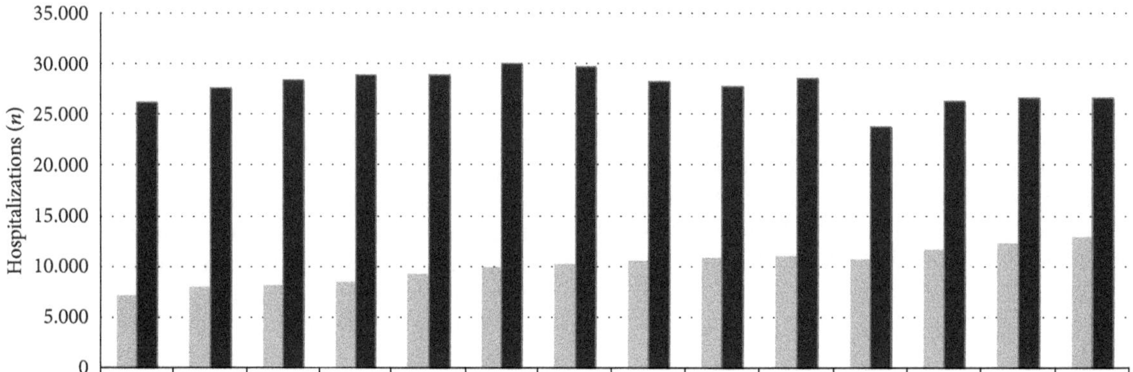

	1998	1999	2000	2001	2002	2003	2004	2005	2006	2007	2008	2009	2010	2011
AMI	7.252	7.989	8.152	8.463	9.236	9.924	10.327	10.613	10.900	11.147	10.724	11.650	12.344	12.947
AIDS	26.132	27.585	28.384	28.879	28.847	30.047	29.630	28.229	27.747	28.639	23.703	26.281	26.602	26.608

FIGURE 2: Annual hospitalizations due to AMI and AIDS (25–49 years).

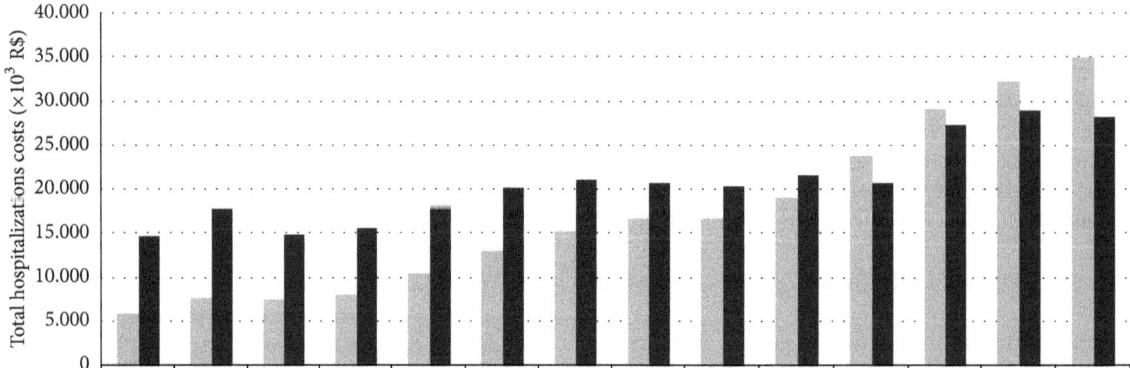

	1998	1999	2000	2001	2002	2003	2004	2005	2006	2007	2008	2009	2010	2011
AMI	5.807	7.699	7.521	8.106	10.403	12.951	15.280	16.668	16.663	19.122	23.927	29.083	32.357	35.113
AIDS	14.713	17.849	14.806	15.650	18.229	20.259	21.145	20.705	20.327	21.642	20.764	27.282	28.939	28.264

FIGURE 3: Annual costs with AMI and AIDS hospitalizations (25–49 years).

hospitalizations costs (92% versus 504% increase for AIDS and AIM, resp.). This cost increase can be due to changes in clinical practice, such as the use of thrombolytic agents and revascularization procedures during admissions.

The total budget of the Brazilian Ministry of Health in 2007 was R$ 44.3 billion and of this total, R$ 23 billion were allocated to reimburse outpatient and inpatient treatment costs. In the same year, the expenses with hospitalizations for HIV/AIDS-related conditions and AIM (25–49 years) were approximately 0.12 and 1.52% of this budget, respectively. Its worth mentioning that, in the same year, spending on antiretroviral treatment totaled 1.5% of the total budget (all age groups).

There are 18 antiretroviral drugs and 37 formulations available in Brazil for the treatment of people living with HIV (for children and adults). Ten of these drugs are produced by multinational companies and eight are locally produced (one private and six state-run Brazilian laboratories). It has been noted that for most of these medications (79%, 11 of 14 antiretroviral drugs) there was a significant reduction in the prices between 2006 and 2007, reaching 50% reduction in some cases [8]. An analysis of the expenditures with the Brazilian antiretroviral drug program suggests that the universal access policy will not be sustainable in long term without compromising investments in other areas [13].

This study has some limitations. Firstly it adds only the indirect evidence that the rising cost of hospitalization for AMI among the low coronary risk may be due to HIV infection and the use of antiretroviral agents. Secondly, it was not possible to compare the costs of AMI in both HIV positive and negative populations, mainly due to the lack of information available in the Brazilian databases. Further work is needed to clarify this important and relevant issue.

5. Conclusion

The prevalence of HIV/AID is still increasing among young adults and all these individuals will have access to long-term antiretroviral treatment in Brazil. There are scientific evidences suggesting an increased incidence of myocardial infarction in this population. Considering the high costs for the treatment of both diseases, health managers and decision-makers should be aware of strengthening preventive measures in order to guarantee the financial sustainability of the treatment in public health units in Brazil.

Conflict of Interests

The authors declare that there is no conflict of interests regarding the publication of this paper.

References

[1] Ministério da Saúde, "Política do programa Nacional DST/AIDS," http://www.aids.gov.br/.

[2] Ministério da Saúde, "Secretaria de Vigilância em Saúde. Programa Nacional de DST e AIDS. Metas e Compromissos Assumidos pelos Estados-Membros na Sessão Especial da Assembléia Geral das Nações Unidas em HIV/AIDS UNGASS-HIV/AIDS," Resposta Brasileira, 2007, http://www.idea.int/political-finance/international-dollars.cfm#_ftn1.

[3] Ministério da Saúde, Programa Nacional de DST/AIDS, "A sustentabilidade do acesso universal a anti-retrovirais no Brasil," Documento elaborado para divulgação durante a 157a Reunião Ordinária do Conselho Nacional de Saúde, 2005.

[4] N. Friis-Møller, C. A. Sabin, R. Weber et al., "Data Collection on Adverse Events of Anti-HIV Drugs (DAD) Study Group. Combination antiretroviral therapy and the risk of myocardial infarction," *New England Journal of Medicine*, vol. 349, no. 21, pp. 1993–2003, 2003.

[5] S. W. Worm, C. Sabin, R. Weber et al., "Risk of myocardial infarction in patients with HIV infection exposed to specific individual antiretroviral drugs from the 3 major drug classes: the data collection on adverse events of anti-HIV drugs (D : A : D) study," *Journal of Infectious Diseases*, vol. 201, no. 3, pp. 318–330, 2010.

[6] F. M. Islam, J. Wu, J. Jansson, and D. P. Wilson, "Relative risk of cardiovascular disease among people living with HIV: a systematic review and meta-analysis," *HIV Medicine*, vol. 13, no. 8, pp. 453–468, 2012.

[7] Health Informations (TABNET)—Brazilian Ministry of Health database, http://www.datasus.gov.br.

[8] F. S. Vieira, "Ministry of Health's spending on drugs: program trends from 2002 to 2007," *Revista de Saúde Pública*, vol. 43, no. 4, pp. 674–681, 2009.

[9] Ministério do Planejamento, Orçamento e Gestão, "Portal de Compras do Governo Federal: ComprasNet," http://www.comprasnet.gov.br.

[10] M. I. Schmidt, B. B. Duncan, G. A. E Silva et al., "Chronic non-communicable diseases in Brazil: burden and current challenges," *The Lancet*, vol. 377, no. 9781, pp. 1949–1961, 2011.

[11] Ministério da Saúde, "DATASUS. Sistema de informações hospitalares. Internações e valor total de internações segundo capítulo CID-10," http://www.datasus.gov.br.

[12] Departamento de DST, AIDS e Hepatites Virais, Ministério da Sáude, http://www.aids.gov.br/pagina/aids-no-brasil.

[13] A. Grangeiro, "Sustentabilidade da política de acesso a medicamentos anti-retrovirais no Brasil," *Revista de Saúde Pública*, vol. 40, pp. 60–69, 2006.

7

Cardiovascular Risk Assessment: A Comparison of the Framingham, PROCAM, and DAD Equations in HIV-Infected Persons

Max Weyler Nery,[1,2] Celina Maria Turchi Martelli,[1,3,4] Erika Aparecida Silveira,[5,6] Clarissa Alencar de Sousa,[1] Marianne de Oliveira Falco,[6] Aline de Cássia Oliveira de Castro,[6] Jorge Tannus Esper,[1] Luis Carlos Silva e Souza,[3] and Marília Dalva Turchi[1,3,4,6]

[1] *Postgraduate Studies Program, Institute of Tropical Pathology and Public Health, Federal University of Goiás, Brazil*
[2] *Department of Medicine, Catholic University of Goiás, Brazil*
[3] *Institute of Tropical Pathology and Public Health, Federal University of Goiás, Brazil*
[4] *National Institute for Health Technology Assessement, Brazil*
[5] *School of Nutrition, Federal University of Goiás, Brazil*
[6] *Postgraduate Studies Program in Health Sciences, School of Medicine, Federal University of Goiás, Brazil*

Correspondence should be addressed to Max Weyler Nery; maxwnery@uol.com.br

Academic Editors: S. C. Fuchs, M. B. Moreira, and B. Oyeledun

This study aims to estimate the risk of cardiovascular disease (CVD) and to assess the agreement between the Framingham, Framingham with aggravating factors, PROCAM, and DAD equations in HIV-infected patients. A cross-sectional study was conducted in an outpatient centre in Brazil. 294 patients older than 19 years were enrolled. Estimates of 10-year cardiovascular risk were calculated. The agreement between the CVD risk equations was assessed using Cohen's kappa coefficient. The participants' mean age was 36.8 years (SD = 10.3), 76.9% were men, and 66.3% were on antiretroviral therapy. 47.8% of the participants had abdominal obesity, 23.1% were current smokers, 20.0% had hypertension, and 2.0% had diabetes. At least one lipid abnormality was detected in 72.8%, and a low HDL-C level was the most common. The majority were classified as having low risk for CV events. The percentage of patients at high risk ranged from 0.4 to 5.7. The PROCAM score placed the lowest proportion of the patients into a high-risk group, and the Framingham equation with aggravating factors placed the highest proportion of patients into the high-risk group. Data concerning the comparability of different tools are informative for estimating the risk of CVD, but accuracy of the outcome predictions should also be considered.

1. Introduction

Highly active antiretroviral therapy (HAART) has significantly reduced morbidity and mortality among AIDS patients in many parts of the world [1, 2]. In addition, broad coverage of HAART is also associated with the reduction in the risk of HIV transmission at the population level [3]. The World Health Organization and the Joint United Nations Program on HIV/AIDS have set an international goal for expanding HAART to 15 million people by 2015 [4]. Brazil has a well-established HIV control program, and HAART has been universally offered to all eligible individuals at no charge since 1996. By 2011, approximately 200,000 HIV-infected patients were receiving antiretroviral therapy (ART), resulting in a remarkable survival benefit in the last decade [5, 6].

HAART has enhanced the life expectancy and improved the quality of life for HIV-infected patients. However, the aging of the population and the cumulative adverse effects caused by long periods of exposure to antiretroviral drugs have markedly increased the prevalence of dyslipidaemia, insulin resistance, impaired glucose metabolism, and abnormal fat distribution among HIV patients [7, 8]. Patients with metabolic syndrome have an increased risk of developing chronic nontransmissible conditions such as diabetes and cardiovascular diseases [9, 10].

Overall, the benefits of HAART in reducing mortality significantly outweigh the risks of metabolic abnormalities. Nevertheless, reducing metabolic abnormalities and identifying groups at high risk for cardiovascular diseases (CVD) are an important part of HIV management. Guidelines about managing dyslipidaemia in the general population [11] and in HIV-infected patients [12, 13] recommend identifying and treating patients at high risk for cardiovascular events. Traditional cardiovascular risk factors, such as smoking, lack of physical activity, and metabolic syndrome, play a very important role in determining cardiovascular events. Assessing and addressing those modifiable risk factors are important for CVD prevention.

Over the past decade, an increasing number of studies have assessed the cardiovascular risk profile of HIV-infected patients [14–22]. The majority of the studies used cardiovascular risk equations developed for a non-HIV-infected population, such as the Framingham or the Prospective Cardiovascular Münster Study (PROCAM) scores. The accuracy of these risk scores for predicting cardiovascular events in HIV-infected patients is not well established. Generally, these scores have been proposed and validated in high-income populations of older patients. In the last decade, a growing number of studies estimated CVD risk in HIV-infected populations, mainly using the Framingham score and less frequently using other cardiovascular risk equations, such as the PROCAM and Systematic Coronary Risk Evaluation (SCORE) equations [14–17, 19–25]. The prevalence of patients at high risk for coronary events in the next 10 years varies largely among these studies, ranging from less than 1% to 21% [15, 16]. These equations were not developed to assess cardiovascular risk in HIV-infected patients, and their accuracy is still uncertain [26, 27].

Presently, there is only one cardiovascular risk score specifically developed for HIV-infected patients [18]. It was based on the results of a large multicentre cohort study (The Data Collection on Adverse Effects on Anti-HIV Drugs Cohort-DAD), conducted mainly in Europe and North America. The DAD equation takes antiretroviral drug exposure into account as a potential risk factor for cardiovascular events. To date, the DAD risk equation has only been applied for CVD risk estimation in one developing country [22]. This study aims to estimate the cardiovascular risk for HIV-infected patients in Brazil using the Framingham, PROCAM, and DAD equations and to compare the results.

2. Methods

This study is a cross-sectional analysis of a cohort of HIV-infected patients (PRECOR study) attending an outpatient public referral centre for infectious diseases in central Brazil. HIV-infected patients between 20 and 75 years old were consecutively enrolled between October 2009 and January 2011. The study protocol was approved by the local Institutional Review Board. The participants showed no clinical evidence of active opportunistic diseases at the time of enrolment.

Clinical and Epidemiological Investigation. At the time of enrolment, all the participants were interviewed and examined by the same cardiologist, a member of the research team. A structured questionnaire that addressed sociodemographic variables and general medical history was used to collect data.

The participants were also asked about the time of their HIV diagnosis, previous opportunistic diseases, antiretroviral exposure, and cardiovascular risk factors. Smoking status was classified as never, former, or current (those who had stopped smoking within the past 30 days were considered current smokers). The participants were considered to have a history of cardiovascular disease if they had a convincing history of myocardial infarction (MI), angina, stroke, peripheral arterial disease, or an intervention for coronary artery disease. Family history was defined as cardiovascular disease in a first-degree male before the age of 55 or in a first-degree female relative before the age of 65.

Arterial blood pressure was measured. The patients on antihypertensive therapy or with systolic blood pressure ≥140 mmHg and/or diastolic blood pressure ≥90 mmHg were classified as having hypertension [28].

Afterward, the participants met with a multidisciplinary research team including nutritionists, a pharmacist, a biomedical professional, anthropometrists, and a physiotherapist. Waist circumference (WC) was measured as the narrowest circumference between the lower rib margin and the anterior superior iliac crest using a standard inelastic anthropometric tape. A WC ≥94 centimetres (cm) for men and ≥80 cm for women was considered a risk factor for CVD [29].

Laboratory Investigation. The participants were advised to fast overnight for 12 h, to avoid alcohol consumption for 3 days prior to blood collection. All of the analyses were performed at the same laboratory.

Serum total cholesterol (TC), high-density lipoprotein (HDL) cholesterol and triglycerides (TG) were assayed. Serum low-density lipoprotein (LDL) cholesterol was estimated using the Friedewald formula when TG was ≤400 mg/dL [30]. Dyslipidaemia was defined as LDL cholesterol ≥160 mg/dL, HDL cholesterol <40 mg/dL for men and <50 mg/dL for women or diabetics or triglycerides ≥150 mg/dL [11, 31].

High sensitivity C-reactive protein (hsCRP) was quantified. hsCRP values <1 mg/L were classified as normal, between 1 and 3 mg/L were classified as intermediate risk, and >3 mg/L were classified as high risk [32].

Diabetes was defined as a fasting serum glucose level greater than 125 mg/dL [33] or a self-reported diagnosis of diabetes and use of specific therapy. The glomerular filtration rate (GFR) was calculated based on the Cockcroft-Gault equation [34]. A GFR below <60 mL/min or a serum creatinine level equal to or higher than 1.5 mg/dL indicated impaired renal function [35].

A urine sample was collected to determine the albumin/creatinine ratio (ACR) [36]. Patients were categorised as having normoalbuminuria (<30 mcg/mg), microalbuminuria (30 to 299 mcg/mg), or clinical albuminuria (>300 mcg/mg) [37].

CD4 counts and the HIV RNA levels were obtained from the patient's medical chart. HAART data were obtained from the patients' medical and pharmaceutical records.

Metabolic syndrome was defined in accordance with the standards of the International Diabetes Federation [29].

Calculation of Cardiovascular Risk. Framingham and PROCAM scores were calculated to predict 10-year CVD risk. DAD equations were used to calculate 5-year CVD risk. The participants with a history of CVD or were older than 75 were excluded from this analysis.

Framingham Equation. The following variables were included in the equation: age, sex, systolic blood pressure, antihypertensive therapy (yes or no), serum TC and HDL-cholesterol values, and current smoking status (yes or no). The 10-year risk of CVD was classified as low (<10%), moderate (10% to 20%), or high (>20%) [38]. The patients with diabetes were classified as high risk [11, 31]. The participants who had low or moderate 10-year risk according to the Framingham equation were also reevaluated based on the presence of aggravating factors: family history of CVD, metabolic syndrome, serum creatinine ≥1.5 mg/dL, hsCRP >3.0 mg/L, or albuminuria >30 mcg/mg. Patients presenting at least one of these aggravating factors were reclassified into the high-risk category for CVD over 10 years (Framingham equation with aggravating factors, according to the IV Brazilian Guideline for Dyslipidemia and Atherosclerosis Prevention) [31].

PROCAM Equation. The following variables were included in the equation: age; sex; known diabetes or fasting blood glucose level ≥120 mg/dL; systolic blood pressure; serum TG, LDL, and HDL-cholesterol levels; current nicotine consumption and family history of CVD. The 10-year risk of acute coronary events was classified as low (<10%), moderate (10% to 20%), or high (>20%) [39].

DAD Equation. The following variables were included in the equation: age; sex; systolic blood pressure; serum CT and HDL-cholesterol level; diabetes; smoking status; family history of CVD; current use of abacavir, indinavir, or lopinavir; and the number of years on indinavir or lopinavir. The 5-year risk of coronary heart disease was classified as low (<1%), moderate (1 to 5%), high (5 to 10%), or very high (>10%) [18].

Statistical Analysis. Normally distributed continuous variables were expressed as means and standard deviations; otherwise, they were expressed as medians and interquartile ranges (IQR). Categorical variables were expressed as percentages with 95% confidence intervals (95% CI). A χ^2 test or Fisher's test was used to compare proportions.

The agreement between the CVD risk equations was assessed using Cohen's kappa coefficient with 95% CIs. The participants at high or very high risk according to the DAD equation were considered high-risk patients for the comparison with the Framingham, Framingham with aggravating factors, and PROCAM equations.

Two-sided P values <0.05 were considered statistically significant. The data were analysed using IBM SPSS Statistics base 18.0 for MAC (Chicago, IL, USA).

3. Results

A total of 335 HIV-infected adults were enrolled during the study period. Clinical and laboratory data were obtained from 299 patients (89.3%). Thirty-six participants (10.7%) were excluded because their laboratory analyses were incomplete. There was a higher proportion of previous intravenous drug users (IDU) among the individuals with incomplete laboratory data ($P < 0.01$). There were no statistically significant differences in sex, age, educational level, or monthly income ($P > 0.05$) between these two groups. Five patients reported a previous cardiovascular event and were excluded, resulting in 294 participants.

Table 1 presents the sociodemographic and clinical characteristics of the 294 participants. The study population was predominantly male (76.9%). The mean age was 36.8 (SD = 10.3), and the ages ranged from 20 to 71 years. Approximately 80% (185/226) of the males were younger than 45, and approximately 90% (59/68) of the females were younger than 55. The majority of the participants (72.4%) had more than 8 years of schooling. A total of 92.2% reported being exposed to HIV through a sexual route; among these participants, 54.1% declared that they were homosexual males or bisexual. Previous IDU was reported by 2.7%.

The median time since receiving the HIV diagnosis was 2.0 years (IQR: 0.7–5.0 years). At least one opportunistic disease in the previous 12 months was reported by 5.8% of those recruited. At the time of enrolment, 54.1% presented an undetectable HIV viral load, and 72.6% had a CD4 count ≥350 cells/mm^3. Overall, 195 (66.3%) out of 294 participants were receiving HAART, with a median duration of 19.0 months (IQR: 5.0–54.0 months) (Table 1).

Figure 1 shows the prevalence of cardiovascular risk factors among the participants. A history of smoking was reported by 46.9% (138/294), and 23.1% (68/294) were current smokers. Seven participants reported a family history of premature atherosclerotic disease. Twenty-three patients had high blood pressure (HBP), and 47.8% of them were receiving antihypertensive therapy. At the time of the physical examination, 55 participants had HBP. In total, 20.0% (59/294) of the participants were considered hypertensive. Abdominal obesity was detected in 47.8% of the participants. The proportion of females with abdominal obesity (82.4%) was higher than the proportion of males (23.0%) ($P < 0.001$).

Most (72.8%) participants had at least one abnormality in their lipid profile. The most common dyslipidaemia was a low HDL-C level, which was found in 61.9% of the participants. The prevalence of isolated hypertriglyceridemia and isolated hypercholesterolemia was 36.4% and 3.5%, respectively. The prevalence of low HDL-C combined with high TG was 46.6%. For 11 participants, LDL cholesterol was not estimated because TG was higher than 400 mg/dL. The mean values

TABLE 1: Sociodemographic and clinical characteristics of 294 HIV-infected patients.

Characteristics	Values	95% CI
Sociodemographic		
Males	226 (76.9)	71.4–81.9
Age, years mean (SD)	36.8 (10.3)	—
Male <45 y	185 (81.9)	76.5–86.5
Female <55 y	59 (86.8)	78.7–94.8
≥8 y schooling	213 (72.4)	63.0–82.9
Exposure categories		
Sexual route	271 (92.2)	81.5–103.8
Homosexual or bisexual[a]	142 (51.4)	43.3–60.6
Previous IDU[b]	7 (2.7)	1.0–5.5
Clinical HIV history		
HIV diagnosis, years median (IQR)	2.0 (0.7–5.0)	—
Opportunistic disease in previous 12 months[c]	16 (5.8)	3.5–8.9
Undetectable HIV viral load[d]	153 (54.1)	48.1–60.2
CD4 ≥350 cells/mm^{3}[e]	207 (72.6)	22.4–32.7
Antiretroviral therapy	195 (66.3)	61.3–71.7
ART duration, months, median (IQR)	19.0 (5.0–54.0)	—

IDU: intravenous drug users; ART: antiretroviral therapy.
[a]18 missing, [b]33 missing, [c]17missing, [d]11 missing, [e]9 missing.
Continuous variables are presented as means (SD), median (IQR), and categorical variables are presented as absolute value and percentage with 95% CI.

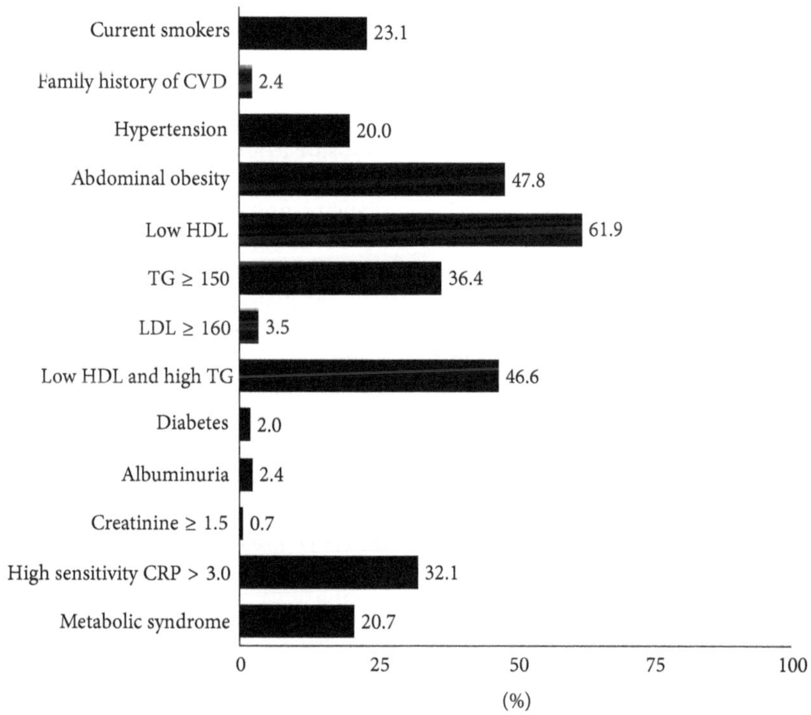

CVD: cardiovascular disease
HDL: high-density lipoprotein
TG: triglycerides
LDL: low-density lipoprotein
CRP: C-reactive protein

FIGURE 1: Prevalence of cardiovascular risk factors among 294 HIV-infected patients.

were 169.5 (SD = 42.7) mg/dL for TC, 42.5 (SD = 11.3) mg/dL for HDL cholesterol, 96.6 (SD = 32.5) mg/dL for LDL cholesterol, and 151.4 (SD = 104.5) mg/dL for TG.

A total of 6 patients (2.0%) were categorised as having diabetes. Seventeen patients had albuminuria, and two had creatinine levels equal to or higher than 1.5 mg/dL. High sensitivity C-reactive protein >3 mg/L was detected in 32.1% of the participants. Sixty-one (20.7%) participants had metabolic syndrome. The prevalence of metabolic syndrome was higher among females (36.8%) than among males (16.0%) ($P < 0.001$).

Table 2 presents the antiretroviral regimens at the baseline interview by 195 patients receiving treatment. Of the participants, 62.6% were taking a combination of zidovudine, lamivudine, and efavirenz. The second most frequent antiretroviral regimen was a combination of zidovudine, lamivudine, and lopinavir boosted by ritonavir (12.8%). Twenty-nine patients (15.1%) were using a regimen containing tenofovir. Fifty-one (26.2%) patients were using a protease inhibitor (PI) regimen; among these participants, 28 were taking a lopinavir regimen (25 were taking a regimen boosted by ritonavir). Additional 6 patients used lopinavir in a previous regimen. The median duration of lopinavir-based therapy was 13.0 months (IQR: 4.0–23.5). One participant was taking abacavir. None of the participants were ever exposed to indinavir.

Figure 2 presents the estimated CVD risk of the 283 HIV-infected patients based on the Framingham, Framingham with aggravating factors, PROCAM, and DAD risk equations. Eleven participants were excluded because they had TG >400 mg/dL. The majority of participants were classified at low risk for future CV events. The percentage of patients classified as having a high risk of future CVD ranged from 0.4 to 5.7 using these four scoring systems.

Framingham Equation. Based on the Framingham equation, 94.0% of the participants were classified as low-risk, 3.2% as moderate-risk, and 2.8% as high-risk patients.

Framingham with Aggravating Factors. Of the participants, 54.4% were classified as low-risk patients, 39.9% as moderate-risk patients, and 5.7% as high-risk patients for CVD. At least one aggravating cardiovascular risk factor was detected in 42.0% of the participants. The most frequent aggravating factor was hsCRP >3.0 mg/L (32.1%), followed by the presence of metabolic syndrome (20.7%). Impaired renal function was identified in 0.7% of the participants, and 2.4% reported a family history of CVD.

PROCAM Equation. Of the participant, 98.2% were classified as low-risk patients, 1.4% as moderate-risk patients, and 0.4% as high-risk patients for CVD.

DAD Equation. Of the participants, 74.2% were classified as low-risk patients, 23.7% as moderate-risk patients, and 2.1% as high-risk patients. None had a very high risk for CVD.

The agreement of the DAD equation with the Framingham equation was 77.4% ($k = 0.23$; 95% CI 0.07–0.39), with the Framingham with aggravating factors was 56.7% ($k = 0.14$; 95% CI 0.02–0.25), and with the PROCAM equation was 75.3% ($k = 0.07$; 95% CI 0.00–0.26). The agreement was good, but low kappa values were detected for all three comparisons (Table 3).

4. Discussion

The present study was conducted in a population of HIV-infected individuals, mainly composed of young adult males, who were clinically stable. One-third of them were naïve to antiretroviral drugs. Less than 3.0% of the patients were at high risk for cardiovascular events over the next 10 years according to equations developed for the general population, such as the Framingham and PROCAM equations. A similar profile was obtained using the DAD equation, which was specifically constructed for HIV patients. When aggravating factors were incorporated into the Framingham equation, as recommended by the Brazilian Guidelines for clinical management, the proportion of the participants classified in the high-risk group increased twofold: almost 40% of the patients were classified in the intermediate-risk group for CV events. Similarly, the DAD equation placed a higher proportion of the patients in the moderate-risk category.

Initially, CVD risk equations were conceived for those over 30 in the general North American and European populations. However, these risk estimations were applied to younger age groups in other settings and, more recently, to people living with HIV [15]. In alignment with our results, other Latin American studies also found a low risk of future CV events using the conventional cardiovascular equations among predominantly male HIV patients in their 30s and 40s [16, 19]. In contrast, a high risk of cardiovascular events was found among older populations, those with greater exposure to antiretroviral drugs, or populations with a higher prevalence of well-known risk factors, such as smoking, diabetes, or hypertension [14, 15, 24].

In our study, the participants were young and had relatively short exposure to antiretroviral drugs. The prevalence of diabetes was low, but the prevalence of abdominal obesity was high, especially among the female participants. Furthermore, most of our patients had low incomes. Obesity and low income were associated with an increased 10-year risk for CVD in a large study conducted in the USA [23]. In addition, aging, abdominal obesity, and the duration of antiretroviral drug exposure are intrinsically associated with the development of diabetes [40], leading to an increased risk for CVD disease in the study population in the near future.

A high triglyceride level is one of the most common lipid abnormalities described among HIV-infected patients [40, 41]. A similar lipid profile was found in the current study and in a previous evaluation in the same setting [42]. One potential disadvantage of using Framingham scores for HIV-infected patients is that triglyceride values are not incorporated into the CVD risk equations. However, the use of elevated triglycerides as a marker for future CVD is still a controversial issue [43].

In the PROCAM equation, triglycerides and LDL levels are incorporated into the risk equation. Nevertheless, for patients with triglyceride levels higher than 400 mg/dL, it is

TABLE 2: Antiretroviral regimen in 195 HIV-infected patients.

Antiretroviral regimen	Class of drug	N (%)	95% CI
ZDV + 3TC + EFZ	2NRTI + 1NNRTI	122 (62.6)	51.9–74.7
ZDV + 3TC + LPV/RTV	2NRTI + 1PI/Booster	25 (12.8)	8.3–18.9
3TC + TDF + EFZ	2NRTI + 1NNRTI	15 (7.7)	4.3–12.7
3TC + TDF + ATV + RTV	2NRTI + 1PI/Booster	5 (2.6)	0.8–5.9
ZDV + 3TC + TDF + LPV + RTV	3NRTI + 1PI/Booster	3 (1.5)	0.3–4.5
ZDV + 3TC + NVP	2NRTI + 1NNRTI	3 (1.5)	0.3–4.5
Others	—	22 (11.3)	7.0–17.0

ATV: atazanavir; ZDV: zidovudine; 3TC: lamivudine; EFZ: efavirenz; LPV: lopinavir; NNRT: nonnucleoside reverse transcriptase inhibitor; NRTI: nonnucleoside reverse transcriptase inhibitor; NVP: nevirapine; PI: protease inhibitor; RTV: ritonavir; TDF: tenofovir.

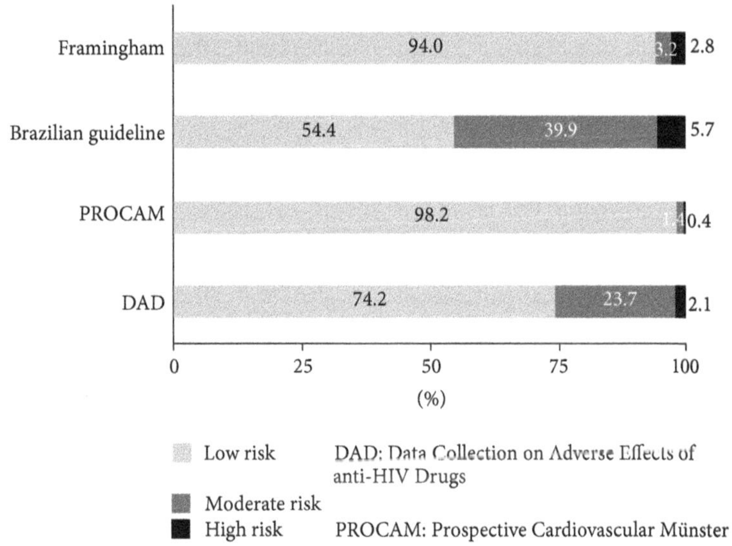

FIGURE 2: Prevalence of estimated CVD risk according to Framingham, Framingham with aggravating factors (Brazilian Guideline for Dyslipidemia and Atherosclerosis Prevention), PROCAM and DAD risk equations for 283 HIV-infected patients.

not possible to estimate LDL levels, which hampers CVD risk calculation. Similar to our results, other studies using PROCAM equations [14, 15, 19, 24, 25] have found a lower percentage of patients with high 10-year risk for CV events compared with the risk estimates using the Framingham equation. In two studies [19, 25], the coefficient of agreement between the PROCAM and Framingham equations was evaluated. In one study [19], the low- and moderate-risk groups were combined to compare the Framingham and PROCAM scores, yielding weak agreement between these equations. Another study found good agreement between these scores [25]. Determining the proportion of patients with high or moderate 10-year cardiovascular risk has clinical and economic repercussions. It has not been determined which of these two equations is more accurate, and the answer most likely will not be determined [27]. Large cohort studies conducted in HIV-infected populations with different clinical and demographic profiles would be needed to approach this question [27].

In the present study, the Framingham equation with aggravating risk factors most likely overestimated the 10-year cardiovascular risk. The percentage of participants in the high-risk group increased from 2.8% to 5.7%, and the percentage of moderate-risk patients increased more than 10 times (from 3.2% to 39.9%), mainly because of the high sensitivity C-reactive protein (hsCRP) values. hsCRP is a nonspecific marker for inflammation and is considered an independent cardiovascular risk predictor [32]. HIV infection itself and opportunistic infections can lead to a proinflammatory state. The accuracy of CRP as a cardiovascular risk predictor has not been well established in HIV-infected populations [44].

Few large cohort studies have investigated the accuracy of the conventional risk equations to predict cardiovascular events in HIV-infected populations [18, 45, 46]. To date, the DAD equation is the only tool for estimating cardiovascular risk developed specifically for an HIV-infected population. In our study, the proportion of patients in the high-risk

TABLE 3: Comparison between CVD risk estimation using different equations (283 patients).

	Cardiovascular risk	Framingham			Brazilian Guideline			PROCAM		
		Low	Moderate	High	Low	Moderate	High	Low	Moderate	High
DAD	Low	210	0	0	126	85	0	210	0	0
	Moderate	56	6	5	28	29	10	65	2	0
	High and very high	0	3	3	0	0	6	3	2	1
Agreement			77.4%			56.7%			75.3%	
Kappa			0.23			0.14			0.07	
95% CI			0.07–0.39			0.02–0.25			0–0.26	

DAD: Data Collection on Adverse Effects of Anti-HIV Drugs; PROCAM: Prospective Cardiovascular Münster; CI: confidence Interval.

group for CV events was low using the DAD equation and conventional risk equations (Framingham and PROCAM). Another study from Thailand found a low prevalence of patients with high CVD risk using the DAD equation and the Framingham equation, with good agreement between these scores [22]. However, the Framingham equation predicted higher CVD risk compared with the DAD equation. In our results, the DAD equation placed a higher proportion of the patients in the moderate category of risk for CVD compared with the Framingham and PROCAM scores; this result has implications for clinical followup and management.

Methodological issues regarding the comparability and applicability of these different CVD risk scores, particularly among people living with HIV, have been thoroughly discussed, most recently by D'Agostino [27]. In addition to the differences in the composition of the cardiovascular risk scores and the differences in the relevant outcomes, the comparison of CVD scores using kappa coefficients may have some limitations. Our findings pointed out good agreement for the risk predictions produced by the DAD equations compared with Framingham or PROCAM in constrast with low statistical kappa estimates. Other studies also found good agreement between different risk systems but calculated low kappa values [22, 25]. This apparent paradox could be explained by the imbalanced distribution of the values and by kappa's dependence on the prevalence of the measured event [47]. However, the clinical significance of these inconsistencies is not completely understood.

5. Conclusions

Comparing different tools that predict the risk of CVD is informative, but these comparisons do not assess the accuracy of the outcome. Because HAART is offered to large cohort of HIV patients in Brazil, it seems promising to address this issue by monitoring patients and CV events using the existing official surveillance system. These data would be valuable for individual clinical management and for economic evaluations from a public health perspective. Large cohort studies including different HIV-infected groups would be necessary to address these questions.

Conflict of Interests

The authors declare that there is no conflict of interests regarding the publication of this paper.

Acknowledgments

The project has received funds from the Brazilian National Research Council (CNPq-Edital Universal) and from the State Foundation for Research Support of Goias (FAPEG/Edital PPS-SUS). Martelli CMT and Turchi MD have received Fellowship Grants (CNPq nos. 306489/2010-4, 306928/2010-8), and they are research members of the National Institute for Health Technology Assessment (IATS).

References

[1] A. Mocroft, B. Ledergerber, C. Katlama et al., "Decline in the AIDS and death rates in the EuroSIDA study: an observational study," *The Lancet*, vol. 362, no. 9377, pp. 22–29, 2003.

[2] T. C. Quinn, "HIV epidemiology and the effects of antiviral therapy on long-term consequences," *AIDS*, vol. 3, supplement 22, pp. S7–S12, 2008.

[3] J. S. Montaner, V. D. Lima, R. Barrios et al., "Association of highly active antiretroviral therapy coverage, population viral load, and yearly new HIV diagnoses in British Columbia, Canada: a population-based study," *The Lancet*, vol. 376, no. 9740, pp. 532–539, 2010.

[4] UNAIDS, *Global AIDS Response Progress Reporting: Monitoring the 2011 Political Declaration on HIV/AIDS: Guidelines on Construction of Core Indicators*, 2012.

[5] I. Dourado, M. A. Veras, D. Barreira, and A. M. de Brito, "AIDS epidemic trends after the introduction of antiretroviral therapy in Brazil," vol. 40, supplement 9-17, pp. 9–17, 2006.

[6] M. Malta, F. I. Bastos, C. M. F. P. da Silva et al., "Differential survival benefit of universal HAART access in Brazil: a nation-wide comparison of injecting drug users versus men who have sex with men," *Journal of Acquired Immune Deficiency Syndromes*, vol. 52, no. 5, pp. 629–635, 2009.

[7] M. P. Dube and J. J. Cadden, "Lipid metabolism in treated HIV infection," *Best Practice & Research*, vol. 25, no. 3, pp. 429–442, 2011.

[8] J. A. Aberg, "Cardiovascular complications in HIV management: past, present, and future," *Journal of Acquired Immune Deficiency Syndromes*, vol. 50, no. 1, pp. 54–64, 2009.

[9] J. H. Stein, "Cardiovascular risk and dyslipidemia management in HIV-infected patients," *Topics in Antiviral Medicine*, vol. 20, no. 4, pp. 129–133, 2012.

[10] S. W. Worm and J. D. Lundgren, "The metabolic syndrome in HIV," *Best Practice & Research Clinical Endocrinology & Metabolism*, vol. 25, no. 3, pp. 479–486, 2011.

[11] J. I. Cleeman, "Executive summary of the third report of the National Cholesterol Education Program (NCEP) expert

panel on detection, evaluation, and treatment of high blood cholesterol in adults (adult treatment panel III)," *Journal of the American Medical Association*, vol. 285, no. 19, pp. 2486–2497, 2001.

[12] M. P. Dubé, J. H. Stein, J. A. Aberg et al., "Guidelines for the evaluation and management of dyslipidemia in human immunodeficiency virus (HIV)-infected adults receiving antiretroviral therapy: recommendations of the HIV Medicine Association of the Infectious Disease Society of America and the Adult AIDS Clinical Trials Group," *Clinical Infectious Diseases*, vol. 37, no. 5, pp. 613–627, 2003.

[13] J. D. Lundgren, M. Battegay, G. Behrens et al., "European AIDS Clinical Society (EACS) guidelines on the prevention and management of metabolic diseases in HIV," *HIV Medicine*, vol. 9, no. 2, pp. 72–81, 2008.

[14] H. Knobel, C. Jericó, M. Montero et al., "Global cardiovascular risk in patients with HIV infection: concordance and differences in estimates according to three risk equations (Framingham, SCORE, and PROCAM)," *AIDS Patient Care and STDs*, vol. 21, no. 7, pp. 452–457, 2007.

[15] G. E. Vrentzos, J. A. Papadakis, E. S. Ganotakis et al., "Predicting coronary heart disease risk using the Framingham and PROCAM equations in dyslipidaemic patients without overt vascular disease," *International Journal of Clinical Practice*, vol. 61, no. 10, pp. 1643–1653, 2007.

[16] E. F. Silva, K. C. Bassichetto, and D. S. Lewi, "Lipid profile, cardiovascular risk factors and metabolic syndrome in a group of AIDS patients," *Arquivos Brasileiros de Cardiologia*, vol. 93, no. 2, pp. 113–118, 2009.

[17] P. Cahn, O. Leite, A. Rosales et al., "Metabolic profile and cardiovascular risk factors among Latin American HIV-infected patients receiving HAART," *Brazilian Journal of Infectious Diseases*, vol. 14, no. 2, pp. 158–166, 2010.

[18] N. Friis-Moller, R. Thiebaut, P. Reiss, R. Weber, A. D. Monforte, S. De Wit et al., "Predicting the risk of cardiovascular disease in HIV-infected patients: the data collection on adverse effects of anti-HIV drugs study," *European Journal of Cardiovascular Prevention and Rehabilitation*, vol. 17, no. 5, pp. 491–501, 2010.

[19] M. M. M. Guimarães, D. B. Greco, R. B. Fóscolo, and L. J. D. C. Machado, "Coronary heart disease risk assessment in HIV-infected patients: a comparison of Framingham, PROCAM and SCORE risk assessment functions," *International Journal of Clinical Practice*, vol. 64, no. 6, pp. 739–745, 2010.

[20] N. Önen, E. Overton, W. Seyfried et al., "Aging and HIV infection: a comparison between older HIV-infected persons and the general population," *HIV Clinical Trials*, vol. 11, no. 2, pp. 100–109, 2010.

[21] C. R. Pullinger, B. E. Aouizerat, C. Gay, T. Coggins, I. Movsesyan, H. Davis et al., "Metabolic abnormalities and coronary heart disease risk in human immunodeficiency virus-infected adults," *Metabolic Syndrome and Related Disorders*, vol. 8, no. 3, pp. 279–286, 2010.

[22] N. Edwards-Jackson, S. J. Kerr, H. V. Tieu et al., "Cardiovascular risk assessment in persons with HIV infection in the developing world: comparing three risk equations in a cohort of HIV-infected Thais," *HIV Medicine*, vol. 12, no. 8, pp. 510–515, 2011.

[23] R. C. Kaplan, L. A. Kingsley, A. R. Sharrett, X. Li, J. Lazar, P. C. Tien et al., "Ten-year predicted coronary heart disease risk in HIV-infected men and women," *Clinical Infectious Diseases*, vol. 45, no. 8, pp. 1074–1081, 2007.

[24] E. M. O. Lima, D. M. Gualandro, P. C. Yu et al., "Cardiovascular prevention in HIV patients: results from a successful intervention program," *Atherosclerosis*, vol. 204, no. 1, pp. 229–232, 2009.

[25] Z. M. Barros, R. A. De Alencar Ximenes, D. B. Miranda-Filho et al., "Comparison between the Framingham and Prospective Cardiovascular of Münster scores for risk assessment of coronary heart disease in human immunodeficiency virus-positive patients in Pernambuco, Brazil," *Metabolic Syndrome and Related Disorders*, vol. 8, no. 6, pp. 489–497, 2010.

[26] N. Friis-Moller and S. W. Worm, "Can the risk of cardiovascular disease in HIV-infected patients be estimated from conventional risk prediction tools?" *Clinical Infectious Diseases*, vol. 45, no. 8, pp. 1082–1084, 2007.

[27] R. B. D'Agostino Sr., "Cardiovascular risk estimation in 2012: lessons learned and applicability to the HIV population," *The Journal of Infectious Diseases*, vol. 205, 3, pp. S362–S367.

[28] SBC/SBH/SBN, "VI diretrizes brasileiras de hipertensão," *Arquivos Brasileiros De Cardiologia*, vol. 95, pp. 1–51, 2010.

[29] P. Zimmet, K. G. MMA, and M. S. Rios, "A new international diabetes federation worldwide definition of the metabolic syndrome: the rationale and the results," *Revista Española de Cardiología*, vol. 58, no. 12, pp. 1371–1376, 2005.

[30] W. T. Friedewald, R. I. Levy, and D. S. Fredrickson, "Estimation of the concentration of low-density lipoprotein cholesterol in plasma, without use of the preparative ultracentrifuge," *Clinical Chemistry*, vol. 18, no. 6, pp. 499–502, 1972.

[31] SBC, "IV diretriz brasileira sobre dislipidemias e prevenção da aterosclerose. Departamento de aterosclerose da sociedade brasileira de cardiologia," *Arquivos Brasileiros de Cardiologia*, vol. 88, 2007.

[32] P. M. Ridker, "Clinical application of C-reactive protein for cardiovascular disease detection and prevention," *Circulation*, vol. 107, no. 3, pp. 363–369, 2003.

[33] American Diabetes, "Standards of medical care in diabetes," *Diabetes Care*, supplement 1, pp. S15–S35, 2004.

[34] D. W. Cockcroft and M. H. Gault, "Prediction of creatinine clearance from serum creatinine," *Nephron*, vol. 16, no. 1, pp. 31–41, 1976.

[35] G. L. Myers, W. G. Miller, J. Coresh, J. Fleming, N. Greenberg, T. Greene et al., "Recommendations for improving serum creatinine measurement: a report from the Laboratory Working Group of the National Kidney Disease Education Program," *Clinical Chemistry*, vol. 52, no. 1, pp. 5–18, 2006.

[36] J. M. Ginsberg, B. S. Chang, R. A. Matarese, and S. Garella, "Use of single voided urine samples to estimate quantitative proteinuria," *The New England Journal of Medicine*, vol. 309, no. 25, pp. 1543–1546, 1983.

[37] M. E. Molitch, R. A. DeFronzo, M. J. Franz et al., "Diabetic nephropathy," *Diabetes Care*, vol. 22, no. 1, pp. S66–S69, 1999.

[38] K. M. Anderson, P. W. F. Wilson, P. M. Odell, and W. B. Kannel, "An updated coronary risk profile. A statement for health professionals," *Circulation*, vol. 83, no. 1, pp. 356–362, 1991.

[39] G. Assmann, P. Cullen, and H. Schulte, "Simple scoring scheme for calculating the risk of acute coronary events based on the 10-year follow-up of the Prospective Cardiovascular Münster (PROCAM) study," *Circulation*, vol. 105, no. 3, pp. 310–315, 2002.

[40] J. P. van Wijk and M. C. Cabezas, "Hypertriglyceridemia, metabolic syndrome, and cardiovascular disease in HIV-infected patients: effects of antiretroviral therapy and adipose tissue distribution," *International Journal of Vascular Medicine*, vol. 2012, 2012.

[41] S. W. Worm, D. A. Kamara, P. Reiss, O. Kirk, W. El-Sadr, C. Fux et al., "Elevated triglycerides and risk of myocardial infarction in HIV-positive persons," *AIDS*, vol. 25, no. 12, pp. 1497–1504, 2011.

[42] M. W. Nery, C. M. Martelli, and M. D. Turchi, "Dyslipidemia in AIDS patients on highly active antiretroviral therapy," *Brazilian Journal of Infectious Diseases*, vol. 15, no. 2, pp. 151–155.

[43] M. Miller, N. J. Stone, C. Ballantyne, V. Bittner, M. H. Criqui, H. N. Ginsberg et al., "Triglycerides and cardiovascular disease: a scientific statement from the American Heart Association," *Circulation*, vol. 123, no. 20, pp. 2292–2333, 2011.

[44] M. Masia, E. Bernal, S. Padilla, M. L. Graells, I. Jarrin, M. V. Almenar et al., "The role of C-reactive protein as a marker for cardiovascular risk associated with antiretroviral therapy in HIV-infected patients," *Atherosclerosis*, vol. 195, no. 1, pp. 167–171, 2007.

[45] N. Friis-Moller, C. A. Sabin, R. Weber, A. d'Arminio Monforte, W. M. El-Sadr, P. Reiss et al., "Combination antiretroviral therapy and the risk of myocardial infarction," *The New England Journal of Medicine*, vol. 349, no. 21, pp. 1993–2003, 2003.

[46] M. May, J. A. C. Sterne, M. Shipley et al., "A coronary heart disease risk model for predicting the effect of potent antiretroviral therapy in HIV-1 infected men," *International Journal of Epidemiology*, vol. 36, no. 6, pp. 1309–1318, 2007.

[47] A. R. Feinstein and D. V. Cicchetti, "High agreement but low kappa: I. The problems of two paradoxes," *Journal of Clinical Epidemiology*, vol. 43, no. 6, pp. 543–549, 1990.

Spatial and Temporal Distribution of Tuberculosis in the State of Mexico, Mexico

Adrian Zaragoza Bastida,[1] Marivel Hernández Tellez,[2] Lilia P. Bustamante Montes,[1] Imelda Medina Torres,[3] Jaime Nicolás Jaramillo Paniagua,[3] Germán David Mendoza Martínez,[4] and Ninfa Ramírez Durán[1]

[1] *Facultad de Medicina, Universidad Autónoma del Estado de México, 50180, Toluca, MEX, Mexico*
[2] *Centro Interamericano de Recursos del Agua, Universidad Autónoma del Estado de México, 50200, Toluca, MEX, Mexico*
[3] *Facultad de Medicina Veterinaria Zootécnia, Universidad Autónoma del Estado de México, 50200, Toluca, MEX, Mexico*
[4] *Departamento de Producción Agrícola y Animal, Universidad Autónoma Metropolitana, 04960, México, DF, Mexico*

Correspondence should be addressed to Ninfa Ramírez Durán, nramirezd@uaemex.mx

Academic Editors: K. Akakura, P. Domingo, and Q. He

Tuberculosis (TB) is one of the oldest human diseases that still affects large population groups. According to the World Health Organization (WHO), there were approximately 9.4 million new cases worldwide in the year 2010. In Mexico, there were 18,848 new cases of TB of all clinical variants in 2010. The identification of clusters in space-time is of great interest in epidemiological studies. The objective of this research was to identify the spatial and temporal distribution of TB during the period 2006–2010 in the State of Mexico, using geographic information system (GIS) and SCAN statistics program. Nine significant clusters ($P < 0.05$) were identified using spatial and space-time analysis. The conclusion is that TB in the State of Mexico is not randomly distributed but is concentrated in areas close to Mexico City.

1. Introduction

Tuberculosis (TB) is an infectious disease, generally chronic, and caused by a group of bacteria: *Mycobacterium tuberculosis, M. africanum, M. bovis, M. microti* and *M. canettii* [1]. The main transmission is from person to person by microdrops generated by coughing or sneezing of a person with active TB [1, 2].

TB is one of the oldest human diseases that still affects large population groups, mainly in marginal areas and comprising vulnerable groups impacted by extreme poverty, malnutrition, and crowded housing. These groups are prone to infection by the tuberculosis bacilli and to acquiring active TB [2, 3].

In Mexico, the National Population Commission (CONAPO) considers a marginal index based on a census of localities according to the global impact of several total measurements or items, such as lack of education (illiteracy, incomplete grade school) and inadequate housing conditions (without water, drainage, bathrooms, electricity, refrigerator [4], and other basic household equipment, houses with earth floors and crowded living conditions). These items can be used to identify geographic areas with greater marginalization (socioeconomic development) and a greater risk from TB infection.

The World Health Organization (WHO) reported in 2010 that there were an estimated 9.4 million incident cases (range 8.9 million–9.9 million) of TB globally, equivalent to 137 cases per 100,000 population, and that 1.1 million of those cases also tested positive for human immunodeficiency virus (HIV). The mortality of HIV-negative patients with TB was estimated at 1.3 million, this being equivalent to 20 deaths per 100,000 people. The incidence of TB patients in Asia was 55% and 30% in Africa; smaller proportions of cases occurred in the Eastern Mediterranean Region (7%), the European Region (4%), and the Americas Regions (3%) [5].

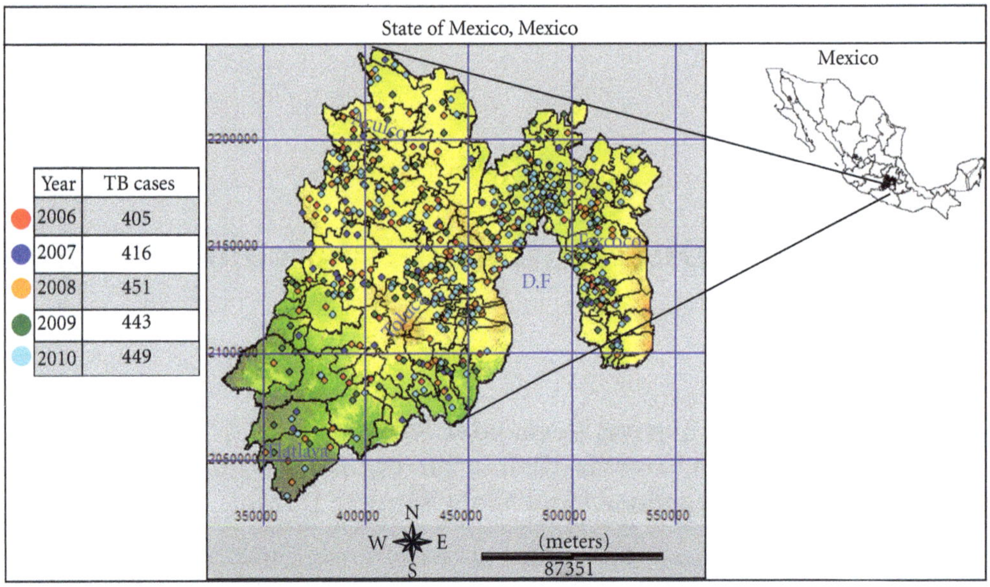

FIGURE 1: Location and geographic distribution of tuberculosis cases during 2006–2010 in the State of Mexico.

In Mexico, 18,848 TB cases (in all clinical forms) were reported in 2010, which is a rate of 16.77 per 100,000 habitants. Of all the cases reported, 15,384 or 13.7 per 100,000 corresponded to lung TB, the mortality rate was 2.14 per 100,000 (in all clinical forms) [6], and the incidence rate was higher in the 60-year-old or 60+-year-old groups of patients, and males had a 1.5 times higher rate than females [3].

In the federal entities, TB presents a well-defined concentration pattern. High incidence rates are present in the western states and the Gulf of Mexico, and lower rates are found in the central states. Tamaulipas and Baja California have double the national rate (13.5 per 100,000 inhabitants). In these states, together with the Veracruz, Chiapas, Nuevo León, Jalisco, Sinaloa, Nayarit, Guerrero, Sonora, Oaxaca, and Chihuahua states, are concentrated 70% of all the identified cases of TB in the country [3].

At present, geographic information systems (GISs) are among the most useful tools in epidemiology, as they can be used to identify geographical areas and population groups with a higher risk of sickness or premature mortality and which therefore require higher preventive care or health information and monitoring of diseases in time and space [7, 8].

Spatial cluster of a disease grouping is one of the most important techniques in epidemiology. In 1995, Kuldorff and Negarwalla developed a new space statistics method called SCAN for the detection and cluster inference in time-space under the likelihood ratio (LLR) hypothesis [8].

SCAN statistics is a spatial-temporal analysis defined by a large number of transposed cylinders; the circular base defines the geographic area with a radius that can vary from zero to a larger distance influenced by the percentage of the population at risk, while the height of the cylinder represents the temporal parameter. The LLR was calculated for each cylinder. The cylinder with the highest LLR was considered to constitute the most probable cluster. A Monte Carlo simulation was used to calculate the P value [9].

In the case of TB, various researchers have used GIS to study this infectious disease. Moonan et al. [10] used GIS to identify the geographic locations of TB transmission and incidence in the United States of America during 1993 to 2000. In India, Tiwarin et al. [11] carried out a geospatial investigation of TB occurrence in the Almora district using GIS and the SCAN statistics program. Nunes [12] in Portugal detected spatial and temporal clusters during 2000–2004 by using SCAN. The above-mentioned authors agree that GIS and SCAN are useful tools for vigilance against TB.

The SCAN statistics program has been used worldwide by various researchers with different lengths of search windows: the most frequently used are 25% and 50% of the population [11]. Sabel et al. [13] added some health determinants in their model, such as age, gender, and margination, as covariants as a form of correction or data adjustment.

The objective of this research was to use the spatial statistics program SCAN and GIS to identify the spatial and temporal distribution of TB during 2006 to 2010 and to determine the geographic locations of higher transmission and incidence of TB in the State of Mexico, Mexico.

2. Materials and Methods

2.1. Study Location. This study used as its research area the State of Mexico, located in the centre of Mexico at 98°35′30″–100°37′00″ west longitude and 18°21′15″–20°17′00″ north latitude, and occupying 22,499.95 km^2, which represents 1.1% of the national territory. It is divided into 125 municipalities that include 4, 341 localities (Figure 1).

According to the II Conteo de Población and Vivienda 2005 (II Population and Housing Census 2005), the State of Mexico had 14,007,495 inhabitants, representing 13.6% of the entire Mexican population and making it the most populated state.

2.2. Data Collection

2.2.1. Population Data. In accordance with the Sistema Nacional de Vigilancia Epidemiológica (Epidemiology Vigilance National Surveillance), tuberculosis cases were reported from 499 localities during the period 2006–2010. Cases in each locality were categorized using a marginalization index [14]: Category 1: very low; Category 2: low; Category 3: medium; Category 4: high; Category 5: very high. The number, age and gender of the inhabitants in each locality were obtained from the II Population and Housing Census 2005 by the "Instituto Nacional de Estadística y Geografía" (INEGI) (National Institute of Statistics and Geography) [15]. Age was classified into five categories: Category 1: 0–4 years old; Category 2: 5–14 years old; Category 3: 15–17 years old; Category 4: 18–59 years old; Category 5: 60 and 60+ years of age. The data for gender was combined with the age categories, and therefore 10 groups of age-gender were created to describe the population of each locality.

2.2.2. Tuberculosis Case Data. The collected cases were diagnosed at several hospitals and healthcare centres and their demographic characteristics were reported to the TB National Registry during 2006–2010. Marginality was obtained from the 2005 marginality index [14] for the locality where each TB case was found. For the statistical strategy, the covariables were age-gender and margination.

2.2.3. Geographic Localization Data. For data analysis, locality with the TB case was used as a geographic unit. The georeference came from the latitude-longitude projection system obtained from the Instituto de Geografía Estadística y Catastral del Estado de México (IGECEM) (Institute of Statistical Geography and Tax Revenue of the State of Mexico) [16].

2.3. Statistical and Geographic Analysis

2.3.1. TB Cluster Detection and Identification. Determination and identification of TB clusters were carried out with the statistics spatial SCAN program and calculated with the SaTScan (V8.0) computer package that obtains statistical significance and the approximate cluster localization. The SaTScan program requires three files for initiation: cases, population, and geography localization files. A Poisson probability model was used with a 25% and 50% search window for high rates: age, gender and, margination index were the covariables.

2.3.2. Geographic Analysis. For the graphic cluster representation, a map was drawn based on the information obtained with the SCAN and the IDRISI Taiga software. A factorial format map of the State of Mexico obtained from the

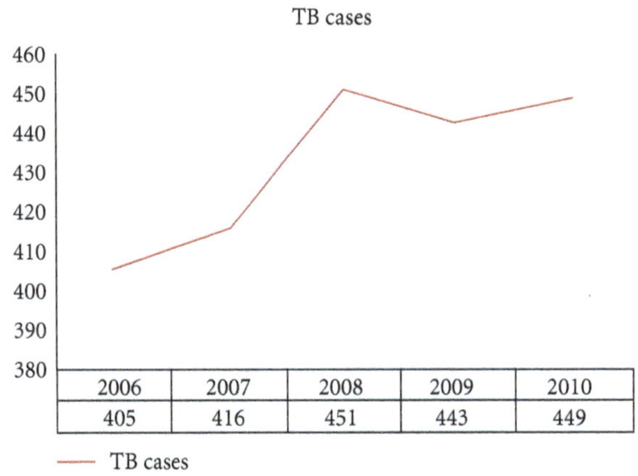

FIGURE 2: Frequency of TB cases in the State of Mexico during the years 2006 to 2010.

IGECEM and a Lansat 7 satellite medium infrared colour image at bands 2, 4, and 7 were used [17].

3. Results

There were 2,164 human TB cases detected from 2006 to 2010, distributed in 499 localities and in 125 municipalities. The municipalities with more than 100 TB cases are Ecatepec de Morelos with 365 (16.9%) cases; Netzahualcóyotl with 172 (7.9%); Naucalpan de Juárez with 153 (7%); Tlalnepantla de Baz with 123 (5.7%); Toluca county with 109 cases (5%). The distribution of the 2,164 cases is shown in Figure 2 with an increment from 405 cases in 2006 up to 449 in 2010.

As mentioned in the methodology section, the 10 "age-gender-margination" groups or categories were found in 499 locations with TB cases. A database with 4990 groups was created. Two analyses were performed using the collected information: the first analysis was spatial and the second was a space-time analysis.

3.1. Spatial Analysis. A search window with a maximum length of ≤50% population with high TB rates was used. A primary cluster and five secondary clusters were identified. The centre of the primary cluster was located in the municipality of Valle de Chalco Solidaridad in the locality of Santa Cruz. The relative risk (RR) was 337.68 with 14 TB cases *versus* the 0.04 expected cases. The second cluster was formed of the municipalities of Acolman, Atenco, Chiautla, Chiconcuac, Ecatepec de Morelos, Papalotla, Tecámac, Teotihuacán, Tepetlaoxtoc, Texcoco, and Tezoyuca. The RR was 1.68 with 423 TB cases and the expected RR was 282.2 cases. The third cluster, in the Atizapán de Zaragoza, Villa Nicolás Romero, and Cuautitlán Izcalli municipalities, had a 215.58 RR with seven TB cases compared to 0.03 expected cases. The 10.75 RR for the fourth cluster with 20 TB cases, located in Huixquilucan and Lerma municipalities, had an expected number of cases of 1.88.

Cluster 5, located in the municipalities of Tlalnepantla de Baz, Tultitlán, Apizapán de Zaragoza, and Cuahutitlán Izcalli,

Table 1: TB clusters with a high RR identified in the State of Mexico using a space analysis and a search window maximum length of ≤50% and ≤25% population, adjusted for age-gender-margination.

Cluster	Loc.[a]	Centre coordinates	Radius (km)	Obs[b]	Exp[c]	RR[d]	LLR[e]	P
Primary cluster								
1	1	19.287 N, 98.933 W	**0**	**14**	0.04	337.68	67.5	0.001
Secondary clusters								
2	23	19.585 N, −98.945 W	13.11	423	282.20	1.62	35.8	0.001
3	3	19.596 N, −99.269 W	4.48	7	0.03	215.58	30.6	0.001
4	3	19.306 N, −99.386 W	6.88	20	1.88	10.75	29.3	0.001
5	5	19.610 N, −99.191 W	5.08	38	8.77	4.39	26.7	0.001
6	4	19.501 N, −99.284 W	5.57	8	0.78	10.24	11.4	0.001

[a]Locations with TB cases, [b]Observed number of cases in cluster, [c]Expected number of cases in cluster, [d]Relative risk of the cluster, [e]Log likelihood ratio.

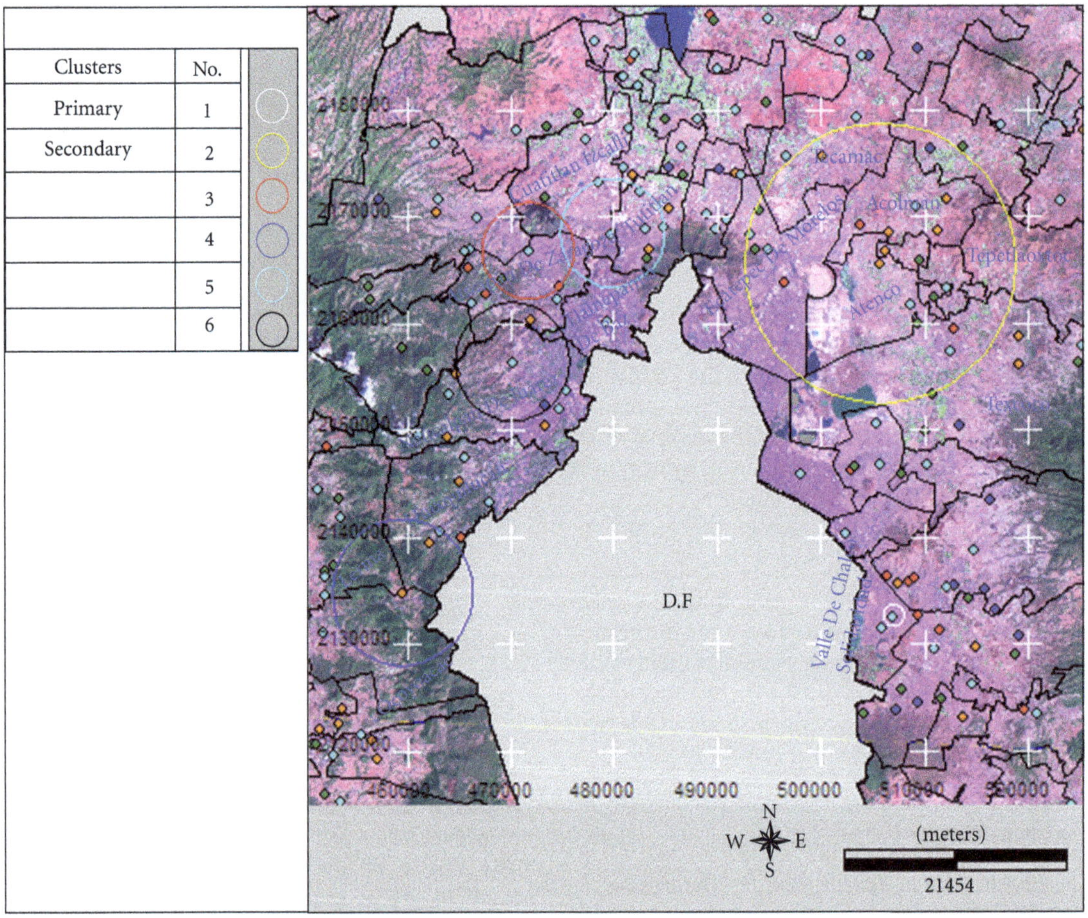

Figure 3: Geography of the identified high TB rate clusters in the State of Mexico detected with a spatial analysis and a search window maximum length of ≤50% and ≤25% population, adjusted for age-gender-margination.

was found to have a 4.39 RR with 38 TB cases compared with the 8.77 expected cases.

The last identified secondary cluster, located in the Tlalnepantla de Baz, Jilotzingo, Atizapán de Zaragoza, and Naucalpan de Juaréz, showed a 10.24 RR with eight TB cases against the 0.78 expected cases.

A maximum l ength of ≤25% search window was used for a population with high TB rates and the results of the analysis were similar to those obtained with a ≤50% search window. General information about the identified clusters is shown in Table 1, and their geography is shown in Figure 3.

3.2. Space-Time Analysis. A primary cluster was identified using a search window maximum of ≤50% population with high TB rates. The cluster centre was located in the Tultitlan, a municipality formed of the Tlalnepantla de Baz, Cuautitlán, Cuautitlán Izcalli, and Atizapán de Zaragoza municipalities. The relative risk (RR) during the 2007–2009

TABLE 2: A cluster with high rates of tuberculosis in the State of Mexico was detected with a spatial-temporal analysis and a search window maximum length of ≤50% and ≤25% risk population, adjusted for age-gender-margination.

Cluster	Loc.[a]	Centre coordinates	Radius (km)	Year	Obs[b]	Exp[c]	RR[d]	LLR[e]	P
Primary cluster									
1	6	19.315 N, −98.928 W	3.49	2006–2008	16	0.2	81.08	54.467248	0.001
Secondary clusters									
2	19	19.585 N, −98.945 W	11.93	2006–2008	267	140.59	2.03	48.880307	0.001
*3	5	19.610 N, −99.191 W	5.08	2007–2009	27	4.39	6.22	26.578700	0.001

[a]Locations with TB cases, [b]Observed number of cases in cluster, [c]Expected number of cases in cluster, [d]Relative risk of the cluster, [e]Log likelihood ratio.
*Cluster detected with a search window maximum length of ≤50% risk population.

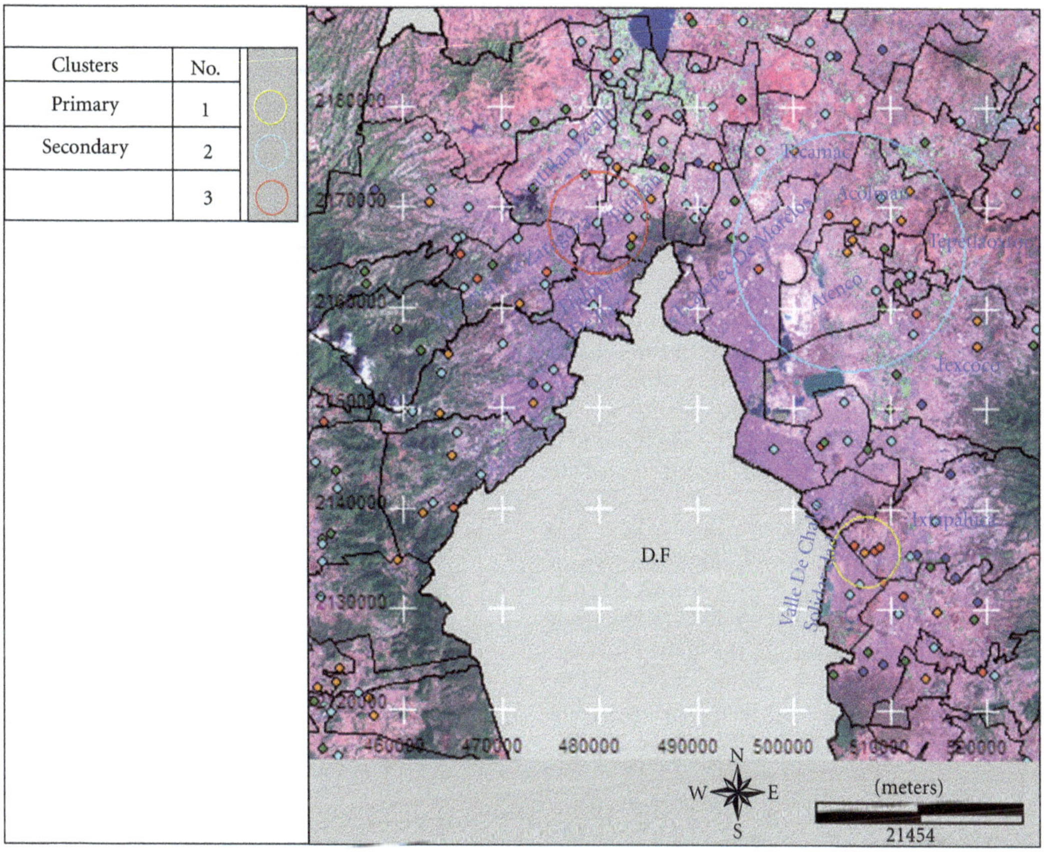

FIGURE 4: Geographic locations of the identified clusters with high rates using a space-time analysis and a search window maximum length of ≤50% and ≤25% population, adjusted for age-gender-margination.

period was 6.22 with 27 TB cases and 4.39 expected cases. Secondary clusters were not identified.

A search window maximum length of ≤25% population was used to identify three significant clusters. The primary cluster was located in the Valle de Chalco Solidaridad, Ixtapaluca, and a small part of Chalco. The RR was 81.08, with 16 TB cases during the period 2008–2006, compared with 0.2 expected cases.

Two secondary clusters were identified. One was similar to that described above using the ≤50% population search window. The other was formed by 11 municipalities: Acolman, Atenco, Chicuautla, Chiconcuac, Ecatepec de Morelos, Papalotla, Tecamac, Teotihuacan, Tepetlaoxtoc, Texcoco, and Tezoyuca. The RR was 2.03 with 267 cases of TB during the years 2006–2008 against expected cases of 140.50. General information about the identified clusters is shown in Table 2 and their geography in Figure 4.

4. Discussion

In the field of epidemiology one of the most important analyses is the detection in space-time of a disease cluster, since a non-control-spreading of the disease takes place and a social or economic factor favours cluster formation. The use of GIS plus spatial statistics has been used to determine spatial distribution patterns of various infectious and noninfectious diseases [18–22]. SCAN, available in the SaTScan V8 software, has been used worldwide to detect various disease clusters, including TB.

GISs plus molecular diagnosis techniques have been used to locate TB clusters and to identify the *Mycobacterium* responsible for the outbreak [10]. Frequently, however, it is not possible to obtain a detailed and complete analysis since the information is mainly based on a positive bacilloscopy.

However, this study obtained data on TB according to age, gender, and marginality index, representing valuable information since the highest rate of this disease occurs in adults of 60 and 60+ years of age [3], in males 1.5 to 1 rate and in marginal groups [2].

With the SCAN statistical results and a 25% and 50% search window population and a spatial analysis ($P \leq 0.05$), six clusters were identified, showing that TB is not randomly distributed in the State of Mexico but in clusters in a spatial pattern. In similar studies by Navaet al. [23] in Acapulco, Mexico, using a different spatial method, clusters were not found. We used two search windows (50% and 25%) in order to find small clusters but identification differences were not seen in cluster identification. These results were in agreement with those reported by Tiwarin et al. [11].

The six identified clusters are located close to and around Mexico City (Federal District), the largest city in the Mexico. The highest incidence rates of TB are found in urban zones [24] in comparison with rural areas. Our results agreed with those reported by Moonan et al. [10]. They found a strong association between the strains of TB clusters and the distance to the centre of urban zones.

Three TB clusters were identified with spatial and temporal analysis using the same search windows; two of these clusters grouped the TB cases from the 2006 to 2008 period, and the cases from 2007 to 2009 were in the third cluster. The three clusters all contained the 2008 TB cases, making it the year with the highest incidence.

Of the three identified clusters, only one is in agreement with those identified with the spatial-only analysis, but the others are located in areas close to the spatial clusters.

The results of the present study are of great importance in TB epidemiological surveys in the State of Mexico. The presence of clusters is valuable to the healthcare system since strategy can be revised accordingly in those areas containing TB clusters.

5. Conclusions

TB is spatially clustered in the State of Mexico, Mexico. Nine clusters were identified using two types of analysis: spatial and spatial-temporal. Such clusters were mainly found in Valle de Chalco Solidaridad, Atenco, Ecatepec de Morelos, Tlalnepantla de Baz, Acolma, Tultitlan, Cuautitlán Izcalli, Atizapán de Zaragoza, Huixquilucan, and Naucalpan de Juárez, all municipalities that are very close to Mexico City (Federal District).

Acknowledgments

The authors extend their thanks to The Health Institute of the State of Mexico for providing the necessary help and support for the study. This work is derived from the thesis for the degree of Doctorate in Sciences of Health, registered in the PNPC-CONACYT, and benefited from the economic contribution of Project SIEA-UAEM 2742/2008U.

References

[1] S. D. Lawn and A. I. Zumla, "Tuberculosis," *The Lancet*, vol. 378, no. 9785, pp. 57–72, 2011.

[2] M. G. Baker, K. Venugopal, and C. P. Howden, *Household Crowding and Tuberculosis*, World Health Organization Regional Office for Europe, Copenhagen, Denmark, 2011.

[3] Secretaría de Salud, *Programa de Acción Específico 2007–2012 Tuberculosis*, Distrito Federal, Mexico.

[4] Consejo Nacional de Población (CONAPO), Índice de Marginación 2005 a nivel localidad, 2005, http://www.conapo.gob.mx/index.php?option=com_content&view=article&id=46&Itemid=194.

[5] World Health Organization (WHO), *Global Tuberculosis Control*, WHO, Geneva, Switzerland, 2010.

[6] Secretaría de Salud, *Dirección General Adjunta del Programas Preventivos del Centro Nacional de Vigilancia Epidemiológica y Control de Enfermedades (CENAVECE)*, Mexico, 2010, http://www.cenave.gob.mx/tuberculosis/PRESENTACION/cifras%20oficiales.asp.

[7] R. Martinez, M. Vidaurre, P. Najera, E. Loyola, and C. Castillo, "SIG-Epi uso de sistemas de información geográfica en epidemiología y Salud Pública," *Boletín Epidemiológico, Organización Panamericana de la Salud*, vol. 22, no. 3, pp. 1–8, 2001.

[8] M. Kulldorff and N. Nagarwalla, "Spatial disease clusters: detection and inference," *Statistics in Medicine*, vol. 14, no. 8, pp. 799–810, 1995.

[9] M. Kulldorff, F. Mostashari, L. Duczmal, W. K. Yih, K. Kleinman, and R. Platt, "Multivariate scan statistics for disease surveillance," *Statistics in Medicine*, vol. 26, no. 8, pp. 1824–1833, 2007.

[10] P. K. Moonan, M. Bayona, T. N. Quitugua et al., "Using GIS technology to identify areas of tuberculosis transmission and incidence," *International Journal of Health Geographics*, vol. 3, article 23, 2004.

[11] N. Tiwari, C. M. S. Adhikari, A. Tewari, and V. Kandpal, "Investigation of geo-spatial hotspots for the occurrence of tuberculosis in Almora district, India, using GIS and spatial scan statistic," *International Journal of Health Geographics*, vol. 5, article 33, 2006.

[12] C. Nunes, "Tuberculosis incidence in Portugal: spatiotemporal clustering," *International Journal of Health Geographics*, vol. 6, article 30, 2007.

[13] C. E. Sabel, J. G. Wilson, S. Kingham, C. Tisch, and M. Epton, "Spatial implications of covariate adjustment on patterns of risk: respiratory hospital admissions in Christchurch, New Zealand," *Social Science and Medicine*, vol. 65, no. 1, pp. 43–59, 2007.

[14] Consejo Nacional de Población (CONAPO), Índice de marginación a nivel localidad, 2005, http://www.conapo.gob.mx/index.php?option=com_content&view=article&id=46&Itemid=194.

[15] Instituto Nacional de Estadística y Geografía (INEGI), Conteo de Población y Vivienda, 2005, http://www.inegi.org.mx/sistemas/consulta_resultados/iter2005.aspx?c=27436&s=est.

[16] Instituto de Geografía Estadística y Catastral del Estado de México (IGECEM), Nomenclator de Localidades del Estado de México, 2009, http://igecem.edomex.gob.mx/descargasgeograficas.htm.

[17] Instituto de Geografía Estadística y Catastral del Estado de México (IGECEM), Divisi6n Política del Estado de México (Metadatos), 2010, http://igecem.edomex.gob.mx/descargasgeograficas.htm.

[18] J. Elias, D. Harmsen, H. Claus, W. Hellenbrand, M. Frosch, and U. Vogel, "Spatiotemporal analysis of invasive meningococcal disease, Germany," *Emerging Infectious Diseases*, vol. 12, no. 11, pp. 1689–1695, 2006.

[19] R. E. Bonilla, "Distribuci6n espacio-temporal de la fiebre dengue en Costa Rica," *Poblaci6n y Salud en Mesoaméroca*, vol. 3, no. 2, pp. 1–9, 2006.

[20] J. E. Oeltmann, J. K. Varma, L. Ortega et al., "Multidrug-resistant tuberculosis outbreak among US-bound Hmong refugees, Thailand, 2005," *Emerging Infectious Diseases*, vol. 14, no. 11, pp. 1715–1721, 2008.

[21] D. C. Wheeler, "A comparison of spatial clustering and cluster detection techniques for childhood leukemia incidence in Ohio, 1996–2003," *International Journal of Health Geographics*, vol. 6, article 13, 2007.

[22] D. I. Gregorio, H. Samociuk, L. DeChello, and H. Swede, "Effects of study area size on geographic characterizations of health events: prostate cancer incidence in Southern New England, USA, 1994–1998," *International Journal of Health Geographics*, vol. 5, article 8, 2006.

[23] E. Nava-Aguilera, Y. López-Vidal, E. Harris et al., "Clustering of mycobacterium tuberculosis cases in Acapulco: spoligotyping and risk factors," *Clinical and Developmental Immunology*, vol. 2011, Article ID 408375, 12 pages, 2011.

[24] R. Graham Barr, A. V. Diez-Roux, C. A. Knirsch, and A. Pablos-Méndez, "Neighborhood poverty and the resurgence of tuberculosis in New York City, 1984–1992," *American Journal of Public Health*, vol. 91, no. 9, pp. 1487–1493, 2001.

9

Beta-Thalassemia in Iran: New Insight into the Role of Genetic Admixture and Migration

Ali Reza Rezaee,[1] Mohammad Mehdi Banoei,[2] Elham Khalili,[3] and Massoud Houshmand[2]

[1] *Department of Animal Science, Faculty of Agriculture, Ferdowsi University of Mashhad, Mashhad, Iran*
[2] *Department of Medical Genetics, National Institute of Genetic Engineering and Biotechnology, Tehran 14155-6343, Iran*
[3] *Department of Genetics, Special Medical Center, Tehran, Iran*

Correspondence should be addressed to Massoud Houshmand, housh62@yahoo.com

Academic Editors: P. Erlich, K. Schlaefer, and K. Spratt

Iran with an area of 1.648 million km^2 is located between the Caspian Sea and the Persian Gulf. The Iranian population consists of multiethnic groups that have been influenced by various invasions and migration throughout history. Studies have revealed the presence of more than 47 different β-globin gene mutations responsible for β-Thalassemia in Iran. This paper is an attempt to study the origin of β-Thalassemia mutations in different parts of Iran. Distribution of β-Thalassemia mutations in Iran shows different patterns in different areas. β-Thalassemia mutations have been a reflection of people and area in correlation with migration and origin of ancestors. We compared the frequencies of β-globin mutations in different regions of Iran with those derived from neighboring countries. The analysis provided evidence of complementary information about the genetic admixture and migration of some mutations, as well as the remarkable genetic classification of the Iranian people and ethnic groups.

1. Introduction

The Iranian population consists of several ethnic groups most of whom are of "Aryan origin." The strategical position of Iran as a crossroad between the west and the eastern civilizations has impressed many to determine the circumstances of gene flow. Thalassemia is the commonest monogenic disorder in the world and globally it is estimated that there are 270 million carriers, of which 80 million are carriers of β-Thalassemia with about 60000 affected children born annually [1]. More than 200 mutations affecting the β-globin gene are now known to result in a phenotype of β-Thalassemia. It affects different ethnic and geographical groups with miscellaneous prevalence in different regions [2, 3]. Association studies for screening the distribution patterns of β-Thalassemia mutations may have a source of information in population genetics science and could be tools as molecular tags in the heredity of human populations. Any geographic distribution of specific mutations may represent information on the place of origin of the genetic change that generated it. Therefore, we are able to analyze specific genetic links between different populations. Since the knowledge of the mutation spectrum present in a population is essential for the molecular diagnosis and prevention of hemoglobinpathies, the knowledge of the ethnical background of a particular area is equally important. Our study provides information on the history and origin of the different β-Thalassemia mutations, population movements, and the relationship between the different affected groups in the country. To improve the construction of a geographical map, results from neighboring countries have also been compared. This paper is based on the reports from the literature together with previously unpublished data collected from the diagnostic service in Iran. Author's efforts have been based on drawing data out from all local, international references, and presented abstracts in national or international congresses. All data (published and unpublished) are classified regarding to different regions and ethnicities and then added to other data (Table 1).

2. Materials and Methods

All materials and methods were used from 150 β-Thalassemia patients from Medical Genetic Laboratory (Special Medical Center, Tehran) and other publication from Iranian β-Thalassemia patients (Akbari, $n = 45$; Drakhshandeh, $n = 96$; Najmabadi, $n = 164$) [4–6].

3. Thalassemia in Iran

Among the eastern Mediterranean region, Iran is one of the major centers for the prevalence of β-Thalassemia. Regarding to high consanguinity among population, it is estimated that there are between two and three million β-Thalassemia carriers and 25,000 patients in Iran. Like many other countries in the region, a large number of Thalassemia patients are β-Thalassemia [7]. Alpha Thalassemia is not as prevalent as β-Thalassemia in Iran [8]. The gene frequency of β-Thalassemia, however, is high and varies considerably between areas. Recent studies have revealed the presence of more than 47 different β-globin gene mutations responsible for β-Thalassemia in Iran. The predominant IVS-II-1 (G > A; beta0) mutation is followed by decreasing order of frequency by the IVS-I-5 (G > C, beta+), the codons 8/9 (+G, beta0), the IVS-I-110 (G > A, beta+), the IVS-I-1 (G > A, beta0), 25 bp deletion (beta0), the IVS-I-6 (T > C, beta+), the codon 5 (-CT, beta0), and codon 39 (C > T, beta0) mutations. This group of mutations covers more than 85% of the total β-Thalassemia defects present in Iran [6, 9]. We compared β-Thalassemia mutations based on geographical area and frequency of mutation. Distribution of β-Thalassemia mutations in Iran shows different pattern in different area. In general, β-Thalassemia mutations have been a reflection of people and area in correlation with migration and origin of ancestors. We evaluated nine regions (A, B, C, . . . , I) which cover all of throughout Iran. Molecular screening revealed distribution pattern of different mutations of β-Thalassemia in 21 provinces (Figure 1, Table 1).

Region A. This region defines northwest of Iran which includes three provinces with common ethnicity, that of the Azeri ethnic group, the IVS-II-1 (G > A), codons 8/9 (+G), IVS-I-110 (G > A), and IVS-I-1 (G > A) mutations are most frequent in this area. Distribution pattern among these three provinces shows differences due to geographical region. IVS-II-1 (G > A) is a frequent mutation in the two northwestern provinces (West and East Azerbaijan provinces), region A-1 and A-2, respectively (Figure 1) [10–12]. There are different patterns of the prevalence of β-globin among the Azeri ethnic group, so that in the north of two provinces (region A-3, Figure 1) codons 8/9 (+G) are the most frequent mutation which has similarity with those in the Northeast of Iran. It is thought that the codons 8/9 (+G) was transferred by the big migration of the Seljuk Turks and the invasion by the Mongols to the north in 1219 . Also, we observed significant differences between East Azerbaijan and West Azerbaijan provinces, respectively. Samplings from the latter province included regions with dominant Kurdish ethnicity which showed that mutations are similar to the Khug region in Kurdistan of Iraq [13]. The pattern in this region is more or less the same as in the Mediterranean regions [10]. IVS-I-110 (G > A) as an East Mediterranean mutation reaches a high frequency in some countries of the Arabian Peninsula, a fact that may be explained by gene flow and founder effect [14]. It decreases from the Northwest to the East and Center and other parts of Iran. Ottoman Empire role in admixture of cultural and social character of areas under their control is apparent. Primary documentation of the empire's relations with other powers is to be found in the archives of thirty-nine nations.

Region B. IVS-II-1 (G > A), codons 8/9 (+G), IVS-I-1 (G > A), and codon 8 (−AA) are the most frequent of the β-globin mutations in areas of Kurdistan [15]. It has been reported that codons 36/37 (−T) have a Kurdish origin that is prevalent in Kurdistan region, an area residing between Iran, Iraq and Turkey. Our study showed a low frequency of codons 36/37 (−T) in comparison to other areas. codon 8 (−AA) is another relative frequent mutation in the β-globin gene among populations who settle in the Northwest and west. Association studies showed this mutation has been observed frequently in the eastern parts of Turkey and Azerbaijan. Codon 8 (−AA) is the most frequent mutation of the β-globin gene in Azerbaijan [16]. The last country separated from Iran during 150 to 200 years ago. Contrary to previous studies, present investigation showed that this mutation is very low in the northwest among the Azeri ethnic group of Iran, so we could suppose a different origin for the two ethnic groups with a common name, or absence of any movement of codon 8 (−AA) toward this region. The first could be true especially due to dissimilarity in the most frequent β-globin mutations between the two regions regard to the evident migration from Azerbaijan to Iran during past century. On the other hand, IVS-II-1 (G > A) with frequency of 31.8% was similar to pervious studies and surrounding regions, also codon 44 (−C) showed frequency of 4.55% among Kurd ethnic group, while Rund et al. reported it as a frequent mutation (31.2%) in the Jews of Kurdistan in north of Iraq [17]. This study showed relative frequency for codon 44 (−C) (4.5%–9.3%) in northwest and West of Iran.

Region C. The area in southwest is near the Arabian Peninsula, IVS-I-1 (G > A), codons 8/9 (+G), IVS-I-110 (G > A), IVS-II-1 (G > A), IVS-I-6 (T > C) and IVS-I-5 (G > C) are frequent mutations that cause 86% of β-Thalassemia. Frequency of all mutations had approximate similarities that showed the population gained mutations from different origins. Land fertility has prepared suitable

Table 1: Frequency of the β-thalassemia mutations among different provinces of the Iran*.

Provinces	Sample size	Mutation														Studied location
		IVS-II-1 (G > A)	IVS-I-5 (G > C)	Codons 8/9 (+G)	IVS-I-110 (G > A)	IVS-I-6 (T > C)	Codons 36/37 (–T)	25 bp del.	IVS-I-1 (G > A)	IVS-II-745 (G > C)	Codon 39 (C > T)	Codon 44 (–C)	Codon 30 (G > C)	Codon 5 (–CT)	Codon 8 (–AA)	
West Azerbaijan	75	**50.7%**[a]	8.0%	16.0%	5.3%	8.0%						9.3%	2.7%			A
East Azerbaijan	80	**32.0%**	2.6%	18.7%	16.0%				22.6%				5.3%			A
Ardebil	142	17.8%	7.0%	**30.0%**	25.4%	2.5%		0.6%	6.3%			6.3%		3.8%		A
Kurdistan	33	**31.8%**	1.5%	13.6%	1.5%	1.5%	1.5%					4.5%			6.0%	B
Khuzestan	208	12.0%	8.6%	17.3%	16.8%	10.5%			**23.3%**							C
Lorestan	65	27.7%	4.6%	10.7%	11.5%		**33.8%**	0.7%		1.6%		0.7%				D
Chaharmahal and Bakhtiari	57		29.8%		10.5%		**31.5%**		24.5%	3.5%		1.7%				D
Bushehr	104	13.0%	7.7%	8.2%	5.8%	1.5%		**24.4%**	9.1%	3.3%	3.3%		3.3%	2.4%		E
Fars	70	**47.1%**	1.4%		1.4%			21.4%		1.4%			1.4%		8.6%	F
Kerman	50	16%	**44%**	12.0%	4.0%											G
Sistan and Baluchistan	224	1.4%	**76.5%**	3.7%	11.1%			0.7%	0.7%		1.4%	0.7%		0.5%		G
Yazd	49	32.5%	**44.8%**	4.0%	6.1%				2.0%			2.0%				G
Hormozgan	70	4.2%	**90.0%**	5.8%												G
Esfahan	205	**29.0%**		26.0%	8.0%	2.9%	17.5%	2.0%			3.9%	4.4%			8.3%	H
Semnan	52	**40.3%**	5.7%	23.3%						3.8%			3.8%			H
Tehran	638	**42.4%**	8.4%	16.6%	7.8%	2.0%			7.5%	0.8%		0.1%	1.5%	1.3%		H
Mazandaran	77	**68.8%**								3.8%		1.3%	6.4%			H
Gilan	65	**49.2%**		10.7%			9.2%						9.2%	3.0%		H
Qazvin	60	**50.0%**	1.6%	5.0%	15.0%	3.3%						3.3%	3.3%		1.6%	H
Hamedan	47	**34.0%**	8.5%	19.1%	8.5%	2.1%			10.6%							H
Khorasan	70	10.0%		**65.7%**	8.5%											I

[a]It has been written in bold the most frequent mutations in each province.

*This table includes data from publishec data in local and international references and unpublished data during routinely diagnostic tests. Also the data is not available for blank areas.

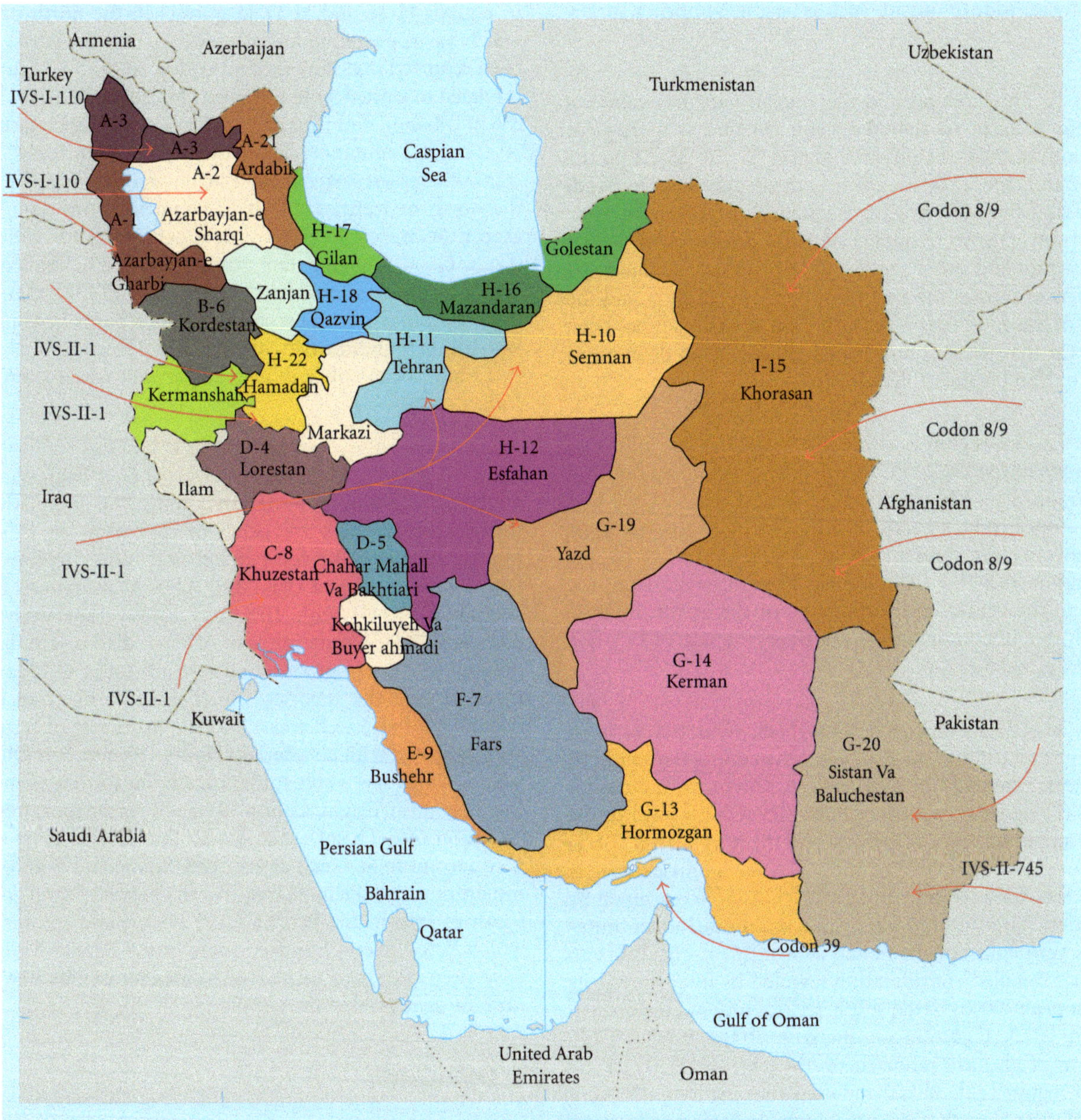

Figure 1: Distribution pattern of different mutations of β-Thalassemia in 21 provinces of Iran.

circumstances for survival for long periods. In fact, many ethnicities have migrated or passed into or through this ancient territory during the past 3000 to 5000 years old [10]. Following the advent of Islam, small and numerically inferior Arab tribes migrated to inland Iran. This migration caused the introduction of mutations such as IVS-I-6 (T > C) [18, 19] which has a frequency as high as 11% in this area that disappeared in other areas with the exception of the northwest where the IVS-I-6 (T > C) could have been introduced through Turkey [20].

IVS-I-1 (G > A) is the most frequent mutation in southwest. IVS-I-1 (G > A) has been described initially as a Mediterranean mutation. This mutation is at high frequency in east of the Mediterranean countries such as Lebanon, Palestine, and Syria [21]. It has been suggested that the Ottoman Empire played an important role in the migration of the IVS-I-1 (G > A) mutation from these countries to Iran during Ottoman rules.

Region D. As it is clear in Figure 1, this region is in the west of central of Iran, and this area belongs to two ethnic of Iranian group, called the Lur and the Bakhtiaris shown as region D-4 and D-5 in Figure 1, respectively. Codons 36/37 (−T) are the most frequent mutation within these groups (31% to 34%) [22]. It could be supposed that the origin of codons 36/37 (−T) is related to the above mentioned area not observed in other areas inside or outside such as near neighboring Turkey [23].

Region E. This area around the Persian Gulf has shown a different pattern, so that the 25 bp deletion is a frequent mutation in this region and region F [24–26]. On the other hand, the 25 bp deletion is most prevalent in Saudi Arabia and Bahrain showing frequencies of 14% and 36%, respectively. Due to frequency of 25 bp deletion within Iran and Bahrain and other regions of the Arabian peninsula as old parts of Iran in the past centuries [14, 27], It is said the origin of this mutation is Asian-Indian as well as, it has been proposed that there is another origin for 25 bp deletion in south of Iran littoral of Persian Gulf.

Region F. This region is in the south and has the following mutations of the β-globin: IVS-II-1 (G > A), 25 bp deletion and codon 8 (−AA), in frequencies of 47.4%, 21.6% and 8.6%, respectively. Overall, IVS-II-1 (G > A) is the most frequent in Iran present in at least two thirds of the population. IVS-II-1 (G > A) has been observed from the north to the center and some parts of the south. Because of high rate of consanguinity marriage, the rate of IVS-II-1 (G > A) is high [24, 26].

Region G. IVS-I-5 (G > C) has been observed as most frequent mutation in the β-globin gene among the southern provinces, especially in southeastern provinces outlined as region G (Figure 1) [6, 28]. Its frequency reduces towards the center and disappears in the west and the north. Also, IVS-I-5 (G > C) is a frequent mutation in Arab countries, mostly in Eastern Asian Arab countries which may be explained by migration. This mutation known as the Asian/Indian mutation is very common in Indian subcontinent and Pakistan [29–31]. Detailed consideration revealed its frequency at its highest peak (90%) in the southern province of Hormozgan (region G-13, Figure 1) on the cost of the Persian Gulf. Yavarian et al. have reported 69.0% for IVS-I-5 (G > C) in this region [32]. Baysal reported that the IVS-I-5 (G > C) allele was introduced to the Arabian Peninsula by gene migration from Baluchistan, a region spanning Southern Iran, Afghanistan, and Pakistan [33]. This paper shows that gene migration from the province of Hormozgan (an economical center) has occurred over a long period during the past centuries [32, 34].

Region H. This area shows that IVS-II-1 (G > A) is the most frequent mutation followed by codons 8/9 (+G). The IVS-II-1 (G > A) allele is observed at variable frequencies in many countries. Chifu et al. declared multiple origins for this mutation [35]. The high frequency and multiple haplotypes indicate that the IVS-II-1 (G > A) mutation is native and one of the oldest β-Thalassemia defects in Iran.

The codons 8/9 (+G) mutation has been frequently observed after the IVS-II-1 (G > A) in most provinces of region H (Table 1), but there is exception like observed data in region H-18 (Table 1, Figure 1, Qazvin province) [36]. Also, the codon 30 (G > C) mutation has high frequency in regions H-16 and H-17 (Figure 1) in the north of Iran, which has appeared in lower frequency in other parts. It has been reported that the origin of codon 30 (G > C) mutation is related to United Arab Emirates [14], its frequency is about 3% in Lebanon and United Arab Emirates. Overall the codon 30 (G > C) mutation has frequency approximately 2% in Iran. Whereas, it seems there is no close relationship between the north of Iran and Arabian countries from population aspect. So we could propose another origin for codon 30 (G > C). Complementary studies showed a frequency of 17.5% for codons 36/37 (−T) in region H-12 [37], that could have relationship with two neighboring regions D-4 and D-5 which this mutation is frequent there. Hence codons 36/37 (−T) have been concentrated in the west toward center of Iran.

Region I. Finally, the codons 8/9 (+G) have been observed as the first β-globin mutation among the population of the north east with a frequency of approximately 65%, the highest frequency in comparison with other regions. The IVS-II-1 (G > A) and IVS-I-110 (G > A) mutations follow codons 8/9 (+G) with 10% and 8.4%, respectively. The codons 8/9 (+G) mutation is of Asian-Indian origin that the invasion and big migration of the Seljuk Turks and Mongol's invasions are the theories which support the transfer of codons 8/9 (+G) to the east and the northeast of Iran. The area indicated with an asterisk (Figure 1) represents Queshm Island, which has a sole mutation similar to that of the east Mediterranean origin. Codon 39 (C > T) is the most frequent mutation of β-Thalassemia among the western parts of the Mediterranean Sea such as Portugal, Spain, and France. This mutation is also the most frequent in Queshm Island, located south of Iran in the Persian Gulf. Portuguese colonial rule which lasted over a hundred years in the Persian Gulf may have been the main way for the entrance of this new gene into the gene pool of the population in this area [38].

4. Discussion

Iran has experienced admixture from various populations throughout history. Invasion and migration have important roles in genetic admixture. Basically, the Iranian people show heterogeneity, as reflected by other studies (unpublished data). The association studies between Turkey and the Arab countries in the East of the Mediterranean Sea have shown large number of β-Thalassemia mutations due to the heterogeneity of the population [32, 34, 39, 40]. We have not observed known mutations which are most frequent in all parts of Iran [9]. Recent studies have confirmed previous conclusions regarding the distribution of codons 8/9 (+G) in Iran [34]. Accordingly, It seems that codons 8/9 (+G) might reflect two circumstances; one connected to the secular trade along the great silk road which extends from Xian in China through the Indian subcontinent to Iran and the Eastern Mediterranean; the other to the invasion of the Mongols (1220 AD) and the Tatars (1380–87 AD), with respect to the prevalence of codons 8/9 (+G) in the Northeast, and toward center and northwest, it may be that the Turkish ethnicity may have affinities with the Oghuz Turk who migrated there from central Asia. The high occurrence of the codons 8/9 (+G) in Eastern Anatolia may also be the cause of its introduction to Turkey from Southern Asia [41].

Zahed reported that 52 mutations in the Arab world, as part of a study that included 13 countries representative of 21 Arabian nations [14], more than 47 observed mutations in the β-globin gene in Iran showed high heterogeneity among the population in comparison with Arabian people in area less than the Arab world. It is proposed that this heterogeneity has been derived originally from a population with an ethnic Aryan background; these results confirm earlier reports from other groups as well as could help to complete information of the population studies [7].

This paper also proposed new theories for the origin of 25 bp deletion, codons 36/37 (−T), and codon 30 (G > C) based on the recent investigations carried out in the southern and western and northern part of Iran, respectively (Regions D and E, Figure 1). It is clear that haplotypes determination could be useful in the case of analyzing the origin of hemoglobin gene, while it is often difficult to distinguish a new mutation or changes in haplotypes due to gene conversion. Up to now, there are not many studies regarding β-globin haplotypes in Iranian population only a few haplotypes analysis has been performed as published and unpublished data which the authors used for their conclusion. Some studies of the haplotypes background showed Iran known as the gate of Asia through which passed the important Silk Road could be attributed to a single and independent mutational event or due to the genetic admixture with other Asian populations like India, China, and Kuwait, the United Arab Emirates (UAE) and areas along the south shore of the Persian Gulf [42, 43].

Comparison of populations and haplotypes analyzed in the Mediterranean types revealed that the same polymorphism is associated with more population in the Iranian Thalassemic population than in the Mediterranean ones, suggesting that the Iranian Thalassemic population is more ancient than the Mediterranean one. On the other hand, the high heterogeneity and miscellaneous mutations among the Iranian population reflect the sociocultural background of this nation that due to a rich cultural education emphasizes fraternity and hospitality and urges population to accept newcomers with open arms. Also, this study can help the researchers doing low cost of test when they know which mutation has high rate in these regions.

Acknowledgments

The authors are very thankful to Dr. Parvin Shariati for her valuable comments and all participants whose collaboration allowed them to carry out this work, as well as their permission to publish it.

References

[1] A. Eleftheriou, *About Thalassemia*, Thalssemia International Federation, 2003.

[2] R. C. Hardison, D. H. K. Chui, B. Giardine et al., "HbVar: a relational database of human hemoglobin variants and thalassemia mutations at the globin gene server," *Human Mutation*, vol. 19, no. 3, pp. 225–233, 2002.

[3] R. C. Hardison, B. Giardine, C. Riemer et al., "HbVar database for human hemoglobin variants and Thalassemia mutations," *Blood Cells, Molecules and Diseases*, vol. 38, no. 2, pp. 167–168, 2007.

[4] M. T. Akbari, P. Izadi, M. Izadyar, K. Kyriacou, and M. Kleanthous, "Molecular basis of Thalassemia intermedia in Iran," *Hemoglobin*, vol. 32, no. 5, pp. 462–470, 2008.

[5] P. Derakhshandeh-Peykar, H. Hourfar, M. Heidari, M. Kheirollahi, and M. Miryounesi, "The spectrum of β-Thalassemia mutations in Isfahan Province of Iran," *Iranian Journal of Public Health*, vol. 37, no. 2, pp. 106–111, 2008.

[6] H. Najmabadi, R. Karimi-Nejad, S. Sahebjam et al., "The β-Thalassemia mutation spectrum in the iranian population," *Hemoglobin*, vol. 25, no. 3, pp. 285–296, 2001.

[7] H. Najmabadi, A. A. Pourfathollah, M. Neishabury, F. Sahebjam, W. Krugluger, and C. Oberkanins, "Rare and unexpected mutations among Iranian β-Thalassemia patients and prenatal samples discovered by reverse-hybridization and DNA sequencing," *Haematologica*, vol. 87, no. 10, pp. 1113–1114, 2002.

[8] M. Garshasbi, C. Oberkanins, H. Y. Law, M. Neishabury, R. Kariminejad, and H. Najmabadi, "α-globin gene deletion and point mutation analysis among Iranian patients with microcytic hypochromic anemia," *Haematologica*, vol. 88, no. 10, pp. 1196–1197, 2003.

[9] A. Merat, M. Haghshenas, Z. M. Pour et al., "β-Thalassemia in Southwestern Iran," *Hemoglobin*, vol. 17, no. 5, pp. 427–437, 1993.

[10] M. Omrani, "Prevalent mutations in β-Thalassemia patients in West Azerbaijan province using ARMS/PCR method," *Uromieh Medical Journal*, vol. 2, no. 14, pp. 117–126, 2003.

[11] M. A. H. Feizi, A. A. H. Feizi, M. Asgharzadeh et al., "Prevalent mutation of β-Thalassemia in Northwesthern region of Iran," *Journal of Yazd Shahid Sadoghi Medical Science University*, vol. 4, no. 12, pp. 39–44, 2005.

[12] S. M. M. Ardebili, S. J. Tabrizi, A. Nikanfar et al., "Prevalent mutation of β-globin gene in the central region of West Azerbaijan province," *Medical Journal of Tabriz Medical Science University*, vol. 64, pp. 67–72, 2004.

[13] N. A. S. Al-Allawi, J. M. S. Jubrael, and M. Hughson, "Molecular characterization of β-Thalassemia in the Dohuk region of Iraq," *Hemoglobin*, vol. 30, no. 4, pp. 479–486, 2006.

[14] L. Zahed, "The spectrum of β-Thalassemia mutations in the Arab populations," *Journal of Biomedicine and Biotechnology*, vol. 2001, no. 3, pp. 129–132, 2001.

[15] A. Fathollah-Pour and R. Naghshi-Zadeian, "Common β-Thalassemia Mutation in the city of Sanandaj," *Scientific Journal of Kurdistan Medical Unversity*, vol. 3, pp. 21–26, 2003.

[16] M. A. Cürük, G. T. Yüregir, C. D. Asadov et al., "Molecular characterization of β-Thalassemia in Azerbaijan," *Human Genetics*, vol. 90, no. 4, pp. 417–419, 1992.

[17] D. Rund, T. Cohen, D. Filon et al., "Evolution of a genetic disease in an ethnic isolate: β-Thalassemia in the Jews of Kurdistan," *Proceedings of the National Academy of Sciences of the United States of America*, vol. 88, no. 1, pp. 310–314, 1991.

[18] A. D. Adekile, L. H. Gu, E. Baysal et al., "Molecular characterization of α-Thalassemia determinants, β-Thalassemia

alleles, and β(S) haplotypes among Kuwaiti Arabs," *Acta Haematologica*, vol. 92, no. 4, pp. 176–181, 1994.

[19] M. A. El-Latif, D. Filon, D. Rund, A. Oppenheim, and M. Kanaan, "The [β+-IVS-I-6 (T → C) mutation accounts for half of the Thalassemia chromosomes in the Palestinian populations of the mountain regions," *Hemoglobin*, vol. 26, no. 1, pp. 33–40, 2002.

[20] A. N. Basak, H. Ozcelik, A. Ozer et al., "The molecular basis of β-Thalassemia in Turkey," *Human Genetics*, vol. 89, no. 3, pp. 315–318, 1992.

[21] M. A. Saleh, L. F. Zahed, and R. S. Talhouk, "The molecular basis of β-Thalassaemia in Lebanon and its neighbouring countries," *Le Journal Médical Libanais*, vol. 44, no. 2, pp. 75–79, 1996.

[22] A. Kiani, Y. Mortezavi, S. Zeinali et al., "Determination of prevalent mutations of β-globin gene in major Thalassemia patients of Lurestan province," *Yakhteh Medical Journal*, vol. 2, no. 8, pp. 88–91, 2006.

[23] G. O. Tadmouri, S. Tüzmen, and A. N. Başak, "Rare β-Thalassemia mutation in a Turkish patient: FSC-36/37 (-T)," *Human Biology*, vol. 69, no. 2, pp. 263–267, 1997.

[24] M. Karimi, A. A. Ghavanini, and M. R. . Kadivar, "Regional mapping of the gene frequency of β-Thalassemia in Fars province, Iran during 1997-1998," *Iranian Journal of Medical Sciences*, vol. 25, no. 3-4, pp. 134–137, 2000.

[25] H. Khodaei, S. Zeinali, and S. Delmaghani, "Moelcular investigation of mutations of β-globin gene in β-Thalassemia patients in Boushehr province," *Journal of Medical South*, vol. 2, no. 3, pp. 83–89, 2000.

[26] M. Karimi, H. Yarmohammadi, S. Farjadian et al., "β-Thalassemia intermedia from Southern Iran: IVS-II-1 (G → A) is the prevalent Thalassemia intermedia allele," *Hemoglobin*, vol. 26, no. 2, pp. 147–154, 2002.

[27] E. Baysal, "Molecular heterogeneity of β-Thalassemia in the United Arab Emirates," *Community Genetics*, vol. 8, no. 1, pp. 35–39, 2005.

[28] E. M. Moghaddam, M. Naroei Nejad, P. Eshghi et al., "Basic of molecular and prenatal diagnosis of Thalassemia in Southeasthern of Iran from 2002 to 2004," *Journal of Mazandaran Medical Science University*, vol. 48, no. 15, pp. 105–111.

[29] S. Agarwal, M. Pradhan, U. R. Gupta, S. Sarwai, and S. S. Agarwal, "Geographic and ethnic distribution of β-Thalassemia mutations in Uttar Pradesh, India," *Hemoglobin*, vol. 24, no. 2, pp. 89–97, 2000.

[30] F. E. E. Vaz, C. B. Thakur, M. K. Banerjee, and S. G. Gangal, "Distribution of β-Thalassemia mutations in the Indian population referred to a diagnostic center," *Hemoglobin*, vol. 24, no. 3, pp. 181–194, 2000.

[31] S. N. Khan and S. Riazuddin, "Molecular characterization of β-Thalassemia in Pakistan," *Hemoglobin*, vol. 22, no. 4, pp. 333–345, 1998.

[32] M. Yavarian, C. L. Harteveld, D. Batelaan, L. F. Bernini, and P. C. Giordano, "Molecular spectrum of β-Thalassemia in the Iranian Province of Hormozgan," *Hemoglobin*, vol. 25, no. 1, pp. 35–43, 2001.

[33] E. Baysal, "Hemoglobinopathies in the United Arab Emirates," *Hemoglobin*, vol. 25, no. 2, pp. 247–253, 2001.

[34] F. Mahboudi, S. Zeinali, A. Merat et al., "The molecular basis of β-Thalassemia mutation in Fars procvince, Iran," *Iranian Journal of Medical Sciences*, vol. 21, no. 3-4, p. 108, 1996.

[35] Y. Chifu, H. Nakashima, H. Hara, E. Yokota, and T. Imamura, "β-Thalassemia major resulting from a compound heterozygosity for the β-globin gene mutation: further evidence for multiple origin and migration of the Thalassemia gene," *Human Genetics*, vol. 89, no. 3, pp. 343–346, 1992.

[36] M. Tafazzoli, I. Normohammadi, F. Zaker et al., "Investigation of β-globin mutations in β-Thalassemia patients in Qazvin province," *Journal of Semnan Medical Science University*, vol. 6, pp. 255–258, 2005.

[37] R. Salehi, M. Salehi, and H. Horfar, "Investigation of frequencies of eight β-Thalassemia mutations among Thalassemia patient in Esfahan provine using ARMS-PCR method," *Journal of Esfahan Medical Faculty*, vol. 23, no. 76, pp. 1–7, 2005.

[38] M. R. Noori-Daloii, N. Moazami, S. Farhangi et al., "β-Thalassemia in Iran: a high incidence of the nonsense codon 39 mutation on the Island of Queshm," *Hemoglobin*, vol. 18, no. 6, pp. 449–453, 1994.

[39] Z. Rahimi, A. V. Raygani, A. Merat et al., "Thalassemic mutations in Southern Iran," *Iranian Journal of Medical Sciences*, vol. 31, no. 2, pp. 70–73, 2006.

[40] M. A. F. El-Hazmi, A. S. Warsy, and A. R. Al-Swailem, "The frequency of 14 β-Thalassemia mutations in the Arab populations," *Hemoglobin*, vol. 19, no. 6, pp. 353–360, 1995.

[41] G. O. Tadmouri, N. Garguier, J. Demont, P. Perrin, and A. N. Başak, "History and origin of β-Thalassemia in Turkey: sequence haplotype diversity of β-globin genes," *Human Biology*, vol. 73, no. 5, pp. 661–674, 2001.

[42] Z. Rahimi, R. Akramipour, R. L. Nagel, A. S. Ahmadi, A. Merat, and F. Bahrehmand, "The β-globin gene haplotypes associated with Hb D-Los Angeles [β121(GH4)Glu → Gln] in Western Iran," *Hemoglobin*, vol. 30, no. 1, pp. 39–44, 2006.

[43] M. Yavarian, M. Karimi, A. Zorai, C. L. Harteveld, and P. C. Giordano, "Molecular basis of Hb H disease in Southwest Iran," *Hemoglobin*, vol. 29, no. 1, pp. 43–50, 2005.

10

Hepatitis C Virus in Arab World: A State of Concern

Mohamed A. Daw[1] and Aghnaya A. Dau[2]

[1] *Department of Medical Microbiology & Immunology, Tripoli Medical Centre, Faculty of Medicine Tripoli, P.O. Box 82668, Tripoli, Libya*
[2] *Department of Vascular Surgery, Tripoli Medical Centre, Faculty of Medicine Tripoli, P.O. Box 82664, Tripoli, Libya*

Correspondence should be addressed to Mohamed A. Daw, madaw@consultant.com

Academic Editors: L. A. Videla and T. Weiss

Hepatitis C virus has been considered to be one of the most important devastating causes of chronic hepatitis, cirrhosis, and hepatic cellular carcinoma. The prevalence of such virus varies greatly over the world. Arab world has a unique geography and consists over nineteen countries who share the same heritage and customs and do speak the same language. In this area, the epidemiology of hepatitis C is not well understandable. Hepatitis C virus was found to be endemic in Arabia. The serostatus of such virus was found to be variable among these countries with uniform patterns of genotypes. Such prevalence varies tremendously according to the risk factors involved. Blood and blood products, haemodialysis, intravenous, and percutaneous drug users, and occupational, habitual, and social behavior were found to be the important factors involved. Hepatitis C will have major social, economic, and even political burdens on such young and dynamic societies. Thus, strategies and clear policy of intervention are urgently needed to combat the consequences of HCV both regionally and at state level of each country.

1. Introduction

Hepatitis C virus has been considered to be one of the most potential pathogens that have hindered the medical community all over the world. Indeed, since its discovery in 1989, hepatitis C virus (HCV) has been recognized as a major cause of chronic liver disease worldwide and due to the surpassing hepatitis B virus [1]. The data reported by WHO estimated that the prevalence of HCV infection is 2.2%, and more than one million new cases were reported annually. Furthermore, an estimated 27% of cirrhosis and 25% of hepato-cellular carcinomas (HCC) worldwide occur in HCV-infected people [2]. Such infection increases tremendously among the developing countries particularly at those categories that were considered to be at a potential risk of acquiring hepatitis C virus.

Arabian compound states are composed of unique geography being the central and transcross of the world. It is composed of more than nineteen countries with more than 350 million; they all speak the same language and mostly they have the same heritage and customs. Indeed it is the whole site of east and south of the Mediterranean basin up to the Atlantic cost in the west and Persian gulf and Indian Ocean south east. The African region is composed of the whole north African countries which are composed of approximately 23% of Africa, though the Asian region composed most of the north west of Asia and composed around 10% of Asia. Such area has over 30% of the world oil revenue, and most of them enjoy great wealth and prosperous capital.

The global epidemiology of HCV varies greatly allover the world, and different studies have shown such variations. Hepatitis C virus was found to be endemic in certain countries, and different studies have confirmed such endemicity [3]. It is important to consider the shortcoming of regional studies are in Arab world. Most of the epidemiological studies carried out individually based upon seroprevalence of HCV among specific groups. These include blood donors, heath care workers, or patients undergoing haemodialysis. Such studies were not representative of the community, they were usually carried out by independent scientists. Even though, some countries lack such studies.

Table 1: Prevalence of hepatitis C virus and its common genotypes among Arab countries.

Region/country	Prevalence (%) of HCV among		Genotypes/subtype	
	Population [M]	Haemodialysis	More frequent	Less frequent
Arabian peninsula region				
Saudi Arabia [Sa]	23.513 (1.7)	55.7	4	1a 1b 3a
Yemen [Ye]	23,701 (2.1)	62.7	4	NA
Oman [Om]	3.2 (1.2)	26.5	4	NA
Bahrain [Bh]	0.656397 (1.7)	29.24	4	1a, 1b
Qatar [Qr]	0.793341 (6.3)	44.6	4	2, 3, 4
UAE	4,496 (2.3)	37	4	3a
Kuwait [Kt]	3.442 (0.8)	71.0	4	1
Sham region				
Iraq [Irq]	23 (3.2)	35.9	4	1a, 1b, 3a
Syria [Sy]	20.056 (1)	48.9	4	1b, 1a, 3a, 5*
Lebanon [Lb],	3.678 (0.7–1)	27	4	1a, 1b, 2, 3
Jordan [Jr]	5.307 (0.65–6.25)	34.6	1a	1b, 4
Gaza Strip	1.5 (2.2)	31.3	4	1, 3a
Nile river region				
Egypt [Eg]	80 (13–22)	40	4	1a 1b 2a
Sudan [Sud]	40.219 (3)	23.7	4	4e, 4c, 4d
North African region				
Libya [Ly]	6,037 (1.2)	20.5	4/1	2a, 2b, 2c, 3a
Tunis [Tu]	10.102 (0.4–0.7)	51	1b	2a 2c 1a
Algeria [Alg]	35.100 (1.8)	63	NA	NA
Morocco [Mo]	35.757 (7.7)	76	1b	2a 2c 1a
Mauritania [Mu]	3.365 (1.8)	68	NA	NA

NA: no data available, *less frequent type.

Nowadays, HCV is responsible for infecting over 20 million in Arab countries, and without immediate and effective intervention, that number is predicted to increase tremendously in the next two decades. The objectives of this paper were to analyze the status of HCV epidemiology among the Arab countries and its variation accordingly and to highlight the future consequences and how to overcome the implications of such infection.

2. Epidemiology of Hepatitis C Virus in Arab World

The Arab world consists of heterogeneous countries with various levels of developments and different approaches of concepts and priorities. Infrastructure of health services is variable among these countries; some of them succeeded in adapting the modern routes of infection prevention; others fail and rarely adapt such recommendations [4]. However, most of them share the concept of bureaucracy and hierarchal among their health services and education [4, 5]. This will make the implementation of international standards indeed difficult to follow or adapt by their institution and health services personnel. HCV infection is a nagging issue in all the Arab countries; the estimated number of infected individuals in the Arab world by such virus reached 25 million with an average prevalence rate of 3.5%. Table 1 shows the universal epidemiology of HCV among general population and patients undergoing haemodialysis and genotypes reported in each country. Such prevalence varies greatly from one region to another and even among the countries of the same region.

2.1. Hepatitis C Virus in Arabian Peninsula Region. Arabian peninsula is unique geographical area a composed 35% of Arab world that it is composed of Saudi Arabia, Yemen, Oman, Qatar, Bahrain, UAE, and Kuwait. Saudi Arabia is the largest country not only in the Arabian peninsula but in the Arab world, and considered to be the richest. Hepatitis C virus is well studied in Saudi Arabia, and its serostatus is known among the different population [6]. The universal prevalence of HCV in the general population ranged from 1.1 to 1.7% [7]. Such prevalence was found to be high among the risk groups such as haemodialysis patients where it ranged from 18.6 to 56%, 40% among the haemophilia patients, and 94.8% among IVDs. The common genotype isolates were genotype 4 followed by rare ones 1a, 1b, and 3a [8–10]. Yemen is the second largest heavily populated and the poorest country in Arabian peninsula; the prevalence of HCV in Yemenis was found to be 1.7% among healthy volunteers though it reached 2.7% among blood donors [11, 12]. Such prevalence reached up to 60% in haemodialysis patients [13]. In the less populated Gulf states, HCV was found to be 0.9 to 1.5% in blood donors

TABLE 2: Categorization of Arab countries according to the prevalence hepatitis C virus.

Category	Prevalence	Country
Low	1–1.9	Libya, Tunis, Oman, Saudi Arabia, Kuwait, Bahrain, Syria, Lebanon
Moderate	2.0–2.9	Algeria, Mauritania, Yemen, Gaza Strip
High	3–3.9	UAE, Iraq, Sudan
Very high	>4	Egypt, Morocco, Qatar, Jordan

of Oman and 26% in haemodialysis patients [14], though it was found to be 40% among haemolytic Bahraini patients with HCV genotypes 4, and 1a and 1b as the commonly prevalent genotypes [15]. In Qatar, the prevalence rate among the general population reached 6.3% and 44.6% in dialysis patients [16–18], though in UAE, the prevalence was found to be 23% among haemodialysis patients, and the predominantly genotypes were 4, 3, and 1 [19]. In Kuwait, HCV is better known, and different studies were carried out to determine the prevalence of HCV as it was found to be 0.8% among the general populations and 71% among haemodialysis patients [20, 21]. The commonest genotypes were genotype 4 followed by genotype 1 [22]. However, it is clear that in the less populated states of Gulf area, detailed studies on HCV are lacking, and the magnitude of such problem is not well documented. Furthermore, the impact of foreign workers on the prevalence of HCV is not known, particularly as most of these workers are coming from regions that are considered to be endemic of HCV. Therefore, it is evident that the prevalence of HCV in Arabian peninsula ranges from to 0.8% to 2.1% among these countries apart from Qatar which reached 6% and that is difficult to explain (such data has to be taken with caution). Over one and half million were infected with HCV as HCV genotype 4 is more prevalent. This makes such region classified within an intermediate range worldwide as shown in Table 2.

2.2. Hepatitis C Virus in Sham Region. This region is composed of Syria, Iraq, Lebanon, Jordan, and the existing Gaza Strip (ancient Palestine). Different studies were carried out in Syria on the prevalence of HCV among different categories [23]. The prevalence of HCV among Syrian was found to be 1% among the general population, though its remarkably high in the risk groups. Among haemodialysis patients it ranged from 24.4 to 88.6%, though it is 3% among health care workers and 60.5% among IDUs, and 1.96% among prostitutes [24]. The commonly isolated genotypes among Syrian people were genotype 4/1b followed by rare ones as 1a, 3a, and unusual genotype 5 was also reported [25].

In Iraq, the prevalence of HCV ranged from 3.21 to 7.1% among the pregnant women and general population of four HCV genotypes, 1a, 1b, and 3a [26, 27]. A study carried out on Iraqi refuges showed further discrepancy in this regard; Chironna et al.; using HCV-RNA analysis found that the prevalence among these refuges was 0.1%, and HCV genotype 4c, d was the commonest [28]. Hence then further studies were needed to clarify the Iraqi serostatus. However, such prevalence was remarkably increased among haemophilia patients as it reached 66.0% [29].

HCV is less frequent among Lebanese; it ranged from 0.16 to 1.22% among healthy volunteers, blood donors, and health care workers, though it was 27% among haemodialysis patients [30]. Genotype 4 was the commonest isolated genotype among the various groups studied followed by genotypes 1a and 1b [31].

The collected data form Jordanian studies was found to be variable and even contradicting. The overall prevalence of HCV among Jordanian people varied from 0.65 to 6.25% depending on the population studied [32]. It was found to be 28% among haemodialysis patients and 40.5% in hemophiliac patients. The predominant genotype was found to be genotype 1a followed by 1b and 4 [33]. However, few studies were coming out from Gaza Strip concerning the prevalence of HCV where it was found to be 2.2%, though the most prevalent genotype was found to be genotype 4 followed by 1 and 3a [34, 35].

Hence then, over two million with 0.7–6% of prevalence were infected in Sham region; the lowest prevalence was reported in Lebanon followed by Syria, Gaza strip, and then Jordan and Iraq, though the HCV genotype 4 was the commonest among all the regions a part from Jordan which do need further elucidation.

2.3. Hepatitis C Virus in Arabian Nile River Region. Sudan and Egypt are the main countries to be considered in this region as they were resting on the Nile River which originated from the Ethiopian mountains to cross Sudan and pass via Egypt to the Mediterranean basin and indeed its one of the oldest ancient civilizations in the world. Hepatitis C virus has been intensively studied in Egypt, and great efforts have been shown in this important area [36]. The prevalence of such virus is reported to be higher in Egypt than in any other country. Indeed, it is a phenomenon that attracted the attention of many researches and scientists not only in Egypt but allover the world [37]. Despite the different speculation which has been postulated, the argument is still going on, and no obvious reason was proofed. The prevalence of HCV among the general populations was variable according to the studies conducted, as it varied from 13 to 22% accordingly [38, 39]. The prevalence of HCV among various groups and categories was intensively studied. It was found to be 14.5% among blood donors, 7.7% among health care workers, 12.1% of rural primary school children, 18.1% of rural villages residents, and 22.1% among army recruitments. It was even higher among risk groups, 70.4% in haemodialysis patients, 54.9% in multitransfused children, and 47.2% in chronic liver disease patients [40, 41]. The predominant HCV genotype among Egyptians was found to be genotype

4, particularly subtype 4a [42]. However, recent studies revealed that other genotypes and subtypes as 1a, 1b, 2a are also present indicating that HCV genotypes are extremely variable [43].

The status of HCV among Sudanese is also obvious as it is reported to be (2.2–3%) among the general population [44, 45]. High-risk population showed a higher prevalence of HCV, and it was found to be 23.7% in haemodialysis patients [46]. The major genotype isolated was genotype 4 with subtypes 4e, 4c, and 4d [47]. This was found to be similar to those genotypes isolated from Egypt.

Hence then, the Nile River region was considered to be the highest endemic area in prevalence of HCV with 15 million infected persons particularly genotype 4 as shown in Table 2. Further studies are needed to explore new methods for prevention and treatment.

2.4. Hepatitis C Virus among North African (Maghreb) Region. The Arabian North African countries include Libya,Tunis, Algeria, Morocco, and Mauritania, (Mauretania). The prevalence of HCV and its genotypes among different populations at Maghreb countries is variable. In Libya, HCV has been intensively studied by Daw and his collaborators over the last ten years; the prevalence of HCV among Libyans was 1.2% though among hemodialysis was 20.2% [48]. Recently, a comprehensive study consisted of 1240 Libyan patients was carried out [49]. Different genotypes were reported in the study; genotype 4 was the commonest (35.7%), followed by genotype 1 (32.6%). According to subtypes, 28% were unclassified as genotype 4, 14.6% were genotype 1b, and some patients were infected with more than one subtype (2.3% genotype 4c/d, 1% genotype 2a/c). Genotype 1 was the commonest among males, while genotype 4 among females. Despite the obvious role of prevention and control of such virus and data available by Libyan researchers, the national authority failed to adapt these regulations at a national level, though every centre has its own way of adapting such recommendations.

Different studies were also carried out in Tunis [50, 51]; the prevalence of HCV reported among Tunisians was 0.4 to 0.7%; the lowest among was the Maghreb countries, though such prevalence was high in haemodialysis patients as it reached 51% [52]. The commonly isolated HCV genotypes among Tunisians were 1b which accounted for 79%, followed by genotypes 1a(5%), 2a(7%), 2b and 3a(3%), and 4a (1%), respectively [53]. In Algeria, a national seroprevalence study was carried out covering healthy blood donors and pregnant women. Prevalence of HCV among these two groups was 0.18 and 0.19%, respectively, though it was 2.5% among the general population [54–56]. However, further studies on genotype and analyzing the serostatus on other risk population as haemodialysis and haemophilia are needed.

In Morocco, the prevalence of HCV was reported to be high. It varies greatly from one study to another. It was found to be 1.93% in a study carried out by Beghdadli et al. [57], while it reached 7.7% in another study by Benouda et al. [58]. Such prevalence was high among haemodialysis as it reached 42.4%, though it was 35.1% within the haemophiliacs patients [59]. The most prevalent genotypes reported among the Moroccans are 1b (47.6%), 2a/2c (37.1%), and 1a (2.8%) [60]. Furthermore, the prevalence of such genotypes varies according to age; genotype 1b is more prevalent among older patients, whereas subtype 2a/2c is mainly found among younger ones.

Despite the clear picture of HCV epidemiology in Libya, Tunis, and to a certain instant in Algeria and Morocco, such data is lacking in Mauritania; anti-HCV was detected in 1.1% among blood donors [61]. It has been assumed it will be the same pattern as the rest of other Maghreb countries though no reported studies in this subject, and hence then, further studies are needed to clarify such assumption.

The epidemiology HCV among the Maghreb countries was found to be variable, and around one million and half people were infected. It is less prevalence among the Tunisian population, followed by Libya with low prevalence, then Algeria and Mauritania which are classified as moderate and later Morocco with a higher prevalence; furthermore HCV genotype 4 is the predominant one among Libyans, though genotype 1 is more common in the rest of Maghreb countries. However, it was difficult to explain such variation as the people in these countries are very interacted and sometimes difficult to differentiate between. This may be related to the nature of the studies we referred to, and hence then, further detailed studies are needed.

3. Factors Associated with Transmission of Hepatitis C Virus in Arabia

The epidemiology of HCV among Arabs is unique in its nature, and varieties of risk factors have been found to be associated with its high prevalence rate. However, the emphasis on these factors may vary from one country to another as shown in Table 3.

3.1. Blood and Blood Products. HCV has been known to be the most common blood-borne virus over the world particularly among the developing countries. Blood and blood products remain a major cause of spread of HCV among Arab countries, and most of them fail to fulfill the criterions of modern blood transfusion system. Different studies have shown the impact of blood transfusion on the status of HCV in these countries. Studies from Jordan showed that HCV infection was detected in 34% of patients who had received blood transfusion, compared to only 16% of those who received no transfusion [62]. The picture in Syria is also damming where 50.4% of HCV-dialyzed patients have previous history of blood transfusion. In Yemen, 80% received blood transfusion were infected with HCV compared with 20% who received no blood [63]. In Libya, a history of blood transfusion was reported in 22.7% of those with HCV [49]. HCV was found to be remarkably high among thalassemia patients who received repeated blood transfusion; it was found to be 67.3% in Iraq, 42.4% in Morocco, 40.7% in Jordan, and 40% in Saudi Arabia [64].

In Arab countries, blood transfusion is still a problem due to the lack of organized infrastructure and highly trained and qualified staff. The main sources, of blood donation are

Table 3: Factors associated with the Transmission of HCV among Arab countries.

Risk factor	Extent of Exposure among each country Low	Moderate	High
Blood transfusion	[NO]	[All in this range]	[NO]
Haemodialysis	[NO]	[NO]	[All in this range]
Nosocomial transmission	[NO]	[NO]	[All in this range]
Health care workers	[NO]	[All in this range]	[NO]
Invasive Medical procedures	[NO]	[All in this range]	[NO]
Dentistry Practice	[NO]	[Lb, Ly, Tu, Sa, UAE, Om, Bh, Qr, Jr, Kt]	[Eg, Ye, Sud, Mo, Mu, Alg, Irq, Sy]
Laboratory services	[NO]	[Lb, Tu, Ly, Jr, Sy, Sa, Bh, Kt, Qr, Om, UAE]	[Mu, Mo, Alg, Sud, Irq, Ye, Eg]
Hospital Waste Handling	[NO]	[Lb, UAE, Sa, Ly, Lb, Bh, Qr, Om, Tu, Jr, Sy, Kt]	[Alg, Mo, Sud, Eg, Ye, Irq, Mu]
IVDA	[NO]	[NO]	[All in this range]
Habitual	[Ly, Tu, Lb, Sa, Jr, Sy]	[Alg, Irq, UAE, Qr, Bh, Kt, Om]	[Eg, Mr, Mo, Ye, Sud]
High risk behavior	[Ly, Sa, Ye, Sud, Mu, Om, Kt]	[Alg, Tu, Eg, Jr, Sy, Lb]	[Mo, Bh, Irq, UAE, Qr,]

Low: <5%, Moderate: 5–20%, High: > 20%, NO: No country in this category.

usually relatives and friends of the patients who come on social pressure and due to the fear of the death of a patient (i.e. relative). Donors usually come in emergency time, and questions about high-risk behaviors are seldom asked [65]. Therefore, resources and organization should be available to recruit altruistic volunteers.

The current data indicate that all the Arab countries undertake anti-HCV screening mandatory in all blood banks, though in some countries, patients may have to pay for such tests. The main concern is the reliability of such tests, and some data indicated that antibody tests for HCV genotypes/subtypes common in Europe and North America are not well applicable on the sera tested from developing countries though most of Arab countries import such tests [66]. Furthermore, rapid tests and some lots of ELISA failed to detect HCV-reactive sera and up to 1% of seronegative blood units tests positive for HCV-RNA using RT-PCR technology [67]. Therefore, even when HCV screening test is performed the risk of becoming infected is still visible. This however makes it necessary to add new molecular tests such as the determination of HCV RNA by nucleic acid technology (HCV-NAT) to the already performed tests in blood donation which should be coupled with meticulous professional assessment to the effectiveness of such tests [68].

The recent uprising in Arab countries which may brought inspiration to Arab citizens left some of health care services in a chaotic situation. In Libya, such crises left an estimated 50.000 killed and over 120.000 injured; screening of blood in war field was mainly limited quick screening tests and sometimes only matching blood groups to save lives [69]. This will have great impact on the prevalence of HCV and the consequence among the infected victims in such country.

Blood transfusion and hospital-associated practice were found to be important risk factors for HCV among Arabian countries. These conditions can be overcome by development of a fair and organized system of blood screening and transfusion. National and international standards should be implemented, and firm revision for such standards and its implantation should be regularly revised. Further, independent or even legal bodies should observe that such implantation and legal action should be taken.

3.2. Haemodialysis Practice. The prevalence of HCV among haemodialysis patients varies greatly from one region to another, and it has been reduced drastically over the years in developed countries. In Japan and UK, it was found to be (1.2%) and (4%), respectively, though in certain African countries, it reached up to 80% as in Senegal [70]. Among Arab countries the picture of serostatus of HCV among HD patient is peculiar. Such prevalence is higher than that in the general population, blood donors, and even among those with other risk factors. Furthermore, it is more complex and varies greatly from one country to another and even among different dialysis centres in the same country [71]. Indeed, the prevalence of HCV among the haemodialysis patients in any Arabic state per se surpasses any other international centres in the developed countries, who follow the strict regulations of HCV prevention in such setting. The prevalence of HCV varies from 20.2% to 76% in such countries, the highest prevalence was reported in Morocco (76%), Kuwait (71%), and Yemen (61%), though the lowest was reported in Libya (21%) as shown in Table 1.

In Arab countries, blood transfusion has played an important role in transmission of HCV in HD patients. Furthermore, dialysis centres are usually overloaded with patients, and there is a shortage of material support (filters), which leads to multiple use of the filter without proper sterilization in some cases. In addition, there is an insufficient number of dialysis machines; the number of patients dialyzed per machine is twice that in developed countries. Clusters of HCV infection have been noticed in many haemodialysis centres as in Syria, Sudan, Morocco, Yemen, Kuwait, and Bahrain which may suggest large outbreaks in such centres due to patient-to-patient transmission via HCWs' hands [72]. Further evidence from CDC's investigators raises one possible way in which inappropriate use of medication vials intended for single person may result in large HCV outbreaks in haemodialysis units. This is however to be confirmed by phylogenetic analysis of subgenomic regions of HCV [73].

Hepatitis C virus in plasma remains viable and detectable after drying and environmental exposure to room temperature for at least 16 hours; therefore, blood-contaminated surfaces and objects can serve as sources for HCV transmission. Generally, such transmission among haemodialysis units is considered to be nosocomial with possible factors being failure to disinfect devices between patients; sharing of a single-use vials of infusions; poor sterile technique; poor cleaning of dialysis machines; poor distance between chairs in addition to dialyser reuse, duration, and frequency of dialysis [74]. HCV can hardly be transmitted during dialysis procedures when state-of-the-art machines are used, where most of these countries offered to have. The prevention of HCV among HD is visible and such risk could be drastically reduced. Erythropoietin should be used to reduce the need of blood in HD patients, and proper nosocomial prevention program should be implemented. This could be advanced and supplemented by training, proper staffing and a sufficient supply of materials and disposables according to the actual need.

3.3. Intravenous Drug Users (IDUs) and Prisoners. Transmission of HCV was strongly associated with intravenous and percutaneous drug users (IDUs). The hepatitis C European network for cooperative research group reported a prevalence of HC of 80% among intravenous drug users (IVDU), 40% in Thailand and up to 74% in Australia [75]. In injecting drug users (IDUs) population there has been increased shifts among addicts from inhalatory to injectable drugs due decrease in quality and availability of heroin. Further, the effect of injecting drugs is more intense and satisfying as HCV is found in a high concentration in spoons and rinsing liquids that could be used in association with needle drug use.

Injecting illegal drugs, sex behavior, and imprisonment are considered to be shameful and unrespectable misconduct among Arabian society. Individuals usually hide and deny such act even if they did it, a state to be taken with caution when taking history of risk factors particularly among blood donors. More than a third of all prisoners and more than 80% of injecting drug users, were positive for antibodies to hepatitis C virus [76]. Alcohol consumption was also found to accelerate the course of chronic hepatitis C. In Arab countries, alcohol is licensed for sale except in Libya and Saudi Arabia. Such important risk factors rarely are covered by Arab researchers; very little data exist regarding the prevalence of injection drug use combined with Alcoholism and imprisonment and its contribution to HCV infection in the Arab world [77]. In Lebanon HCV among IDU was found to be 52.8%, with no difference in marital status, and in prisoners, it was found to be (3.4%); tattooing was also associated with HCV [78]. In Syria, the prevalence of HCV among Syrian prisoners was found to be 60.5 among IDUs and 1.96 among prostitutes [79]. A study in Saudi Arabia showed that intravenous drug addicts have 14% of exposure rate [80]; another study in Libya found that HCV was 15% among IDUs [49].

Such behaviors are significant factors for HCV infection, and this may become one of the prison system major health concerns over the next two decades. Suggesting that measures to minimize the spread of hepatitis within these groups are essential and education programs seem to be most appropriate way to minimize such risk [81]. This emphasizes that the time has come for national and regional policy makers, researchers, and clinicians among Arab countries to take prisons as important health risks and never to be considered as disadvantaged population.

3.4. Occupational Transmission of HCV. Hepatitis C virus has been known to be an important nosocomial pathogen, and several outbreaks have been linked to breaches in standard precautions for blood-borne infections during nursing procedures or interventions such as colonoscopy surgery and dialysis [82]. In Arab countries where HCV infection is endemic in the general population, hospitalization and invasive procedures do appear to be significant risk factors for HCV infection. Different studies have shown that the prevalence of HCV among HCW was reported to be 3% in Syria, 0.4% in Lebanon. In Egypt, health-care-related risk factors contributed immensely in HCV infection particularly those aged over 20 years old. Surgical practice such as suture was associated with (32.3%), IV catheters (11.7%), though urinary catheter (5.2%), and it was much higher in dental practice as it reached (62.2%) [83].

The occupational transmission was better studied and the picture was more obvious in the North African region. In Libya, the commonest predisposing factor reported was mainly medical-related transmission of HCV, such as hospitalization and/or surgical procedure risk which accounted for 33%, and history of dental procedure for 15.5%, when compared with other risk factors [69]. The prevalence of HCV among Libyan children has an immense increase in 1998, where 420 children have found to be coinfected by both HCV and HIV in a short period of time with no evidence of vertical transmission [84]; this unusual increase in the prevalence of HCV among Libyan children was associated with Bulgarian nurses saga. However, such scrutiny is still under a major scientific dispute among scientists [85].

In Tunis, 51% of HCV cases were reported to be nosocomial rather than transfusion related. In Algeria, occupational exposure seems to be an important risk factor for HCV transmission [54]. Needle stick injuries represented 81% among the health care personnel in Algerian hospitals mainly due the mismanagement of health care waste produced in the hospital environment [57]. Hence then, strict adherence to the international standard precaution should be adapted on a national level allover Algeria.

The assessment of sharps use in Arab countries indicates that injections sometimes were given in a way that may harm the patient. Determinants of these unsafe injection practices include the lack of single-use injecting devices, the lack of awareness of the risk of HCV and HIV infection associated with unsafe injections, and the absence of sharps waste management [86]. Infection control practices in health care settings needs to be reviewed and improved to prevent nosocomial and iatrogenic transmission of HCV (and other blood-borne pathogens). All health care workers should regard patients as infected with a transmissible blood-borne agent.

3.5. Habitual and Community-Associated Factors. Community has been considered to be an important source for hepatitis C, and up to 50% of individuals deny exposure to any of these known risk factors where, infection is often designated as community acquired. Different habitual and biosocial behaviors have reflected on the endemicity of HCV among Arab countries. Indeed children and young adults in Arab countries have a relatively high HCV prevalence, although it is less than in the older population, which suggests that HCV transmission continues in these communities [87]. A variety of contributing factors may be involved, and it becomes imminent that strategies should be implemented to overcome such potential risks. Unsafe use of unsterilized injection is a major risk factor of HCV in Arab communities. It is likely that injections given in rural communities by both traditional and nontraditional health care providers are an important cause of HCV transmission, particularly in countries like Egypt, Sudan, Mauritania, Morocco, Algeria, Iraq, and Yemen. The importance of combating this ubiquitous risk in prevention programs cannot be overstated. A study carried out by World Health Organization (WHO) on the global use of injection has shown that most of the Arab countries have serious problems in using injection in their communities. Eastern Mediterranean region D which mainly includes Egypt, Iraq, Morocco, Yemen, and Sudan has the highest injection per person associated with lack of sterilization. Interestingly, injection practices are safer in sub-Saharan African than in these countries [88]. The same study have also shown that African region which included among the states studied Algeria and Mauritania has also shown a high incidence of unsafe use of injection both health care settings and among community [88]. Furthermore, there is an ongoing speculation that the use of parenteral antischistosomal therapy campaigns contributed to the establishment of a large reservoir of HCV infection in Nile River region [89].

Habitual and social behaviors have been found to influence HCV infection in Arab countries. Circumcision, one of the potential culturally influenced exposures to HCV in the community, occurred too frequently. Males over the age of 20 had been circumcised either by informal health care providers or by community physicians or nurses who were more likely to be infected with HCV than those circumcised by surgeons [83, 90]. Interestingly, marriage was found to be another strong risk for HCV. In UAE, increased prevalence of HCV among spouses was detected with longer duration of marriage being an important risk factor, such infection was passed to children at an early stage [91]. A major logistic-regression model study carried out in Egypt found that the association of HCV in spouses could be the result of sexual transmission or common exposures. Furthermore, they have reported that spouses of patients with HCV have an increased risk for acquiring HCV, and this risk increases with age and is proportional to the duration of marriage [92]. However, unique community-acquired exposures such as smoking goza pipes, shaving by a community barber, ears piercing which common practice among Arab communities were never reported as a cause HCV infections [83, 93]. Elucidating the relative contribution of various modes of transmission of blood-borne viruses could help to direct our efforts towards appropriate intervention strategies in order to achieve viral hepatitis prevention and control. Community centres and counseling institutions should be established in order to understand and facilitate to overcome such existing risk factors. This will help persons in need by modifying behaviors and highlighting risk factors in the setting in which the patient is identified and could be referred to such a convenient community centers.

4. Strategies and Preventive Measures to Control HCV Infection in Arab Countries

Indeed, the status of HCV among Arabic countries should be a worrying issue to all sectors involved in public health, particularly those who are in close contact with patients and strategists who should plan for new healthy look of the Arabic societies [5], despite that there is clear difference among the Arab countries regarding the prevalence and the problematic issues of HCV, which should be eventually taken in consideration regarding the prevention of HCV at each country. Major measures should be implemented as illustrated in Table 4. These include immediate primary intervention (short-run) strategies and long-run prevention strategies. Such prevention strategies should target reduction of transmission of HCV, particularly among those at risk of acquiring the virus. Risk-reduction counseling and HCV screening program were directed to specific population as suggested by Centre for Disease Control (CDC) which may include persons at long-term dialysis, chronic liver diseases patients, health care workers after needle stick injury, and children of HCV-positive mothers [94]. Preventive measures should be directed towards individuals or populations at specific settings such IDUs/STD and prisoners. Hospitals and health care centers should adapt universal and specific infection control programs targeting not only the status of nosocomial infection per se but also particularly those units or persons who were more prone to HCV infection.

Specific prevention programs should take place by adapting better cleansing and standard sterilization methods to stop nosocomial and iatrogenic transmission of HCV. Patient-care practices associated with higher HCV prevalence among chronic hemodialysis units should be identified, and recommendations and precautions in these settings should be adapted. This includes routinely wearing gloves; restricting the use of common supplies, instruments, and medications for multiple patients; prohibiting the use of mobile carts within treatment areas to store or distribute medications and clean supplies [95, 96].

Further programs should include obligatory advanced laboratory screening methods for blood and blood products and reduction of number of transfusion-related transmissions and promote judicious injection and parenteral medications among doctors and patients. Once patients are found to have hepatitis C, they need to be counseled and

TABLE 4: Preventive and combat strategy programs for hepatitis C virus in Arab countries.

(1) Immediate continuous prevention strategies
- (A) *Universal prevention planning*
  - (i) Well-planned educational programs regarding the risk of HCV both at the community and health institutions levels
  - (ii) Implementation of international and national guidelines regarding the prevention of HCV particularly at special hospital settings as blood banks and haemodialysis units and high risk groups at the community
  - (iii) Strict adherence to such guidelines and regular assessment to its applications
  - (iv) Introducing specific patient-care practices
- (B) *Special settings prevention programs*
  - (i) Blood and blood products, HCV screening program and using thioproprin, haemovigilance
  - (ii) Haemodialysis; strict adherence to nosocomial prevention program; review practices to ensure they are consistent with recommendations and applied routinely,
  - (iii) Laboratory and health care; improving laboratory testing, better sterilization, safer injection, and less exposure to blood products

(2) Long-run preventive strategies
- (A) *Universal preventive planning*
  - (i) Vigilance and health alert programs which should report any problem and allow to interfere at any time
  - (ii) Elucidation is needed for better prevention, screening, and updating HCV treatment
  - (iii) Prevention of HCV infection progress
  - (iv) Eradicate the massive use of unsafe medical procedures
- (B) *Special settings preventive planning*
  - (i) Injecting drug users
  - (ii) HIV-HCV coinfected patients
  - (iii) Prisoners inmates

(3) Research planning and priorities

Well-designed research programs should be established both at country level and regional levels which may include
  - (i) Population-based surveillance studies
  - (ii) Evaluation of safety and efficacy of antiviral therapy for HCV alone and with other coinfected viruses particularly HIV
  - (iii) Further evaluation of iatrogenic causes of HCV transmission

clinically evaluated, to reduce the risk of transmission and stop the progression of the disease, respectively. Patients with chronic HCV are susceptible to HAV, or HBV infections should be vaccinated particularly among the Arab countries as the prevalence of these two viruses is high [97]. Further HCV is considered to be an opportunistic disease in persons with HIV infection [98]. Hence then, the safety and efficacy of antiviral therapy INF-& and/or INF-& plus ribavirin for HCV coinfected patients must be evaluated scientifically through clinic trial in Arab world [99]. The implementation of new antiviral treatment and the role of genotyping also have be assessed and appropriate strategies for management of end-stage liver diseases have to be rigorously investigated [100].

4.1. Implications for the Future Challenges. Hepatitis C virus is a serious ongrowing problem in Arab countries, and it has great social-economic impacts which may touch the future of the young generation and influence the infrastructure of such dynamic states. Despite the great capital and natural resources that this nation has, none of these countries have shown meticulous and clear national or regional scientific plans to combat the future damage that HCV may cause. Prevalence of HCV is destined to increase further among Arab countries which should be an alarming issue for further measures. A recent forecast modeling study for prediction of hepatitis C seropositivity among Libyans has shown that in 2020 the HCV will increase by threefold [101]. Another modeled incidence study from Egypt showed that the prevalence of HCV is expected to be continuing at a rate of ≈6.9/1,000 persons per year, indicative of possibly ongoing hyperepidemic transmission in this region [93]. This will have an immense effect on the Arab society with great social clinical and economic implications. Hence then, radical improvement in local infection control measures capable of limiting viral spread among general population should be implemented. Further prospective studies in various population groups are needed in most of the Arabia to generate reliable data on the clinical significance of HCV and its genotypes to hamper such rigorous implications.

Conflict of Interests

The authors declare that they have no conflict of interests. All the authors have read and approved the final paper and contributed immensely in the study. M. A. Daw is a

Professor of Clinical Microbiology and Acting Physician of Internal Medicine, a leading expert in nosocomial infection and epidemiology, and Editor-in-Chief of *Libyan Journal of Medicine*—PubMed indexed. A. A. Dau is a Consultant and Lecturer in Department of Surgery, with a great interest in surgery-associated infection (http://www.hepatitis.ly/; http://www.ljm.org.ly/).

References

[1] C. W. Shepard, L. Finelli, and M. J. Alter, "Global epidemiology of hepatitis C virus infection," *The Lancet Infectious Diseases*, vol. 5, no. 9, pp. 558–567, 2005.

[2] M. J. Alter, "Epidemiology of hepatitis C virus infection," *World Journal of Gastroenterology*, vol. 13, no. 17, pp. 2436–2441, 2007.

[3] W. Sievert, I. Altraif, H. A. Razavi et al., "A systematic review of hepatitis C virus epidemiology in Asia, Australia and Egypt," *Liver International*, vol. 31, supplement 2, pp. 61–80, 2011.

[4] M. A. Daw and S. Shawky, "Going beyond the curriculum to promote medical education and practice (multiple letters)," *Saudi Medical Journal*, vol. 23, no. 1, pp. 116–117, 2002.

[5] M. Daw and E. Elkhammas, "Libyan medical education; time to move forward," *Libyan Journal of Medicine*, vol. 3, no. 1, pp. 1–3, 2008.

[6] Z. A. Memish, B. A. Knawy, and A. El-Saed, "Incidence trends of viral hepatitis A, B, and C seropositivity over eight years of surveillance in Saudi Arabia," *International Journal of Infectious Diseases*, vol. 14, no. 2, pp. e115–e120, 2010.

[7] T. A. Madani, "Hepatitis C virus infections reported over 11 years of surveillance in Saudi Arabia," *Transactions of the Royal Society of Tropical Medicine and Hygiene*, vol. 103, no. 2, pp. 132–136, 2009.

[8] E. I. Azhar, G. A. Jamjoom, A. K. Al-Ghamdi et al., "Hepatitis C virus infection among patients on hemodialysis in jeddah: a single center experience," *Saudi Journal of Kidney Diseases and Transplantation*, vol. 14, no. 1, pp. 84–89, 2011.

[9] M. A. Al Balwi, "Prevalence of mixed hepatitis C virus (HCV) genotypes among recently diagnosed dialysis patients with HCV infection," *Saudi Journal of Kidney Diseases and Transplantation*, vol. 22, no. 4, pp. 712–716, 2011.

[10] A. J. Alzahrani, "Analysis of hepatitis C virus core antigenemia in Saudi drug users," *Saudi Medical Journal*, vol. 26, no. 10, pp. 1645–1646, 2005.

[11] N. A. Haidar, "Prevalence of hepatitis B and hepatitis C in blood donors and high risk groups in Hajjah, Yemen Republic," *Saudi Medical Journal*, vol. 23, no. 9, pp. 1090–1094, 2002.

[12] T. A. Sallam, C. Y. W. Tong, L. E. Cuevas, Y. A. Raja'a, A. M. Othman, and K. R. Al-Kharsa, "Prevalence of blood-borne viral hepatitis in different communities in Yemen," *Epidemiology and Infection*, vol. 131, no. 1, pp. 771–775, 2003.

[13] S. B. Selm, "Prevalence of hepatitis C virus infection among hemodialysis patients in a single center in Yemen," *Saudi Journal of Kidney Diseases and Transplantation*, vol. 21, no. 6, pp. 1165–1168, 2010.

[14] A. Alnaqdy, A. Alfahdi, M. Alkobaisi, and G. Z. Kaminski, "Prevalence of autoantibodies in patients with hepatitis C virus infection in Oman," *Annals of Saudi Medicine*, vol. 23, no. 3-4, pp. 127–131, 2003.

[15] S. H. S. Al-Dhahry, P. N. Aghanashinikar, M. K. Al-Hasani, M. R. Buhl, and A. S. Daar, "Prevalence of antibodies to hepatitis C virus among Omani patients with renal disease," *Infection*, vol. 21, no. 3, pp. 164–167, 1993.

[16] A. M. Lema and E. A. Cox, "Hepatitis C antibodies among blood donors in Qatar," *Vox Sanguinis*, vol. 63, no. 3, p. 237, 1992.

[17] O. Abboud, A. Rashid, and S. Al-Kaabi, "Hepatitis C virus infection in hemodialysis patients in qatar," *Saudi Journal of Kidney Diseases and Transplantation*, vol. 6, no. 2, pp. 151–153, 1995.

[18] A. K. John, S. Al-Kaabi, A. John, R. Singh, and M. Derbala, "Audit of state-funded antiviral treatment for chronic hepatitis C in Qatar," *Eastern Mediterranean Health Journal*, vol. 16, no. 11, pp. 1121–1127, 2010.

[19] M. S. Alfaresi, "Prevalence of hepatitis C virus (HCV) genotypes among positive UAE patients," *Molecular Biology Reports*, vol. 38, no. 4, pp. 2719–2722, 2011.

[20] R. Ameen, N. Sanad, S. Al-Shemmari et al., "Prevalence of viral markers among first-time Arab blood donors in Kuwait," *Transfusion*, vol. 45, no. 12, pp. 1973–1980, 2005.

[21] K. El-Reshaid, M. Kapoor, T. Sugathan, S. Al-Mufti, and N. Al-Hilali, "Hepatitis C virus infection in patients on maintenance dialysis in kuwait: epidemiological profile and efficacy of prophylaxis," *Saudi Journal of Kidney Diseases and Transplantation*, vol. 6, no. 2, pp. 144–150, 1995.

[22] A. S. Pacsa, S. Al-Mufti, T. D. Chugh, and G. Said-Adi, "Genotypes of hepatitis C virus in Kuwait," *Medical Principles and Practice*, vol. 10, no. 1, pp. 55–57, 2001.

[23] B. Othman and F. Monem, "Prevalence of antibodies to hepatitis C virus among hemodialysis patients in damascus, syria," *Infection*, vol. 29, no. 5, pp. 262–265, 2001.

[24] B. M. Othman and F. S. Monem, "Prevalence of hepatitis C virus antibodies among intravenous drug abusers and prostitutes in Damascus, Syria," *Saudi Medical Journal*, vol. 23, no. 4, pp. 393–395, 2002.

[25] N. Antaki, A. Craxi, S. Kamal et al., "The neglected hepatitis C virus genotypes 4, 5 and 6: an international consensus report," *Liver International*, vol. 30, no. 3, pp. 342–355, 2010.

[26] A. R. Omer, J. I. Salih, and A. A. Al-Nakshabandi, "Frequency of blood-borne viral infections among leukemic patients in central Iraq," *Saudi Medical Journal*, vol. 32, no. 1, pp. 55–61, 2011.

[27] W. A. Al-Kubaisy, A. D. Niazi, and K. Kubba, "History of miscarriage as a risk factor for hepatitis C virus infection in pregnant Iraqi women," *Eastern Mediterranean Health Journal*, vol. 8, no. 2-3, pp. 239–244, 2002.

[28] M. Chironna, C. Germinario, P. L. Lopalco, F. Carrozzini, S. Barbuti, and M. Quarto, "Prevalence rates of viral hepatitis infections in refugee Kurds from Iraq and Turkey," *Infection*, vol. 31, no. 2, pp. 70–74, 2003.

[29] W. A. Al-Kubaisy, K. T. Al-Naib, and M. A. Habib, "Prevalence of HCV/HIV co-infection among haemophilia patients in Baghdad," *Eastern Mediterranean Health Journal*, vol. 12, no. 3-4, pp. 264–269, 2006.

[30] N. Irani-Hakime, J. P. Aoun, S. Khoury, H. R. Samaha, H. Tamim, and W. Y. Almawi, "Seroprevalence of hepatitis C infection among health care personnel in Beirut, Lebanon," *American Journal of Infection Control*, vol. 29, no. 1, pp. 20–23, 2001.

[31] Z. Mahfoud, K. Kassak, K. Kreidieh, S. Shamra, and S. Ramia, "Distribution of hepatitis C virus genotypes among injecting drug users in Lebanon," *Virology Journal*, p. 7, article 96, 2010.

[32] F. A. Al Quadan, "Prevalence of anti hepatitis C virus among the hospital populations in Jordan," *New Microbiologica*, vol. 25, no. 3, pp. 269–273, 2002.

[33] S. Bdour, "Hepatitis C virus infection in Jordanian haemodialysis units: serological diagnosis and genotyping," *Journal of Medical Microbiology*, vol. 51, no. 8, pp. 700–704, 2002.

[34] A. E. K. Y. El-Ottol, A. A. Elmanama, and B. M. Ayesh, "Prevalence and risk factors of hepatitis B and C viruses among haemodialysis patients in Gaza strip, Palestine," *Virology Journal*, vol. 7, article 210, 2010.

[35] B. M. Ayesh, S. S. Zourob, S. Y. Abu-Jadallah, and Y. Shemer-Avni, "Most common genotypes and risk factors for HCV in Gaza strip: a cross sectional study," *Virology Journal*, vol. 6, article 105, 2009.

[36] O. A.S. Wasfi and N. A. Sadek, "Prevalence of hepatitis B surface antigen and hepatitis C virus antibodies among blood donors in Alexandria, Egypt," *Eastern Mediterranean Health Journal*, vol. 17, no. 3, pp. 238–242, 2011.

[37] M. Yahia, "Global health: a uniquely Egyptian epidemic," *Nature*, vol. 474, no. 7350, supplement, pp. S12–S13, 2011.

[38] A. Tabll, S. Shoman, H. Ghanem, M. Nabil, N. G.B. El Din, and M. K. El Awady, "Assessment of human cytomegalovirus co-infection in Egyptian chronic HCV patients," *Virology Journal*, vol. 8, article 343, 2011.

[39] A. Paez Jimenez, N. Sharaf Eldin, F. Rimlinger et al., "HCV iatrogenic and intrafamilial transmission in Greater Cairo, Egypt," *Gut*, vol. 59, no. 11, pp. 1554–1560, 2010.

[40] M. Talaat, N. El-Sayed, A. Kandeel et al., "Sentinel surveillance for patients with acute hepatitis in Egypt, 2001-04," *Eastern Mediterranean Health Journal*, vol. 16, no. 2, pp. 134–140, 2010.

[41] M. I. Hanafi, A. M. Mohamed, M. S. Kassem, and M. Shawki, "Needlestick injuries among health care workers of University of Alexandria Hospitals," *Eastern Mediterranean Health Journal*, vol. 17, no. 1, pp. 26–35, 2011.

[42] A. M. Ahmed, M. S. Hassan, A. Abd-Elsayed, H. Hassan, A. F. Hasanain, and A. Helmy, "Insulin resistance, steatosis, and fibrosis in Egyptian patients with chronic Hepatitis C virus infection," *Saudi Journal of Gastroenterology*, vol. 17, no. 4, pp. 245–251, 2011.

[43] G. Esmat, M. Hashem, M. El-Raziky, W. El-Akel, S. El-Naghy, and N. El-Koofy, "Risk factors for hepatitis C virus acquisition and predictors of persistence among Egyptian children," *Liver International*, vol. 10, pp. 1478–3231, 2011.

[44] E. I. Elhawary, G. F. Mahmoud, M. A. El-Daly, F. A. Mekky, G. G. Esmat, and M. Abdel-Hamid, "Association of HCV with diabetes mellitus: an Egyptian case-control study," *Virology Journal*, vol. 8, article 367, 2011.

[45] H. M. Mudawi, "Epidemiology of viral hepatitis in Sudan," *Clinical and Experimental Gastroenterology*, vol. 1, pp. 9–13, 2008.

[46] M. A. A. Abou, Y. M. Eltahir, and A. S. Ali, "Seroprevalence of Hepatitis B virus and Hepatitis C virus among blood donors in Nyala, South Dar Fur, Sudan," *Virology Journal*, vol. 6, article 146, 2009.

[47] G. I. Gasim, H. Z. Hamdan, S. Z. Hamdan, and I. Adam, "Epidemiology of hepatitis B and hepatitis C virus infections among hemodialysis patients in Khartoum, Sudan," *Journal of Medical Virology*, vol. 84, no. 1, pp. 52–55, 2012.

[48] H. M. Y. Mudawi, H. M. Smith, I. A. Fletcher, and S. S. Fedail, "Prevalence and common genotypes of HCV infection in sudanese patients with hepatosplenic schistosomiasis," *Journal of Medical Virology*, vol. 79, no. 9, pp. 1322–1324, 2007.

[49] M. A. Daw, M. A. Elkaber, A. M. Drah, M. M. Werfalli, A. A. Mihat, and I. M. Siala, "Prevalence of Hepatitis C virus antibodies among different populations of relative and attributable risk," *Saudi Medical Journal*, vol. 23, no. 11, pp. 1356–1360, 2002.

[50] H. A. Elasifer, Y. M. Agnnyia, B. A. Al-Alagi, and M. A. Daw, "Epidemiological manifestations of hepatitis C virus genotypes and its association with potential risk factors among Libyan patients," *Virology Journal*, vol. 7, article 317, 2010.

[51] S. Yalaoui, H. L. Ben Nejma, M. M. Azzouz et al., "Detection of hepatitis C virus in the general population of Tunisia," *Bulletin de la Société de Pathologie Exotique*, vol. 91, no. 2, article 177, 1998.

[52] M. Ben Halima, Z. Arrouji, A. Slim, and S. Ben Redjeb, "Serotyping of hepatis C virus in Tunisia," *Tunis-Medindustrie*, vol. 76, no. 6-7, pp. 200–203, 1998.

[53] K. Ayed, Y. Gorgi, T. Ben Abdallah et al., "Hepatitis C virus infection in hemodialysis patients from Tunisia: national survey by serologic and molecular methods," *Transplantation Proceedings*, vol. 35, no. 7, pp. 2573–2575, 2003.

[54] A. Djebbi, H. Triki, O. Bahri et al., "Genotypes of hepatitis C virus circulating in Tunisia," *Epidemiology and Infection*, vol. 130, no. 3, pp. 501–505, 2003.

[55] National Travel Network and Centre (NaTHNaC), Country information, Algeria, Tunisia and Morocco, 2009.

[56] S. Rouabhia, R. Malek, H. Bounecer et al., "Prevalence of type 2 diabetes in algerian patients with hepatitis C virus infection," *World Journal of Gastroenterology*, vol. 16, no. 27, pp. 3427–3431, 2010.

[57] B. Beghdadli, O. Ghomari, M. Taleb et al., "Personnel at risk for occupational blood exposure in a university hospital in West Algeria," *Sante Publique (Vandoeuvre-lès-Nancy, France)*, vol. 21, no. 3, pp. 253–261, 2009.

[58] A. Benouda, Z. Boujdiya, S. Ahid, R. Abouqal, and M. Adnaoui, "Prevalence of hepatitis C virus infection in Morocco and serological tests assessment of detection for the viremia prediction," *Pathologie Biologie*, vol. 57, no. 5, pp. 368–372, 2009.

[59] P. Cacoub, V. Ohayon, S. Sekkat et al., "Epidemiologic and virologic study of hepatitis C virus infection in Morocco," *Gastroenterologie Clinique et Biologique*, vol. 24, no. 2, pp. 169–173, 2000.

[60] S. Sekkat, N. Kamal, B. Benali et al., "Prevalence of anti-HCV antibodies and seroconversion incidence in five haemodialysis units in Morocco," *Nephrologie et Therapeutique*, vol. 4, no. 2, pp. 105–110, 2008.

[61] B. B. Lo, M. Meymouna, M. A. Boulahi et al., "Prevalence of serum markers of hepatitis B and C virus in blood donors of Nouakchott, Mauritania," *Bulletin de la Société de pathologie exotique (1990)*, vol. 92, no. 2, pp. 83–84, 1999.

[62] M. Al-Sheyyab, A. Batieha, and M. El-Khateeb, "The prevalence of hepatitis B, hepatitis C and human immune deficiency virus markers in multi-transfused patients," *Journal of Tropical Pediatrics*, vol. 47, no. 4, pp. 239–242, 2001.

[63] M. A. Bajubair, A. A. Elrub, and G. Bather, "Hepatic viral infections in Yemen between 2000–2005," *Saudi Medical Journal*, vol. 29, no. 6, pp. 871–874, 2008.

[64] I. Al-Fawaz, S. Al-Rasheed, M. Al-Mugeiren, A. Al-Salloum, M. Al-Sohaibani, and S. Ramia, "Hepatitis E virus infection in patients from Saudi Arabia with sickle cell anaemia and β-thalassemia major: possible transmission by blood transfusion," *Journal of Viral Hepatitis*, vol. 3, no. 4, pp. 203–205, 1996.

[65] Z. M. Al-Hawsawi, "Prevalence of hepatitis C virus antibody," *Annals of Saudi Medicine*, vol. 20, no. 5-6, pp. 488–489, 2000.

[66] M. J. Grijalva, R. F. Chiriboga, H. Vanhassel, and L. Arcos-Teran, "Improving the safety of the blood supply in Ecuador through external performance evaluation of serological screening of blood donors," *Journal of Clinical Virology*, vol. 34, no. 2, supplement, pp. S47–S52, 2005.

[67] S. L. Stramer, S. A. Glynn, S. H. Kleinman et al., "Detection of HIV-1 and HCV infections among antibody-negative blood donors by nucleic acid-amplification testing," *The New England Journal of Medicine*, vol. 351, no. 8, pp. 760–768, 2004.

[68] J. Coste, H. W. Reesink, C. P. Engelfriet et al., "Implementation of donor screening for infectious agents transmitted by blood by nucleic acid technology: update to 2003," *Vox Sanguinis*, vol. 88, no. 4, pp. 289–303, 2005.

[69] A. A. Dau, S. Tloba, and M. A. Daw, "Characterization of wound infections among injured patients during Libyan conflict," *Eastern Mediterranean Health Journal*. In press.

[70] M. Rahnavardi, S. M. Hosseini Moghaddam, and S. M. Alavian, "Hepatitis C in hemodialysis patients: current global magnitude, natural history, diagnostic difficulties, and preventive measures," *American Journal of Nephrology*, vol. 28, no. 4, pp. 628–640, 2008.

[71] M. Al-Jamal, A. Al-Qudah, K. F. Al-Shishi, A. Al-Sarayreh, and L. Al-Quraan, "Hepatitis C virus (HCV) infection in hemodialysis patients in the south of Jordan," *Saudi Journal of Kidney Diseases and Transplantation*, vol. 20, no. 3, pp. 488–492, 2009.

[72] A. S. Abdulkarim, N. N. Zein, J. J. Germer et al., "Hepatitis C virus genotypes and hepatitis G virus in hemodialysis patients from Syria: identification of two novel hepatitis C virus subtypes," *American Journal of Tropical Medicine and Hygiene*, vol. 59, no. 4, pp. 571–576, 1998.

[73] A. Karkar, "Hepatitis C in dialysis units: the Saudi experience," *Hemodialysis International*, vol. 11, no. 3, pp. 354–367, 2007.

[74] S. Sekkat, N. Kamal, B. Benali et al., "Prevalence of anti-HCV antibodies and seroconversion incidence in five haemodialysis units in Morocco," *Nephrologie et Therapeutique*, vol. 4, no. 2, pp. 105–110, 2008.

[75] T. Diaz, D. C. Des Jarlais, D. Vlahov et al., "Factors associated with prevalent hepatitis C: differences among young adult injection drug users in lower and upper Manhattan, New York City," *American Journal of Public Health*, vol. 91, no. 1, pp. 23–30, 2001.

[76] L. E. Thorpe, L. J. Ouellet, R. Hershow et al., "Risk of hepatitis C virus infection among young adult injection drug users who share injection equipment," *American Journal of Epidemiology*, vol. 155, no. 7, pp. 645–653, 2002.

[77] A. González Quintela, R. Alende, A. Aguilera et al., "Hepatitis C virus antibodies in alcoholic patients," *Revista Clinica Espanola*, vol. 195, no. 6, pp. 367–372, 1995.

[78] K. Kassak, Z. Mahfoud, K. Kreidieh, S. Shamra, R. Afifi, and S. Ramia, "Hepatitis B virus and hepatitis C virus infections among female sex workers and men who have sex with men in Lebanon: prevalence, risk behaviour and immune status," *Sexual Health*, vol. 8, no. 2, pp. 229–233, 2011.

[79] B. M. Othman and F. S. Monem, "Prevalence of hepatitis C virus antibodies among intravenous drug abusers and prostitutes in Damascus, Syria," *Saudi Medical Journal*, vol. 23, no. 4, pp. 393–395, 2002.

[80] A. J. Alzahrani, D. M. Dela Cruz, O. E. Obeid, H. A. Bukhari, A. A. Al-Qahtani, and M. N. Al-Ahdal, "Molecular detection of hepatitis B, hepatitis C, and torque teno viruses in drug users in Saudi Arabia," *Journal of Medical Virology*, vol. 81, no. 8, pp. 1343–1347, 2009.

[81] S. Allwright, F. Bradley, J. Long, J. Barry, L. Thornton, and J. V. Parry, "Prevalence of antibodies to hepatitis B, hepatitis C, and HIV and risk factors in Irish prisoners: results of a national cross sectional survey," *British Medical Journal*, vol. 321, no. 7253, pp. 78–82, 2000.

[82] A. Mele, E. Spada, L. Sagliocca et al., "Risk of parenterally transmitted hepatitis following exposure to surgery or other invasive procedures: results from the hepatitis surveillance system in Italy," *Journal of Hepatology*, vol. 35, no. 2, pp. 284–289, 2001.

[83] M. Habib, M. K. Mohamed, F. Abdel-Aziz et al., "Hepatitis C virus infection in a community in the Nile Delta: risk factors for seropositivity," *Hepatology*, vol. 33, no. 1, pp. 248–253, 2001.

[84] L. Perrin, "More than 30% HCV prevalence in the HIV-1 El-Fateh children hospital outbreak is a key for both elucidation and public health measures," *Libyan Journal of Medicine*, vol. 2, no. 2, pp. 55–56, 2007.

[85] O. Bagasra, M. Alsayari, R. Bullard-Dillard, and M. A. Daw, "The Libyan HIV outbreak how do we find the truth?" *Libyan Journal of Medicine*, vol. 2, no. 2, pp. 57–62, 2007.

[86] A. M. Hauri, G. L. Armstrong, and Y. J. F. Hutin, "The global burden of disease attributable to contaminated injections given in health care settings," *International Journal of STD and AIDS*, vol. 15, no. 1, pp. 7–16, 2004.

[87] N. Arafa, M. El Hoseiny, C. Rekacewicz et al., "Changing pattern of hepatitis C virus spread in rural areas of Egypt," *Journal of Hepatology*, vol. 43, no. 3, pp. 418–424, 2005.

[88] Y. J. F. Hutin, A. M. Hauri, and G. L. Armstrong, "Use of injections in healthcare settings worldwide, 2000: literature review and regional estimates," *British Medical Journal*, vol. 327, no. 7423, pp. 1075–1078, 2003.

[89] M. R. Rao, A. B. Naficy, M. A. Darwish et al., "Further evidence for association of hepatitis C infection with parenteral schistosomiasis treatment in Egypt," *BMC Infectious Diseases*, vol. 2, no. 1, article 29, 2002.

[90] P. K. Drain, D. T. Halperin, J. P. Hughes, J. D. Klausner, and R. C. Bailey, "Male circumcision, religion, and infectious diseases: an ecologic analysis of 118 developing countries," *BMC Infectious Diseases*, vol. 6, article 172, 2006.

[91] R. M. Kumar and S. Shahul, "Role of breast-feeding in transmission of hepatitis C virus to infants of HCV-infected mothers," *Journal of Hepatology*, vol. 29, no. 2, pp. 191–197, 1998.

[92] R. M. Kumar, P. M. Frossad, and P. F. Hughes, "Seroprevalence and mother-to-infant transmission of hepatitis C in asymptomatic Egyptian women," *European Journal of Obstetrics Gynecology and Reproductive Biology*, vol. 75, no. 2, pp. 177–182, 1997.

[93] F. D. Miller and L. J. Abu-Raddad, "Evidence of intense ongoing endemic transmission of hepatitis C virus in Egypt," *Proceedings of the National Academy of Sciences of the United States of America*, vol. 107, no. 33, pp. 14757–14762, 2010.

[94] Centers for Disease Control and Prevention, "Recommendations for prevention and control of hepatitis C virus HCV infection and HCV-related chronic disease," *MMWR—Recommendations and Reports*, vol. 47, pp. 1–39, 1998.

[95] M. J. Alter, "Prevention of spread of hepatitis C," *Hepatology*, vol. 36, no. 5, pp. S93–S98, 2002.

[96] G. Shimokura, F. Chai, D. J. Weber et al., "Patient-care practices associated with an increased prevalence of hepatitis

c virus infection among chronic hemodialysis patients," *Infection Control and Hospital Epidemiology*, vol. 32, no. 5, pp. 415–424, 2011.

[97] D. Lavanchy, "Hepatitis B virus epidemiology, disease burden, treatment, arid current and emerging prevention and control measures," *Journal of Viral Hepatitis*, vol. 11, no. 2, pp. 97–107, 2004.

[98] M. S. Sulkowski, E. E. Mast, L. B. Seeff, and D. L. Thomas, "Hepatitis C virus infection as an opportunistic disease in persons infected with human immunodeficiency virus," *Clinical Infectious Diseases*, vol. 30, no. 4, pp. S77–S84, 2000.

[99] J. Hu, K. Doucette, L. Hartling, L. Tjosvold, and J. Robinson, "Treatment of hepatitis C in children: a systematic review," *PLoS ONE*, vol. 5, no. 7, Article ID e11542, 2010.

[100] T. Kanda, F. Imazeki, and O. Yokosuka, "New antiviral therapies for chronic hepatitis C," *Hepatology International*, vol. 4, no. 3, pp. 548–561, 2010.

[101] A. Shabash, M. Habas, A. Alhajrasi, A. Furarah, A. Bouzedi, and M. Daw, "Forecast modeling for prediction of hepatitis B and Hepatitis C seropositivity among Libyan population," *Clinical Microbiol Infection*, vol. 16, supplement 2, article 120, 2010.

11

A Meta-Analysis of Tea Drinking and Risk of Parkinson's Disease

Feng-Jiao Li, Hong-Fang Ji, and Liang Shen

Shandong Provincial Research Center for Bioinformatic Engineering and Technique, Shandong University of Technology, Zibo 255049, China

Correspondence should be addressed to Hong-Fang Ji, jhf@sdut.edu.cn and Liang Shen, shen@sdut.edu.cn

Academic Editors: S. Hunot and J. L. Labandeira-García

Background. Many studies have reported an association between tea drinking and Parkinson's disease (PD). Our purpose is to summarize the available information and evaluate the risk of PD associated with tea drinking. *Methods.* We searched all publications in English language on the association of tea drinking and PD risk published up to December 2010. The pooled analysis was performed with Review Manager 5.0. *Results.* In total, eight articles including 1418 cases and 4250 controls were included in the meta-analysis. The pooled odds ratio (95% CI) was 0.85 (0.74–0.98), which suggests the protective effect of tea drinking in PD risks. Moreover, the summary OR (OR: 0.83, 95% CI = 0.69–0.99) for drinkers of ≤1 cup of tea per day versus nonconsumers and that (OR: 0.96, 95% CI = 0.73–1.27) for drinkers of >1 cups of tea per day versus nonconsumers showed that there was not an apparent dose-response relationship. No indication for publication bias was found. *Conclusions.* This meta-analysis showed that tea drinking can lower the risk of PD, while no apparent dose-response relationship was found. Further effort is needed to fully understand the mechanism underlying the beneficial effect of tea consumption in lowering PD risk.

1. Introduction

Parkinson's disease (PD) is a common neurodegenerative disorder, and, with the accelerated aging of human society, the prevalence of PD is expected to rise steadily in future [1, 2]. Despite the pathogenesis of PD is not fully elucidated, many epidemiological factors, such as coffee drinking and smoking, have been demonstrated to lower the risk of PD [3–5]. Tea is one of the most popular beverages worldwide, and the effects of tea consumption on PD risk have attracted much attention in recent years [6–17], as the tea components, such as flavonoids, caffeine, and theanine, have been proven to be neuroprotective in animal models of PD. Many studies have found that tea drinking can lower the risk of PD [6–10, 12–15], while this beneficial effect of tea is not observed in other reports [11, 16]. The purpose of the present study was to perform a meta-analysis to provide a comprehensive conclusion on the association between tea drinking and PD risk, which has important implications for the prevention and treatment of this disease.

2. Methods

2.1. Information Retrieval. We identified procurable published studies in English through a computerized MEDLINE search from 1966 to December 2010 and also the relational document links. We used the following medical subject headings and free text words to search the PubMed database: (TEA) AND (PARKINSON OR PD) AND (CASE-CONTROL OR CASE-REFERENT OR RETROSPECTIVE OR COHORT OR FOLLOW-UP OR INCIDENCE OR PROSPECTIVE OR EPIDEMIOLOG). We also examined conference proceedings; the references in the articles retrieved through the computerized search.

2.2. Selection Criteria. The identified studies must meet the following criteria: (i) the original data includes the number of PD cases studied and the odds ratio (OR) or relative risk (RR), (ii) its corresponding 95% confidence interval (CI) is for highest versus non-/lowest level of tea intake, and (iii) these studies must define the outcome of interest as incident PD based on clearly stated diagnostic criteria or identified through diagnostic codes with additional confirmation. In total, eight published articles were included in the meta-analysis [8–15]. The details of search strategy and study selection processes were shown in Figure 1.

2.3. Data Extraction and Meta-Analysis. We extracted information from each paper including first author, year, and

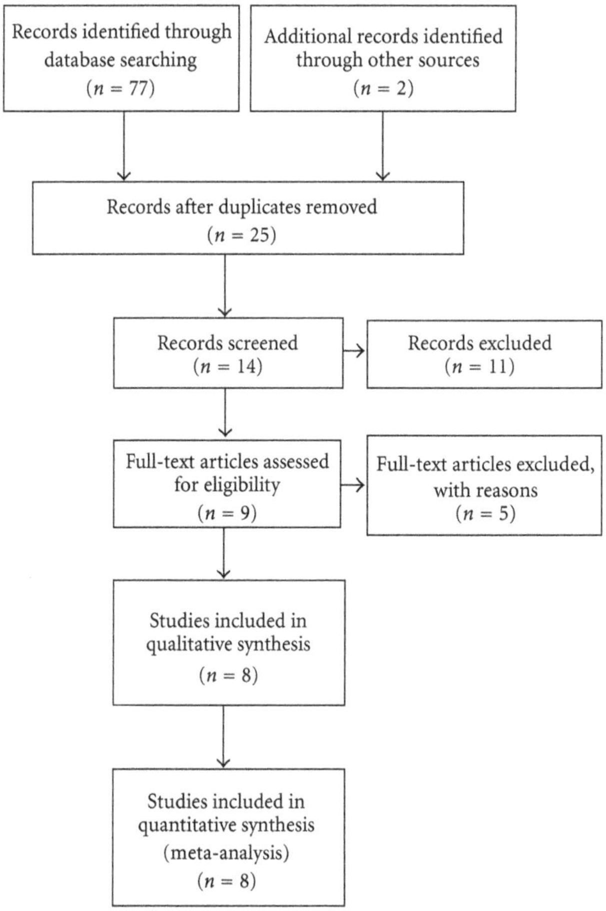

FIGURE 1: Selection of studies for inclusion in the present meta-analysis.

country of publication, the number of cases and controls, the adjusted RRs or ORs, and 95% CI. We examined possible heterogeneity in the identified result. If the P value >0.10, it means that the study does not have statistical significance. We used the fixed effect model to calculate the summary OR and its 95% CI across homogeneous studies and used the random effect model to calculate the summary OR and its 95% CI across heterogeneous studies. Egger's weighted regression method was employed to evaluate P value for publication bias. Finally, stratified analyses were conducted to examine the differences by cups of drinking. Statistical computation was performed using the Review Manager 5.0 statistical software.

3. Results

3.1. Tea Drinking and PD Risks. The eight case-control studies (including 1418 cases and 4250 controls) which met the eligibility criteria were conducted in 5 countries between 1966 and 2010. Table 1 with the extracted information present the relative risk for each of studies along with their summary OR derived from the meta-analysis. Figure 2 presents the forest plot of comparison of tea drinkers versus non-consumers. There was statistically heterogeneity among the eight results ($P = 0.04$). The analyses compared exposed with unexposed for tea drinking, and the overall summary OR based on all studies indicated that tea drinking can protect PD (summary OR = 0.85, 95% CI = 0.85–0.98) with eight cases.

3.2. The Dose Effect Relationship of Tea Drinking and PD Risks. Among the eight studies that included in our present analysis, three reported the results for drinkers of ≤1 and >1 cup of tea per day versus non-consumers. [14, 16, 18]. The information according to the number of cups of tea drinking daily was included in Table 2. It can be seen that, for drinkers of ≤1 cup of tea per day versus non-consumers, the summary OR (OR: 0.83, 95% CI = 0.69–0.99) showed a protective effect against PD (Figure 3). For drinkers of >1 cup of tea per day versus non-consumers, the summary OR (OR: 0.96, 95% CI = 0.73–1.27) also showed a protective effect (Figure 4). According to the present results, we concluded that there was not an apparent dose-response relationship.

3.3. Publication Bias. Figure 5 shows the funnel plot of tea drinking and the risk of PD, in which, the logOR from each study is plotted on the horizontal axis, and its standard error is plotted on the vertical axis. Inspection of the Begg funnel plot did not find the presence of publication bias because the logORs plotted against their standard errors yielded a symmetric distribution.

TABLE 1: Tea drinking and PD risk.

Author	Year of publication	Country	Cases		Controls		Relative risk	95% CI
			N	n	N	n		
Haack et al. [8]	1981	USA	237	223	474	456	0.63	[0.31, 1.29]
Ho et al. [9]	1989	China	34	21	105	70	0.81	[0.36, 1.80]
Fall et al. [10]	1999	Sweden	113	64	263	174	0.67	[0.43, 1.05]
Preux et al. [11]	2000	France	140	40	280	54	1.67	[1.04, 2.68]
Paganini-Hill [12]	2001	USA	395	182	2320	1126	0.91	[0.73, 1.12]
Morano et al. [13]	1994	Spain	74	6	148	6	2.09	[0.65, 6.71]
Chan et al. [14]	1998	China	215	113	313	196	0.66	[0.46, 0.94]
Checkoway et al. [15]	2002	USA	210	72	347	145	0.73	[0.51, 1.04]
Total			1418		4250		0.85	[0.74, 0.98]

Test for heterogeneity among all studies: $Q = 15.03$ based on 7 degrees of freedom $P = 0.04$. Summary OR was based on fixed effect models. N : number of cases/controls, n : number of tea drinkers in cases/controls.

Study or subgroup	Odds ratio M-H, fixed, 95% CI
Chan et al. [14]	0.66 [0.46, 0.94]
Checkoway et al. [15]	0.73 [0.51, 1.04]
Fall et al. [10]	0.67 [0.43, 1.05]
Haack et al. [8]	0.63 [0.31, 1.29]
Ho et al. [9]	0.81 [0.36, 1.8]
Morano et al. [13]	2.09 [0.65, 6.71]
Paganini-Hill [12]	0.91 [0.73, 1.12]
Preux et al. [11]	1.67 [1.04, 2.68]
Total (95% CI)	0.85 [0.74, 0.98]

Total events

Heterogeneity: $\chi^2 = 15.03$, $df = 7$ $(P = 0.04)$, $I^2 = 53\%$

Test for overall effect: $Z = 2.3$ $(P = 0.02)$

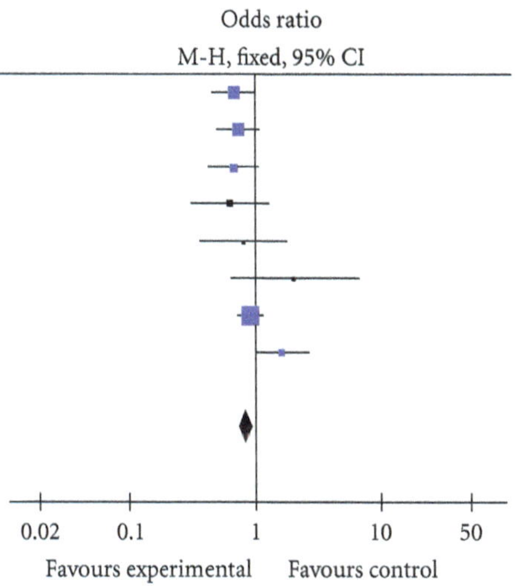

FIGURE 2: Pooled estimate of OR and 95% CI of PD risk for tea drinking. Blue diamonds indicate adjusted OR in each study. Open diamonds are pooled OR. Horizontal line represents 95% CI. Studies are ordered by alphabetical order of last name of first author.

4. Discussion

As we know, PD is a common neurodegenerative disorder in middle- and old-aged crowd. The etiology of PD has long been thought to involve many factors, and there were five major hypotheses regarding the pathogenesis of PD, such as the theory of genetic factors, the theory of environmental factors, immunity doctrine, apoptosis theory, and the oxidative stress theory [18–22]. In oxidative stress theory, oxidative stress contributes to the cascade leading to dopamine cell degeneration in PD. Oxidative stress can impair altered ubiquitination and degradation of proteins directly, which have been implicated as key to dopaminergic cell death in PD, and products of oxidative damage (e.g., 4-hydroxynonenal) can damage the 26S proteasome [23].

Tea is one of the most ancient and popular beverages consumed around the world. There are many important substances in tea leaves, such as polyphenols, methylxanthine, caffeine, different lipids, amino acids, mineral substances, and volatile compounds. The demonstrated health benefits of tea include weight loss, preventing heart disease and cancer, and so forth [24]. For example, epigallocatechin gallate (EGCG), one of the most important antioxidant ingredients of green tea, is responsible for green tea's weight loss effect by increasing metabolism and the body's ability to burn fat [25]. Polyphenols in tea have been proven to inhibit tumor cell proliferation and induce apoptosis [26, 27]. Moreover, in in vitro study and experimental animal model, it has been identified that tea drinking can obviously reduce the formation of molecular products of various small lipid peroxidation and induce antioxidative enzyme activities [28].

In recent years, there were more and more studies devoted to exploring the effects of tea consumption on PD risk. Many studies reported that tea drinking can lower the risk of PD [6–10, 12–15], while this protective effect of tea is not demonstrated by other groups [11, 16]. With the aim to evaluate the association between tea drinking and PD risk, a meta-analysis was conducted based on published studies. The estimated summary OR is 0.85, which donates that tea

Table 2: The dose effect relationship of tea drinking and PD risk.

Author	Year of publication	Country	Cases N	Cases n	Controls N	Controls n	Relative risk	95% CI
Drinkers of ≤1 cup per day of tea versus non-consumers studies								
Fall et al. [10]	1999	Sweden	113	57	263	143	0.85	[0.55, 1.33]
Paganini-Hill [12]	2001	USA	395	132	2320	892	0.80	[0.64, 1.01]
Checkoway et al. [15]	2002	USA	210	61	347	110	0.88	[0.61, 1.28]
Total			718		2930		0.83	[0.69, 0.99]
Drinkers of >1 cups per day of tea versus non-consumers studies								
Fall et al. [10]	1999	Sweden	113	7	263	31	0.49	[0.21, 1.16]
Paganini-Hill [12]	2001	USA	395	50	2320	234	1.29	[0.93, 1.79]
Checkoway et al. [15]	2002	USA	210	11	347	35	0.49	[0.24, 0.99]
Total			718		2930		0.96	[0.73, 1.27]

N: number of cases/controls, n: number of tea drinkers in cases/controls.

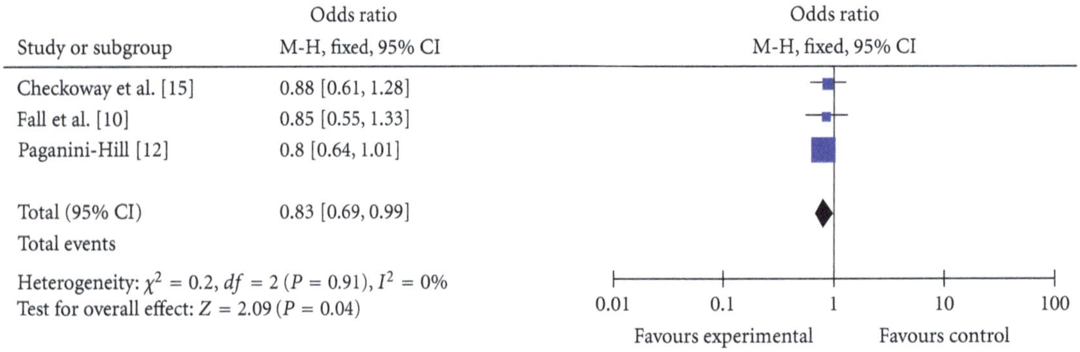

Figure 3: Pooled estimate of OR and 95% CI of PD risk for tea drinking of ≤1 cup per day. Blue diamonds indicate adjusted OR in each study. Open diamonds are pooled OR. Horizontal line represents 95% CI. Studies are ordered by alphabetical order of the last name of first author.

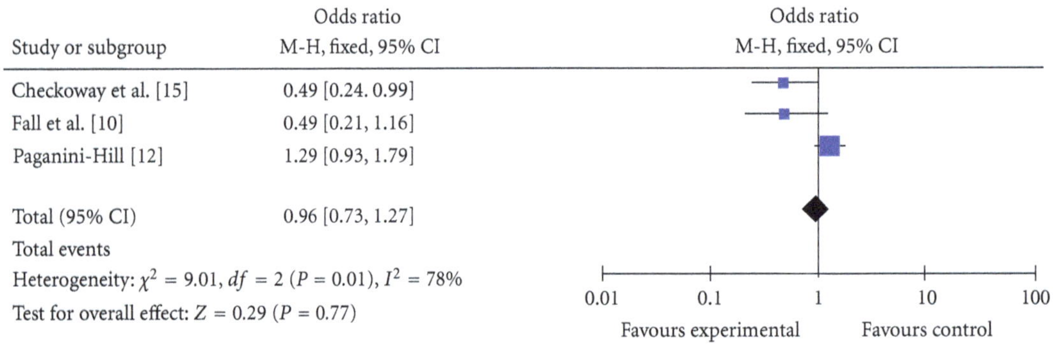

Figure 4: Pooled estimate of OR and 95% CI of PD risk for tea drinking of >1 cups per day. Blue diamonds indicate adjusted OR in each study. Open diamonds are pooled OR. Horizontal line represents 95% CI. Studies are ordered by alphabetical order of the last name of first author.

drinking can decrease the risk of PD. This is consistent with the results of the similar study by Quintana et al. [6] and, thus, further confirms the relation of tea consumption and PD. The mechanisms underlying the protective effects of tea drinking against PD risk should be multiple. In recent years, many natural products have been proposed to be multipotent agent to combat neurodegenerative diseases [29–32]. Firstly, through synthesizing the studies in vitro and experimental animal model and the epidemiological studies we collected, we can infer that the antioxidant effect of tea components, especially polyphones, should be the predominant mechanism of tea against PD. Tea polyphones, such as EGCG, have been found to exhibit neuroprotective effect and the mechanism of the neuroprotection may involve three aspects: antioxidant, anti-inflammatory and iron-chelating activities [29, 33, 34]. Secondly, many other biological activities of tea components may contribute to the beneficial effect of tea in lowering PD risk. For instance, it was found that

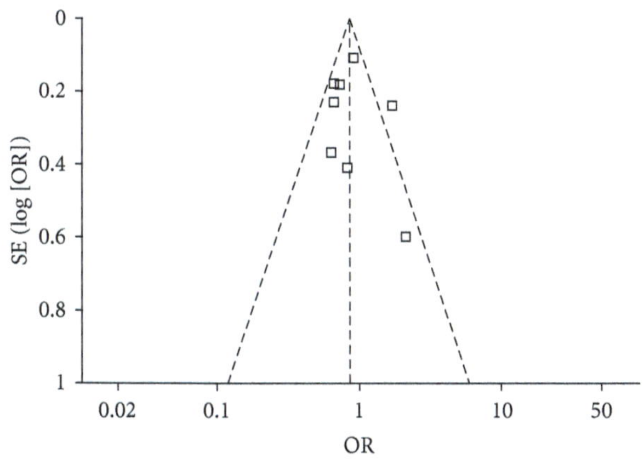

FIGURE 5: Funnel plot of tea drinking and the risk of PD. The log OR from each study is plotted on the horizontal axis, and its standard error is plotted on the vertical axis.

theanine can protect the brain by promoting the secretion of dopamine [35]. Caffeine has been demonstrated to be an adenosine A2A receptor antagonist that may enhance locomotor activity in animal models of PD and improve motor function in patients with PD [36]. In addition, Tan et al. proposed that flavonoids in tea with their anti-inflammatory effects on the cardiovascular system may help ward off PD by increasing circulation to the brain [16].

Moreover, according to the present meta-analysis, we did not find an apparent dose-response relationship as expected. It may arise from the following factors: (i) black tea and green tea differ markedly in the nature of their polyphenols [37, 38], while there were only few studies reporting stratified results according to the types of tea and (ii) the contents of the bioactive compounds in tea may fluctuate because of differences in producing areas, materials, and manufacturing [37, 38].

There were heterogeneity and limitations in our study. Firstly, the population studied in the included references was small and their location was not widespread, which make us unable to perform analysis on race. Secondly, other factors with possible influence on disease progression such as anti-Parkinsonian drugs, food supplements, or alcohol consumption were not considered. Thirdly, there were only few studies reporting stratified results according to specific types of tea (black or green) and the gender of the population studied. If more data is available in future for performing stratified analyses according to the types of tea, through comparing the components of the specific types of tea, we can identify the most important compounds, which will be of significance to the prevention and treatment of PD.

To summarize, our findings indicate that tea drinking can protect against PD, which leads human to value the impact of lifestyle on health. Despite the mechanisms behind this association should be multiple, in view of the widely accepted pathogenic role of oxidative stress in PD and the well-documented antioxidant potential of bioactive tea components, the antioxidant activity is expected to be an important aspect. Further effort is encouraged to fully understand the comprehensive mechanism underlying the beneficial effect of tea consumption in lowering PD risk.

Acknowledgment

This work was supported by the National Natural Science Foundation of China (Grant nos. 30800184 and 30700113).

References

[1] M. H. Polymeropoulos, C. Lavedan, E. Leroy et al., "Mutation in the alphasynuclein gene identified in families with Parkinson's disease," *Science*, vol. 276, no. 5321, pp. 2045–2047, 1997.

[2] A. E. Lang and A. M. Lozano, "Parkinson's disease," *The New England Journal of Medicine*, vol. 339, no. 15, pp. 1044–1053, 1998.

[3] K. Wirdefeldt, H. O. Adami, P. Cole, D. Trichopoulos, and J. Mandel, "Epidemiology and etiology of Parkinson's disease: a review of the evidence," *European Journal of Epidemiology*, vol. 26, supplement 1, pp. S1–S58, 2011.

[4] M. A. Hernán, B. Takkouche, J. J. Gestal-Otero, and F. Caamaño-Isorna, "A meta-analysis of coffee drinking, cigarette smoking, and the risk of Parkinson's disease," *Annals of Neurology*, vol. 52, no. 3, pp. 276–284, 2002.

[5] G. H. Cao, E. Sofic, and R. L. Prior, "Antioxidant capacity of tea and common vegetables," *Journal of Agricultural and Food Chemistry*, vol. 44, no. 11, pp. 3426–3431, 1996.

[6] J. L. B. Quintana, M. F. Allam, A. S. del Castillo, and R. F. C. Navajas, "Parkinson's disease and tea: a quantitative review," *Journal of the American College of Nutrition*, vol. 28, no. 1, pp. 1–6, 2009.

[7] A. Ascherio, S. M. Zhang, M. A. Hernán et al., "Prospective study of caffeine consumption and risk of Parkinson's disease in men and women," *Annals of Neurology*, vol. 50, no. 1, pp. 56–63, 2001.

[8] D. G. Haack, R. J. Baumann, and H. E. McKean, "Nicotine exposure and parkinson disease," *American Journal of Epidemiology*, vol. 114, no. 2, pp. 191–200, 1981.

[9] S. C. Ho, J. Woo, and C. M. Lee, "Epidemiologic study of Parkinson's disease in Hong Kong," *Neurology*, vol. 39, no. 10, pp. 1314–1318, 1989.

[10] P. A. Fall, M. Fredrikson, O. Axelson, and A. K. Granérus, "Nutritional and occupational factors influencing the risk of Parkinson's disease: a case-control study in southeastern Sweden," *Movement Disorders*, vol. 14, no. 1, pp. 28–37, 1999.

[11] P. M. Preux, A. Condet, C. Anglade et al., "Parkinson's disease and environmental factors: matched case-control study in the Limousin region, France," *Neuroepidemiology*, vol. 19, no. 6, pp. 333–337, 2000.

[12] A. Paganini-Hill, "Risk factors for Parkinson's disease: the Leisure World cohort study," *Neuroepidemiology*, vol. 20, no. 2, pp. 118–124, 2001.

[13] A. Morano, F. J. Jiménez-Jiménez, J. A. Molina, and M. A. Antolin, "Risk-factors for Parkinson's disease: case-control study in the province of Caceres, Spain," *Acta Neurologica Scandinavica*, vol. 89, no. 3, pp. 164–170, 1994.

[14] D. K. Chan, J. Woo, S. C. Ho et al., "Genetic and environmental risk factors for Parkinson's disease in a Chinese population," *Journal of Neurology Neurosurgery and Psychiatry*, vol. 65, no. 5, pp. 781–784, 1998.

[15] H. Checkoway, K. Powers, T. Smith-Weller, G. M. Franklin, W. T. Longstreth, and P. D. Swanson, "Parkinson's disease risks associated with cigarette smoking, alcohol consumption, and

caffeine intake," *American Journal of Epidemiology*, vol. 155, no. 8, pp. 732–738, 2002.

[16] L. C. Tan, W. P. Koh, J. M. Yuan et al., "Differential effects of black versus green tea on risk of Parkinson's disease in the Singapore Chinese health study," *American Journal of Epidemiology*, vol. 167, no. 5, pp. 553–560, 2008.

[17] J. Zayed, S. Ducic, G. Campanella et al., "Environmental factors in the etiology of Parkinson's disease," *Canadian Journal of Neurological Sciences*, vol. 17, no. 3, pp. 286–291, 1990.

[18] M. J. Volles, S. J. Lee, J. C. Rochet et al., "Vesicle permeabilization by protofibrillar α-synuclein: implications for the pathogenesis and treatment of Parkinson's disease," *Biochemistry*, vol. 40, no. 26, pp. 7812–7819, 2001.

[19] H. H. Liou, M. C. Tsai, C. J. Chen et al., "Environmental risk factors and Parkinson's disease: a case-control study in Taiwan," *Neurology*, vol. 48, no. 6, pp. 1583–1588, 1997.

[20] W. D. Le, D. B. Rowe, J. Jankovic, W. Xie, and S. H. Appel, "Effects of cerebrospinal fluid from patients with Parkinson disease on dopaminergic cells," *Archives of Neurology*, vol. 56, no. 2, pp. 194–200, 1999.

[21] V. Viswanath, Y. Wu, R. Boonplueang et al., "Caspase-9 activation results in downstream caspase-8 activation and bid cleavage in 1-methyl-4-phenyl-1,2,3,6-tetrahydropyridine-induced Parkinson's disease," *Journal of Neuroscience*, vol. 21, no. 24, pp. 9519–9528, 2001.

[22] S. Bharath, M. Hsu, D. Kaur, S. Rajagopalan, and J. K. Andersen, "Glutathione, iron and Parkinson's disease," *Biochemical Pharmacology*, vol. 64, no. 5-6, pp. 1037–1048, 2002.

[23] P. Jenner, "Oxidative stress in Parkinson's disease," *Annals of Neurology*, vol. 53, no. 3, pp. S26–S36, 2003.

[24] C. S. Yang and J. M. Landau, "Effects of tea consumption nutrition health," *Journal of Nutrition*, vol. 130, no. 10, pp. 2409–2412, 2000.

[25] Y. H. Kao, H. H. Chang, M. J. Lee, and C. L. Chen, "Tea, obesity, and diabetes," *Molecular Nutrition and Food Research*, vol. 50, no. 2, pp. 188–210, 2006.

[26] N. P. Seeram, S. M. Henning, Y. Niu, R. Lee, H. S. Scheuller, and D. Heber, "Catechin and caffeine content of green tea dietary supplements and correlation with antioxidant capacity," *Journal of Agricultural and Food Chemistry*, vol. 54, no. 5, pp. 1599–1603, 2006.

[27] J. D. Lambert and C. S. Yang, "Mechanisms of cancer prevention by tea constituents," *Journal of Nutrition*, vol. 133, supplement 10, pp. 3262S–3267S, 2003.

[28] G. C. Yen and H. Y. Chen, "Antioxidant activity of various tea extracts in relation to their antimutagenicity," *Journal of Agricultural and Food Chemistry*, vol. 43, no. 1, pp. 27–32, 1995.

[29] H. F. Ji and H. Y. Zhang, "Multipotent natural agents to combat Alzheimer's disease. Functional spectrum and structural features," *Acta Pharmacologica Sinica*, vol. 29, no. 2, pp. 143–151, 2008.

[30] H. F. Ji and L. Shen, "Berberine: a potential multipotent natural product to combat Alzheimer's disease," *Molecules*, vol. 16, no. 8, pp. 6732–6740, 2011.

[31] H. F. Ji, X. J. Li, and H. Y. Zhang, "Natural products and drug discovery: can thousands of years of ancient medical knowledge lead us to new and powerful drug combinations in the fight against cancer and dementia?" *EMBO Reports*, vol. 10, no. 3, pp. 194–200, 2009.

[32] L. Shen, H. Y. Zhang, and H. F. Ji, "A theoretical study on Cu(II)-chelating properties of curcumin and its implications for curcumin as a multipotent agent to combat Alzheimer's disease," *Journal of Molecular Structure: THEOCHEM*, vol. 757, no. 1–3, pp. 199–202, 2005.

[33] O. Weinreb, S. Mandel, T. Amit, and M. B. H. Youdim, "Neurological mechanisms of green tea polyphenols in Alzheimer's and Parkinson's diseases," *Journal of Nutritional Biochemistry*, vol. 15, no. 9, pp. 506–516, 2004.

[34] H. F. Ji and H. Y. Zhang, "Theoretical evaluation of flavonoids as multipotent agents to combat Alzheimer's disease," *Journal of Molecular Structure: THEOCHEM*, vol. 767, no. 1–3, pp. 3–9, 2006.

[35] H. S. Cho, S. Kim, S. Y. Lee, J. A. Park, S. J. Kim, and H. S. Chun, "Protective effect of the green tea component, L-theanine on environmental toxins-induced neuronal cell death," *NeuroToxicology*, vol. 29, no. 4, pp. 656–662, 2008.

[36] A. Kachroo, L. R. Orlando, D. K. Grandy, J. F. Chen, A. B. Young, and M. A. Schwarzschild, "Interactions between metabotropic glutamate 5 and adenosine A2A receptors in normal and parkinsonian mice," *Journal of Neuroscience*, vol. 25, no. 45, pp. 10414–10419, 2005.

[37] L. Shen, "Tea intake and liver diseases," *Hepatology*, vol. 53, no. 1, pp. 373–374, 2011.

[38] A. Crozier, I. B. Jaganath, and M. N. Clifford, "Dietary phenolics: chemistry, bioavailability and effects on health," *Natural Product Reports*, vol. 26, no. 8, pp. 1001–1043, 2009.

Epidemiological Patterns of Varicella in the Period of 1977 to 2012 in the Rijeka District, Croatia

Vjekoslav Bakašun and Đana Pahor

Public Health Institute, 51000 Rijeka, Croatia

Correspondence should be addressed to Vjekoslav Bakašun; vjekoslav.bakasun@ri.t-com.hr

Academic Editor: Huibert Burger

The incidence and distribution of reported varicella cases in the Rijeka District (RD), Croatia (323,130 inhabitants in 1990 and because of the new administrative distribution 305,505 inhabitants in 1991), from 1977 to 2012 are presented. During this period, varicella is continuously present in the RD and these epidemics appear practically every other year. The highest incidence of 1642 per 100,000 inhabitants was registered in 1987. High incidence was also registered during the interepidemic years, while the lowest 247 per 100,000 inhabitants was registered in 2001. Children between the ages of 5 and 9 years were mostly infected, while 87.7% of the 78,883 registered cases were in those up to 14 years. Varicella manifests most intensively during winter and spring, with a peak in March and April. Males are not significantly more affected (51.1%) than females (48.9%). In the observed period, there was not a single reported case of death connected with the varicella disease.

1. Introduction

Varicella (chickenpox) is generally perceived to be a common contagious predominantly childhood disease with relatively benign morbidity. Children aged 5 to 9 have the highest incidence. It is endemic in large urban centres with superimposed epidemics every 2 to 3 years. Varicella occur all year round, but in temperate climates it is typically more frequent in the late winter and early spring time [1, 2].

Varicella did not arouse much attention during earlier years when measles, mumps, and rubella were uncontrolled, and data on its incidence were rarely published. Because vaccination programs have resulted in decreased rates of measles, mumps, and rubella, varicella now ranks as the most common exanthema of childhood. Therefore the control of varicella now draws greater attention. Vaccine has been developed and in the last twenty years it has been used in national childhood vaccination programs in some countries. In Croatia, varicella vaccination has not yet been made a part of the programme of vaccination [1]. The individual varicella vaccination of children is being conducted by certain paediatricians in the private sector, but that data is not available. One can only assume that the number of vaccinated children remains rather insignificant. Showing varicella epidemiological characteristics in the prevaccination period is considered useful, due to their probable changes following the introduction of the vaccine.

The purpose of this paper is to present the epidemiological characteristics of reported cases of varicella in the Rijeka District (RD), Croatia, during the period of 1977 to 2012.

2. Material and Methods

The Rijeka District had 321,007 inhabitants in 1990. Because of territorial administrative changes this region has become smaller, and the number of population has been reduced since 1991 (305,505 inhabitants) [3]. Since July 1976 the reporting of varicella cases has become compulsory. It has been done by post on official forms by general practitioners employed in the Health Centres. Until 1991 there was no private primary health care practice, which since then has been introduced. Today about three-quarters of these doctors are practicing it. As the obligation is general, some cases were reported by other doctors (mostly specialists of infectious diseases). As

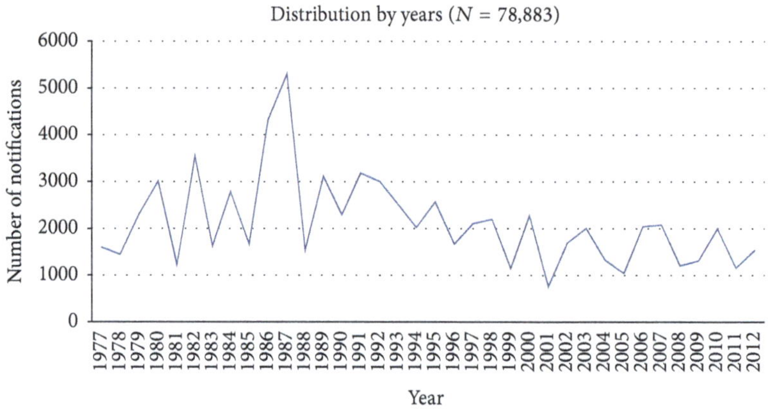

Figure 1: Notification of varicella in RD 1977–2012.

registering was introduced in the middle of 1976, the data analysis in this work began with year 1977.

Reporting has been based on clinical symptoms and signs in patients visited by doctors only. The reports were collected and for the period 1977–2012 were processed and analysed by the Department of Epidemiology, Public Health Institute of Rijeka District (PHI). The official statistics do not include the data about hospitalization and complications in varicella patients.

3. Results

There were 78,883 cases of varicella reported in the RD during the thirty-five-year period (1977–2012) of observation. The yearly average was 2,254 cases. Figure 1 shows that varicella is continuously present in the area and that epidemics appear practically every other year. The incidence was high during the interepidemic period, too. The lowest incidence of 247 per 100,000 inhabitants was registered in 2001, while the highest incidence of 1,642 per 100,000 was registered in 1987.

Figure 2 shows the number of cases according to month of report for the total period of observation and demonstrates the seasonality of varicella infection. The highest incidence is registered in the winter (peak in January) and spring months (peaks in March and April). The number of registered cases is small during the summer months, while the smallest number is registered during September.

Out of the total of registered cases, 51.1% were males and 48.9% were females. The age distribution of the registered cases (Table 1) shows that the highest proportion (41.2%) was in the age group of 5–9 years, followed by the age group of 0–4 years (26.5%) and age group of 10–14 years (20.0%). The majority of cases—87.7%—were in the age group of up to 14 years, while 5.3% of cases were in the age group of 20 years.

Figure 3 gives a more detailed analysis of the registered varicella cases among children and adolescents aged 0–19 years. The cases presented account for 94.7% of all registered cases. High frequencies are recorded from the age of two till eleven, being highest and almost equal in the age of four, five, and six.

Table 1: Age-specific incidence rate of reported varicella cases, RD, 1977–2012 ($N = 78{,}883$).

Age group	Number of reported cases	Age-specific incidence rate 0/0000
0	552	22.0
1–4	20017	200.1
5–9	30961	263.2
10–14	12402	97.7
15–19	7279	52.7
20–29	3356	9.0
30–39	3095	7.7
40–49	929	2.3
50–59	152	0.002
60 and over	140	0.002

In the period under observation not a single case of death connected with varicella disease was reported.

4. Discussion

Prior to introduction of compulsory reporting of varicella cases in 1976, epidemiological characteristics and patterns in RD had not been available.

Varicella is the most commonly notified communicable disease as almost everyone is infected before reaching adulthood. The clinical diagnosis of a typical varicella case is simple, and we consider that yet many cases have still not been reported [2]. The number of reported cases depends partly on the legal duty, but also on the attitude of responsible general practitioners. Probably underreporting of the disease is due to it being so mild in many children whose parents recognised it and did not consult the primary health doctor or perhaps sought a consultation for only the index case in a family and not for subsequent cases [4].

In order to achieve better reporting of varicella in the RD, two actions were done. The first is through education. The epidemiologist from the PHI in Rijeka teaches epidemiology

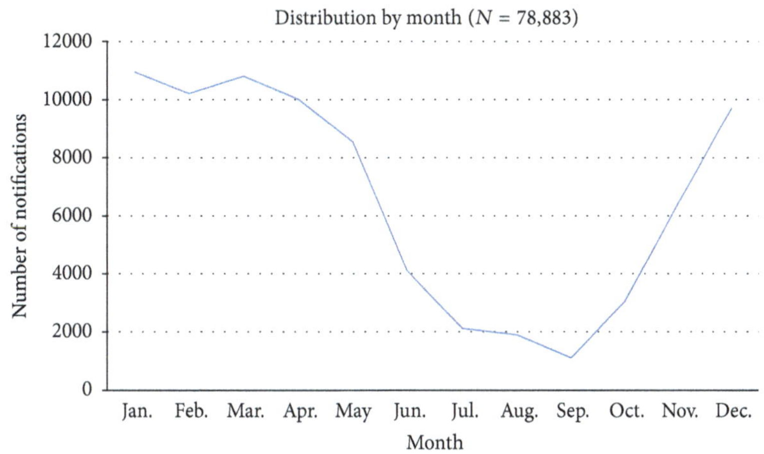

FIGURE 2: Notification of varicella in RD 1977–2012.

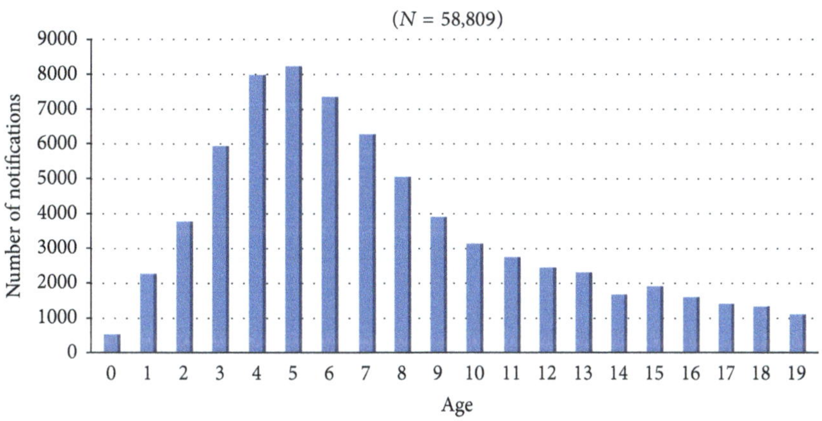

FIGURE 3: Incidence rate of reported varicella cases by the age of 0–19, 1977–2012.

at the Faculty of Medicine, University of Rijeka, where he informs the students about the obligatory reporting of infectious diseases (including varicella). The second is a close cooperation between the Department of Epidemiology of the PHI and general practitioners. The result of such a long period of cooperation is a very good reporting of all infectious diseases.

Because of this, it is assumed that the number of reported cases of varicella in the RD is very close to the actual number of the manifested cases. There were 111,435 children born in RD during the period of observation (yearly average was 3,183), while there were 78,883 registered varicella cases (yearly average was 2,254). Comparing the number of children with the number of registered varicella cases, it can be concluded that 70,8% (probably even more) of children develop typical symptoms and manifest a clinical form of varicella.

The data in Figure 1 displays the decrease of the number of registered varicella cases in the last twenty years. It cannot be proven, but that is a probable consequence of the privatisation of Primary Health Service after 1993. Those doctors, although required, tend to report in lesser numbers those who are infected with infectious diseases.

According to the data available, varicella is evidently endemically present in the RD, and an epidemic is registered nearly every other year, and interepidemic periods are characterised with relatively high incidences.

Clinical reporting scheme in the RD ranged from 247 to 1,642 per 100,000 inhabitants, with a yearly average rate of 945 per 100,000. The average rate is nearly 50 per cent higher, and the maximum is two times higher than the one registered in England and Wales practically in the same period [5] and compared to Slovenia [6, 7].

The analysis of the data indicates that on average 0.72% of the population in RD contract varicella each year. In England and Wales this average was 0.5% in the same period [5].

Varicella is most frequent in this area during the winter and spring months, that is a typically seasonal distribution in the temperate zone. A considerable fall in the registered cases during February is believed to be due to the fact that this month is three days shorter than the two immediately preceding and following it. It is also a result of the winter school holidays in RD, which temporarily break the chain of infections in schools. However, the exclusion from class of the sick, once the disease appeared, did not break the chain of infection.

There is very small prevalence (1.04 : 1.0) of registered cases in males compared to females. The same was noted by other authors as well [1, 5].

The highest incidence of infection is between the ages of 5 and 9 years, which is a known characteristic of varicella [1, 2]. There were 87.7% of cases registered in the 0–14-year age group. This conforms with the findings elsewhere [1, 2, 8–10]. A detailed observation according to age in the RD shows that the most affected are preschool children in the fourth, fifth, and sixth year of life. It can be explained by the fact that many children of that age attend kindergartens, so that starting the elementary school does not represent a greater stimulus for the spreading of the disease.

Officially, there have been no reported cases of varicella related deaths. The authors will do a follow-up research and try to get a hold of the hospital documentation and verify this data.

To conclude, one can only question oneself. In the light of the fact that the varicella were uniformly not serious, one can ask oneself whether or not there are any reasons to use a vaccine to prevent it. After all, the natural immunity acquired by overcoming varicella leaves behind a lifelong immunity. The time span from the introduction of the vaccine has been too short to determine the duration of the immunity acquired by vaccination. Only the decades to follow will be showing the success of the vaccines used for varicella prevention.

Conflict of Interests

The authors declare that there is no conflict of interests regarding the publication of this paper.

References

[1] R. J. Whitney, "Varicella-zoster virus," in *Principles and Practice of Infectious Diseases*, G. L. Mandell, J. E. Bennett, and R. Dolin, Eds., pp. 1963–1969, Churchill Livingstone Elsevier, 7th edition, 2010.

[2] S. R. Preblud, W. A. Orenstein, and K. J. Bart, "Varicella: clinical manifestations, epidemiology and health impact in children," *Pediatric Infectious Disease*, vol. 3, no. 6, pp. 505–509, 1984.

[3] Anonimus, *Zdravstveno-Statistički Ljetopis Primorsko-Goranske Županije Za 2012*, Zavod za Javno Zdravstvo Rijeka, Rijeka, Croatia, 2013.

[4] R. E. Hote-Simpson, "Infectiousness of communicable diseases in the household (measles, chickenpox, and mumps)," *The Lancet*, vol. 2, no. 12, pp. 549–554, 1952.

[5] C. A. Joseph and N. D. Noah, "Epidemiology of chickenpox in England and Wales, 1967–85," *British Medical Journal*, vol. 296, no. 6623, pp. 673–676, 1988.

[6] M. Sočan, A. Kraigher, and L. Pahor, "Epidemiology of varicella in Slovenia over a 20-year period (1979–98)," *Epidemiology and Infection*, vol. 126, no. 2, pp. 279–283, 2001.

[7] M. Socan and M. Blaško, "Surveillance of varicella and herpes zoster in Slovenia, 1996 –2005," *Eurosurveillance*, vol. 12, pp. 13–16, 2007.

[8] S. Deguen, N. P. Chau, and A. Flahault, "Epidemiology of varicella in France (1991–1995)," *Journal of Epidemiology and Community Health*, vol. 52, supplement 1, pp. 46S–49S, 1998.

[9] J. C. Bramley and I. G. Jones, "Epidemiology of chickenpox in Scotland: 1981 to 1998," *Communicable Disease and Public Health*, vol. 3, no. 4, pp. 282–287, 2000.

[10] A. M. Ross and D. M. Fleming, "Chickenpox increasingly affects preschool children," *Communicable Disease and Public Health*, vol. 3, no. 3, pp. 213–215, 2000.

13

Breast Cancer in Young Brazilian Women: Challenge for the Oncology Care

Angela Andréia Franca Gravena,[1] Catia Milene Dell Agnolo,[2] Tiara Cristina Romeiro Lopes,[2] Marcela de Oliveira Demitto,[2] William Augusto de Mello,[1] Deise Helena Pelloso Borghesan,[1] Sheila Cristina Rocha Brischiliari,[1] Maria Dalva de Barros Carvalho,[1] and Sandra Marisa Pelloso[1,2]

[1] *Postgraduate Health Sciences Program, Maringa State University, Colombo Avenue 5790, 87020-900 Maringa, PR, Brazil*
[2] *Department of Nursing, Postgraduate Nursing Program, Maringa State University, Nossa Senhora da Glória Street, 56-A Jardim, São Jorge, 87080-620 Maringa, PR, Brazil*

Correspondence should be addressed to Catia Milene Dell Agnolo; catiaagnolo@gmail.com

Academic Editor: H. Anton-Culver

Objective. To investigate and compare aspects of breast cancer in young women (<40 years old) with older women (>40 years old). *Methods.* Retrospective, cross-sectional, analytical, and exploratory study based on data from 2009 to 2012 obtained from the Breast Cancer Information System (SISMAMA) and the Unified Health System Information Data (DATASUS). The studied population consisted of women ($n = 31.195$) with malignant breast cancer. The analysed variables were education level, race, nodule detection at the clinical examination or image studies, presence of palpable axillary lymph nodes, surgical approach, and tumor histological type and grade. *Results.* There was increasing detection of breast cancer cases in young women among the studied years. Young women had more palpable lymph nodes (OR 1.28, 95% CI: 1.18–1.39), ductal carcinoma as the most frequent histologic type (OR 1.36, 95% CI: 1.22 to 1.53), and grades II and III tumor (OR 16.01 , 95% CI: 13.30 to 19.28). The lesion detection by clinical examination was higher in women <40 years (OR 1.34, 95% CI: 1.24 to 1.45). *Conclusion.* Although there are early detection measures related to breast cancer, they are not the usual practice of the young female public, suggesting the need for a review of existing public policies in the country.

1. Introduction

Breast cancer has high prevalence and is among the leading causes of death worldwide. In Brazil, data from the National Cancer Institute (INCA) project 57,120 new cases of breast cancer in 2014, accounting for 20.8% of new cancers in women [1]. Data from the International Agency for Research on Cancer show that 1.38 million new breast cancer cases are diagnosed each year, representing more than 23% of all cancers among women [2].

Over the past 20 years, Public Health Policies were created with the aim of preventing cancer of the cervix and early detection of breast cancer, diseases whose actions are considered priority for the Health [3]. The National Policy for Cancer Care has tightened controls of breast cancer and cervical cancer as fundamental in the state and municipal health plans [4, 5] consolidating the existing political component. The recent National Plan of Policies for Women (PNPM) of the federal government, launched in 2013, proposes the reduction of cancer mortality in the female population, as well as promoting increased access to quality mammography in the public health system, ensuring detection and treatment in adequate time. Expanding access to breast cancer treatments and psychosocial support to women was also proposed [1].

In Brazil, the Ministry of Health recommends a mammography at least every two years for women 50–69 years of age [1, 3] and the annual clinical breast exam for women 40–49 years of age. For women considered to be at high risk of breast cancer (with family history of breast cancer in first-degree relatives), clinical breast exam and a mammogram every year starting at the age of 35 are recommended [3].

Although breast cancer occurs most often in women over the age of 50, several reports have been published suggesting an increase in the incidence and mortality in young women in different world populations [6]. In young women breast cancer is the leading cause of death in both western and developing countries [7], representing 5% to 7% of cases in some series [8].

Studies suggest that early breast cancer differs from breast cancer in the usual age, regarding etiology, tumor behavior, and prognosis [9–12]. These features can be partly explained by the fact that women under the age of 35 usually have more advanced breast cancer at diagnosis, a higher prevalence of axillary lymph node involvement, less differentiated tumors with a higher proliferation rate and a higher rate of recurrence of cancer [13].

The public service prioritizes screening for women over the age of 50, and breast cancer in young women is still poorly understood in Brazilian women. To our knowledge this study is the first attempt to analyze aspects related to breast cancer in young women. Thus the present study aimed to investigate and compare aspects of breast cancer in young women (<40 years) with older women cancer.

To our knowledge this study was the first analysis of some clinical and biological aspects of breast cancer in young women (<40 years) in Brazil. Thus, the present study aimed to investigate and compare some demographic, clinical, and biological aspects of young patients with breast cancer compared with older women.

2. Methods

This is a retrospective, cross-sectional, analytical, and exploratory study, based on available epidemiological data of women with malignant breast cancer registered in the database of the Information System of Breast Cancer (SISMAMA) and the Unified Health System Data (DATASUS) of the Brazilian Ministry of Health [14, 15]. The SISMAMA is an important tool for official information and provision of computerized data related to screening and diagnostic confirmation of breast cancer in Brazil (Ordinance 779 of 2008) [16].

The studied population consisted of Brazilian women with malignant breast cancer diagnosed between January 2009 and December 2012, separated into two groups according to the age at the diagnosis: young women (less than 40 years) and older women (more than 40 years).

The following variables were evaluated: education (<8 and ≥8 years), race (black and nonblack), lesion detection (clinical breast examination or image study), palpable lymph nodes (presence or absence), histological type (ductal carcinoma or others) and degree (grades I or II and III) of the lesions, and surgical approach (simple or radical mastectomy).

Statistical tests were performed to evaluate demographic, clinical, and pathological characteristics in the two studied groups. The data analyses were performed using the TabWin (DATASUS) and Excel (Microsoft) software. For bivariate analysis statistical program Epi Info version 3.5.1 was used.

As the data was obtained from public domain databases, it was not necessary to refer the project to the Research Ethics Committee; however, the researchers followed all ethical provisions of Resolution CNS 466/2012 published by the Brazilian National Council of Health.

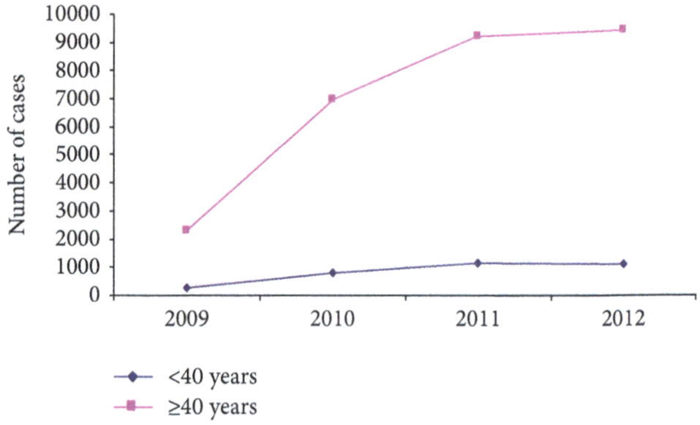

FIGURE 1: Number of cases of breast cancer in Brazilian women from January 2009 to December 2012.

3. Results

A total of 31.195 cases of breast cancer were identified in Brazil between 2009 and 2012. Of this total, 3.039 (10.6%) occurred in women younger than 40. The number of cases of breast cancer increased between the years 2009 and 2012 for both groups of women (Figure 1).

It was observed that women younger than 40 years with less than 8 years of educational background were less likely to develop breast cancer than women with more than 8 years of education (OR 0.62, $P < 0.001$) (Table 1).

The lesion detection by the clinical breast examination as well as the presence of palpable axillary lymph nodes was more common in women <40 (OR 1.34, $P < 0.001$ and OR 1.28, $P < 0.001$) (Table 1).

The most frequent histological type was ductal carcinoma compared to other histological types (10.9% versus 8.2%). According to the histological grade, younger women had 16.01 times more likely to develop grades II and III tumors than the older women ($P < 0.001$) (Table 1).

4. Discussion

The definition of young women with breast cancer is still controversial in the literature, with different authors defining different ages as young, varying from 30 to 45 years [9, 17–19]. In this study those less than 40 were considered as young women.

To our knowledge this is the first study of the clinical and biological aspects of breast cancer in Brazilian young women.

The total number of breast cancer cases found in this study was 31.195. An increase in the number of cases was identified between the years 2009 and 2012, similar to a research conducted in the United States that found an

TABLE 1: Characteristics of breast cancer in Brazilian women from January 2009 to December 2012.

Variables	Age group <40 N (%)	Age group ≥40 N (%)	OR (IC 95%)	*P* value
Number of cases	3309 (10.6)	27886 (89.4)		
Education level				
<8 years	353 (8.1)	4049 (91.9)	0.62 (0.54–0.70)	<0.001
≥8 years	843 (12.4)	5961 (87.6)	1.0	
Lesion detection				
Clinical breast exam	2210 (11.5)	16939 (88.5)	1.34 (1.24–1.45)	<0.001
Image study	973 (8.8)	9993 (91.2)	1.0	
Palpable axillary lymph node				
Presence	1124 (11.9)	8316 (88.1)	1.28 (1.18–1.39)	<0.001
Absence	1635 (9.5)	15494 (90.5)	1.0	
Histological type				
Ductal carcinoma	2145 (10.9)	17468 (89.1)	1.36 (1.22–1.53)	<0.001
Others	397 (8.2)	4413 (91.8)	1.0	
Histological degree				
Grade I	150 (7.2)	1932 (92.8)	1.0	<0.001
Grade II or III	1621 (11.1)	13014 (88.9)	16.01 (13.30–19.28)	
Surgical approach				
Simple mastectomy	121 (13.6)	769 (86.4)	1.0	0.1305
Radical mastectomy	354 (11.6)	2686 (88.4)	0.84 (0.67–1.05)	

increased incidence of breast cancer with metastases in young women (aged 25–35) at the diagnosis (1.53 per 100.000 in 1976 to 2.90 per 100.000 in 2009), without a corresponding increase in older women [20].

The same increasing incidence of breast cancer among young women across the years was registered in Shanghai/China [21], France [22], and Spain [3].

Over the past decade the incidence of breast cancer is increasing among young women, worrying about public health factor. This increase in rates of breast cancer will have important implications for the costs of health services. Hospitalizations in the public health system for breast cancer and cervical cancer are those that require more spending on admissions and are related to loss of user productivity as well. In the period 2008–2011 the costs of hospitalization were 136 million [23].

The treatment of breast cancer also involves public spending. Mastectomy represented the largest spending of about 12 million dollars in the years 2008–2011. Chemotherapy was responsible for 564 million, totaling R$ 712 million spent in treatment, equivalent to 11.87% of total spending for all types of cancer. The expenses with prevention, promotion, and early detection totaled 176 million [23].

For individuals with cancer the government provides sickness benefits and sometimes disability retirement, expensive for public service [24].

The diagnosis and treatment of cancer have social, economic, physical, emotional/psychological, and sexual repercussions for individuals who receive this diagnosis and their families [25].

Study conducted in 2013 women with mastectomies reported that younger patients had to stop working due to cancer treatment, which gave them higher financial difficulties and poor quality of life related to vitality, social, and emotional aspects [26].

The increased incidence of breast cancer in young women should not be attributed to an improvement in the diagnostic methods, as young women are not included in public policies of screening.

Thus, the reduction in delayed diagnosis of breast cancer in our country implies the revision of the current official recommendations for the start of mammographic screening and adherence to this policy of public health.

The trend is that new cases of the disease diagnosed in advanced stages remain emerging from younger women attending public health services. A discussion should be made about the cost-effectiveness of implementation of mammography as a screening option for younger women in Brazil [27].

Mammography is less sensitive and specific for breast cancer screening in women under the age of 35, due to the higher breast density [17]. According to Johnstone et al. [28], the mammography is normal in 90% of the breast cancers in young women. In the present study it was observed that younger women detect the cancer more frequently by the clinical examination (11.5%) compared to imaging tests (8.8%). Trufelli et al. (2008) [29] found that a palpable nodule is the main complaint of the consultation (75.4%).

The clinical breast examination is recommended in Brazil only for women aged 40–49 [3]. Based on the recommendations established by the technical guidelines of the Ministry of Health, the inclusion of other diagnostic methods for breast cancer in young Brazilian women, such as the clinical examination of breast before the age of 40, or even the use of ultrasound examination of breasts, and public policies that encourage the achievement of self-examination for young women [3], is suggested. These techniques would help in early diagnosis of breast cancer in young women, by presenting different clinical aspects of breast cancer in usual age [17, 18, 30, 31].

Regarding clinical characteristics, the presence of palpable axillary lymph nodes was higher in women younger than 40. Other authors have obtained similar results [18, 31, 32]. A survey of women with breast cancer under the age of 30 found that in 90% of cases the first signal was a clinically palpable nodule, with an average size of 3.5 cm [32]. Higher rates of involvement of axillary lymph nodes are described in patients under the age of 40 compared with older patients [33]. A Nepal study with 944 breast cancer patients admitted to a University Hospital between November 1997 and October 2012 identified that axillary lymph nodes were positive in 73% of younger patients (<40 years) and 59% of older patients ($P = 0.002$) [31]. These findings suggest that breast cancer in young women is more aggressive, with the involvement of axillary lymph nodes at diagnosis indicating the severity of the disease in this age group.

Similarly to other studies, the most frequent histological type of breast cancer in young women was ductal carcinoma [31, 34, 35]. Bouzid et al. (2013) [17], in an analytical retrospective survey conducted in Tunisia with breast cancer women younger than 35, identified that the infiltrating ductal carcinoma was present in 95% of cases.

Although the histological type most often found in young women has been infiltrating ductal carcinoma, it is known that the breast cancer manifests more aggressively at this age [36]. What explains the aggressiveness of breast cancer in young women is the histological grade of the lesion [18, 34, 37, 38]. In the present study, younger women were 16.01 times more likely to develop grades II and III tumors than older women. Bouzid et al. (2013) [17] found that grades II and III tumors were present in 41.1% and 37.1% of cases, respectively. Dimitrakakis et al. (2013) [30] when comparing groups of women with cancer at age less than 25 with breast cancer women aged more than 25 noted that the first group exhibited a higher histological grade.

Breast cancer prognosis is poorer in young women than in older women [17, 30, 39, 40]. It is usually characterized by recurrence rate between 20 and 30%, higher incidence of advanced histological grade, advanced stage at diagnosis, more frequent BRCA1 mutations [41], and higher rate of cell proliferation [39, 42].

Freedman and Partridge (2013) [4] asserted that the reasons for the biological differences for breast cancer at different ages are poorly understood. However mutations in BRCA1 may explain some of the types of high-grade triple negative cancer observed in young women.

There is no scientific evidence that lower educational background is a protective factor for breast cancer. However, one can assume that, in Brazil, by socioeconomic and cultural reasons, this population consumes less animal fat, eats more vegetables, and has longer breastfeeding.

This study has some limitation. It was retrospective and missing data from Public Health Agencies is a problem, making the understanding of the real scenario of the breast cancer in Brazilian young women difficult.

Early detection of breast cancer appears to be of utmost importance to support public policies that address women's health, the implementation of screening programs, and to provide data for clinical research. The trend is that new cases of the disease, diagnosed in advanced stages, continue emerging from younger women attending public health services. Further studies of the breast cancer in young women are needed.

5. Conclusion

There was an increase in cases of breast cancer in young women among the studied years. Young women with breast cancer had more palpable axillary lymph nodes, ductal carcinoma as the most frequent histological type, and more advanced tumor grade when compared with older women. An important finding of this study was the identification that the clinical examination was the main tool of breast cancer diagnosis in younger women. Clinical protocols and public policies that encourage this form of detection for young women are advisable in Brazil.

In this sense, we suggest a review of existing public policies in the country, besides conducting new studies to assess the real impact of the use of mammography as a screening in women in general, even those who have low risk of breast cancer, considering the other risk factors, as well as deploy other methods of screening in younger women, aiming at a reduction in the prevalence of breast cancer in Brazil.

Conflict of Interests

The authors declare that there is no conflict of interests regarding the publication of this paper.

References

[1] Brasil, Ministério da Saúde, *Estimativa de 2014, Incidência de câncer no Brasil*, Instituto Nacional de Câncer, Ministério da Saúde, 2013.

[2] J. Ferlay, H. R. Shin, F. Bray, D. Forman, C. Mathers, and D. M. Parkin, "Cancer Incidence and Mortality Worldwide: IARC Cancer Base," GLOBOCAN 2008, no. 10, International Agency for Research on Cancer, Lyon, France, 2010.

[3] M. Pollán, R. Pastor-Barriuso, E. Ardanaz et al., "Recent changes in breast cancer incidence in Spain, 1980–2004," *The Journal of the National Cancer Institute*, vol. 101, no. 22, pp. 1584–1591, 2009.

[4] R. A. Freedman and A. H. Partridge, "Management of breast cancer in very young women," *The Breast*, vol. 22, pp. 176–179, 2013.

[5] Brasil. Ministério da Saúde. Portaria 2439, de 08 de dezembro de 2005, "Institui a Política Nacional de Atenção Oncológica: Promoção, Prevenção, Diagnóstico, Tratamento, Reabilitação e Cuidados Paliativos, a ser implantada em todas as unidades

federadas, respeitadas as competências das três esferas de gestão," Diário Oficial [da] Republica Federativa do Brasil. Brasília, DF, 2005 Dez 09; Seção 1, fls.80-81.

[6] S. Santos, *Câncer de mama em mulheres jovens: incidência, mortalidade e associação com os polimorfismos dos genes NQO1, CYP17 e CYP19 [Tese]*, Escola Nacional de Saúde Pública Sérgio Arouca, Rio de Janeiro, Brazil, 2013.

[7] American Cancer Society, *Breast Cancer Facts & Figures 2011 e 2012*, American Cancer Society, Atlanta, Ga, USA, 2012.

[8] D. F. Hayes, "Follow-up of patients with early breast cancer," *New England Journal of Medicine*, vol. 356, no. 24, pp. 2505–2513, 2007.

[9] M. A. Bollet, B. Sigal-Zafrani, V. Mazeau et al., "Age remains the first prognostic factor for loco-regional breast cancer recurrence in young (<40 years) women treated with breast conserving surgery first," *Radiotherapy and Oncology*, vol. 82, no. 3, pp. 272–280, 2007.

[10] C. K. Anders, R. Johnson, J. Litton, M. Phillips, and A. Bleyer, "Breast cancer before age 40 years," *Seminars in Oncology*, vol. 36, no. 3, pp. 237–249, 2009.

[11] H. Fredholm, S. Eaker, J. Frisell, L. Holmberg, I. Fredriksson, and H. Lindman, "Breast cancer in young women: poor survival despite intensive treatment," *PLoS ONE*, vol. 4, no. 11, Article ID e7695, 2009.

[12] J. Tichy, E. Lim, and C. Anders, "Breast cancer in adolescents and young adults: a review with a focus on biology," *Journal of the National Compreensive Cancer Network*, vol. 11, pp. 1060–1069, 2013.

[13] G. M. Swanson, S. Z. Haslam, and F. Azzouz, "Breast cancer among young African-American women: a summary of data and literature and of issues discussed during the "Summit Meeting on Breast Cancer Among African American Women," Washington, DC, September 8–10, 2000," *Cancer*, vol. 97, no. 1, pp. 273–279, 2003.

[14] Brasil, DATASUS, Ministério da Saúde, Departamento de Informática do SUS, Informações de saúde, Estatísticas vitais, http://www2.datasus.gov.br/DATASUS/index.php?area=0205.

[15] Brasil, Ministério da Saúde, DATASUS, Informações de saúde, Epidemiologia e Morbidade, http://www2.datasus.gov.br/DATASUS/index.php?area=0203.

[16] Brasil, Ministério da Saúde, Portaria 779/31 de dezembro de 2008, http://dtr2001.saude.gov.br/sas/PORTARIAS/Port2008/PT-779.htm.

[17] N. Bouzid, R. Lahmar, S. Tebra, and N. Bouaouina, "Cancer du sein chez la femme jeune de moins de 35 ans en Tunisie: étude rétrospective à propos de 124 cas," *Gynécologie Obstétrique & Fertilité*, vol. 41, pp. 356–360, 2013.

[18] H. Boufettal, M. Noun, and N. Samouh, "Breast cancer in young patient in Morrocco," *Cancer Radiotherapy*, vol. 14, no. 8, pp. 698–703, 2010.

[19] G. Coulombe, S. Tyldesley, C. Speers et al., "Is mastectomy superior to breast-conserving treatment for young women?" *International Journal of Radiation Oncology Biology Physics*, vol. 67, no. 5, pp. 1282–1290, 2007.

[20] R. Johnson, F. Chien, and A. Bleyer, "Incidence of breast cancer with distant involvement among women in the United States, 1976 to 2009," *The Journal of the American Medical Association*, vol. 309, no. 8, pp. 800–805, 2013.

[21] Q. Wu, E. Vogtmann, W. Zhang et al., "Cancer incidence among adolescents and young adults in urban Shanghai, 1973–2005," *PLoS ONE*, vol. 7, no. 8, Article ID 42607, 2012.

[22] A. M. Fontenoy, C. Leux, S. Delacour-Billon et al., "Recent trends in breast cancer incidence rates in the Loire-Atlantique, France: a decline since 2003," *Cancer Epidemiology*, vol. 34, no. 3, pp. 238–243, 2010.

[23] Brasil. Ministério da Saúde. Secretária de Vigilância em Saúde. Departamento de Análise da Situação de Saúde. Departamento de Informática do Sistema Único em Saúde (DataSus). Sistema de Informações Hospitalares do SUS, (SIH/SUS), 2012.

[24] Instituto Nacional de Câncer, "Direitos sociais da pessoa com câncer/Instituto Nacional de CÂNCER Jose Alencar Gomes da Silva. Coordenação Geral de ações estratégicas. Divisão de comunicação social," INCA, Rio de Janeiro, Brazil, 3rd edition, 2012.

[25] J. S. Gomes, H. K. Lichtenfels, A. C. B. Kolankiewicz et al., "Qualidade de vida na oncologia: uma revisão bibliográfica," *Revista Contexto e Saúde*, vol. 10, no. 20, pp. 463–472, 2011.

[26] V. L. A. Furlan, M. Sabrino-Neto, L. E. F. Abla et al., "Qualidade de vida e autoestima de pacientes mastectomizadas submetidas ou não a reconstrução de mama," *Revista Brasileira de Cirurgia Plástica*, vol. 28, no. 2, pp. 264–269, 2013.

[27] C. A. Martins, R. M. Guimarães, R. L. P. D. Silva et al., "Evolução da mortalidade por câncer de mama em mulheres jovens: desafios para uma política de atenção oncológica," *Revista Brasileira de Cancerologia*, vol. 59, no. 3, pp. 341–349, 2013.

[28] P. Johnstone, E. Moore, R. Carillo, and C. Goepfert, "Yield of mammography in selected patients age <30 years," *Cancer*, vol. 91, pp. 1075–1078, 2001.

[29] D. Trufelli, V. Miranda, M. Santos et al., "Análise do Atraso no Diagnóstico e Tratamento do Câncer de mama em Hospital Público," *Revista da Associação Médica Brasileira*, vol. 54, no. 1, pp. 72–76, 2008.

[30] C. Dimitrakakis, A. Tsigginou, F. Z. S. Marinopoulos et al., "Breast cancer in women aged 25 years and younger," *Obstetrics and Gynecology*, vol. 121, no. 6, pp. 1235–1240, 2013.

[31] B. Thapa, Y. Singh, P. Sayami, U. Shrestha, R. Sapkota, and G. Sayami, "Breast cancer in young women from a low risk population in Nepal," *Asian Pacific Journal of Cancer Prevention*, vol. 14, no. 9, pp. 5095–5099, 2013.

[32] E. B. Vargas, A. R. Bau, and V. R. A. Vargas, "Analise dos diagnósticos das doencas da mama de mulheres jovnes que apresentaram queixas mamarias," *Revista Brasileira de Mastologia*, vol. 19, no. 4, pp. 141–145, 2009.

[33] C. S. Foo, D. Su, C. K. Chong et al., "Breast cancer in young Asian women: study on survival," *ANZ Journal of Surgery*, vol. 75, no. 7, pp. 566–572, 2005.

[34] A. Khanfir, M. Frikha, F. Kallel et al., "Le cancer du sein de la femme jeune dans le sud tunisien," *Cancer/Radiothérapie*, vol. 10, pp. 565–571, 2006.

[35] H. Bakkali, C. Marchal, A. Lesur-Schwander, and J. L. Verhaeghe, "Le cancer du sein chez la femme de 30 ans et moins," *Cancer/Radiothérapie*, vol. 7, pp. 153–159, 2003.

[36] C. S. Fassarella, A. A. B. Bueno, B. C. S. Ramos, and F. G. S. Toste, "O impacto da notícia de neoplasia de mama em mulheres jovens: revisão de literatura," *Revista Rede de Cuidados em Saúde*, vol. 7, no. 1, pp. 1–10, 2013.

[37] A. Sidoni, A. Cavaliere, G. Bellezza, M. Scheibel, and E. Bucciarelli, "Breast cancer in young women: clinicopathological features and biological specificity," *Breast*, vol. 12, no. 4, pp. 247–250, 2003.

[38] S. Jmor, H. Al Sayeh, S. D. Heyes, S. Paynes, I. Miller, and A. Ah-Seea, "Breast cancer in women aged 35 and under: prognosis

and survival," *Journal Royal College of Surgeons Edinburgh*, vol. 47, no. 6, pp. 693–699, 2002.

[39] A. Kwong, P. Cheung, S. Chan, and S. Lau, "Breast cancer in Chinese women younger than age 40: are they different from their older counterparts?" *World Journal of Surgery*, vol. 32, no. 12, pp. 2554–2561, 2008.

[40] G. Cancello, P. Maisonneuve, N. Rotmensz et al., "Prognosis and adjuvant treatment effects in selected breast cancer subtypes of very young women (<35 years) with operable breast cancer," *Annals of Oncology*, vol. 21, no. 10, pp. 1974–1981, 2010.

[41] M. A. Maggard, J. B. O'Connell, K. E. Lane, J. H. Liu, D. A. Etzioni, and C. Y. Ko, "Do young breast cancer patients have worse outcomes?" *Journal of Surgical Research*, vol. 113, no. 1, pp. 109–113, 2003.

[42] S. Aebi and M. Castiglione, "The enigma of young age," *Annals of Oncology*, vol. 17, no. 10, pp. 1475–1477, 2006.

14

Determinants of Bone Strength Estimated by Calcaneal Ultrasonography in Inuit Women from Nuuk (Greenland)

Alexandra-Cristina Paunescu,[1] Pierre Ayotte,[1,2] Sylvie Dodin,[1] Éric Dewailly,[1] Gert Mulvad,[3] Henning S. Pedersen,[4] and Suzanne Côté[1]

[1] *Axe Santé des Populations et Pratiques Optimales en Santé, Centre de Recherche du CHU de Québec, Québec, QC, Canada G1V 2M2*
[2] *Laboratoire de Toxicologie, Institut National de Santé Publique du Québec, 945 Avenue Wolfe, Québec, QC, Canada G1V 5B3*
[3] *Center of Primary Health Care, Queen Ingrid's Hospital and Greenland Center for Health Research, University of Greenland, Nuuk 3900, Greenland*
[4] *Medical Centre, Dronning Ingrids Hospital, Nuuk 3900, Greenland*

Correspondence should be addressed to Pierre Ayotte; pierre.ayotte@inspq.qc.ca

Academic Editor: Noriko Yoshimura

This study was conducted to identify determinants of bone strength estimated by quantitative ultrasonography (QUS) at the calcaneus of Greenlandic Inuit women. A total of 153 Inuit women from Nuuk, aged from 49 to 64 years, participated in the first QUS measurement (year 2000) with an *Achilles Lunar* instrument (speed of sound (SOS); broadband ultrasound attenuation (BUA); stiffness index (SI)). A second measurement was performed two years later (year 2002) in 121 participants. Several factors known to be associated with bone strength were recorded at baseline for 118 of them. Determinants of QUS parameters were identified using an automatic (stepwise) selection of variables in linear regression. Significant determinants of baseline QUS measurements were age and body weight for all QUS parameters, height for BUA and SI, and hormone replacement therapy (HRT) use for SI. Significant predictors of follow-up QUS measurements were baseline QUS values, the smoking status and HRT use for all QUS parameters, omega-3/omega-6 PUFA content ratio of erythrocytes membrane phospholipids (BUA and SI), and menopausal status (BUA). Several modifiable dietary factors, such as a diet rich in omega-3 PUFAs and lifestyle factors (i.e., smoking, taking HRT), were shown to determine QUS parameters after a follow-up of two years.

1. Introduction

Inuit populations live in extreme climatic conditions and exhibit specific lifestyle and dietary habits, in particular their traditional diet that comprises large amounts of fish and marine mammal meat and fat [1]. Few data are available on the determinants of bone fragility in Inuit living in circumpolar regions. Bone fragility significantly increases the risk of osteoporotic fracture following minimal trauma, which may have serious public health consequences (mortality, morbidity, and health care costs), especially when the event occurs at a later age [2].

Studies conducted during the 70's reported that Inuit experience an earlier onset and a greater bone loss with age, compared to U.S. Caucasians [3–6]. Furthermore, cortical bone thickness in Inuit was also reported to be lower than in Caucasians [5–8]. Thickness values follow a decreasing trend from Mongoloid groups of Umnak-Kodiak on the Bering Sea going eastward to Greenland, with a breaking point between Inupiaq and Yupik Inuit [9]. Histological analyses of the femur revealed that the Inuit possesses more osteons per surface unit than U.S. Caucasians, although osteons are similar in size [6]. The osteon remodeling pattern in Inuit also seems to differ from that in other populations [8, 10, 11]. In a descriptive cross-sectional study among peri- and postmenopausal Inuit women from Nuuk (capital of Greenland), Côté et al. reported lower values of bone parameters measured by quantitative ultrasonography (QUS) at the right calcaneus compared to values obtained in southern Québec women. Mean values for broadband ultrasound attenuation (BUA), speed of sound (SOS), and the stiffness index (SI) were, respectively, 4%, 1.4%, and 9.5% lower in Greenlandic Inuit women compared to the southern Quebec women [12].

Several hypotheses have been raised to explain the osteological features of Inuit, including their diet rich in animal proteins, phosphorus, and nitrogen and low in calcium [3, 4], genetic factors, low sun exposure, and cultural factors [13]. A low dietary calcium intake, smoking, and the chronic use of oral steroids have been identified as major risk factors for low BMD at the calcaneus of Alaska Natives [14]. The shift toward a Western diet was associated with a significant reduction in vitamin D status in Inuit from Nuuk compared to Inuit with a more traditional diet living outside the capital [15], which may have an impact on bone health. The omega-3 PUFAs from marine food, such as eicosapentaenoic acid (EPA) and docosahexaenoic acid (DHA) and an elevated omega-3/omega-6 polyunsaturated fatty acids (PUFAs) content ratio in phospholipids of erythrocyte membranes were associated with increased BUA values in Inuit women from Nuuk [16]. In the study by Côté et al., age and plasma concentration of a mono-ortho substituted polychlorinated biphenyl congener (PCB 156), displaying some dioxin-like (DL) activity, was negatively associated with calcaneal QUS parameters in Inuit women from Nuuk, whereas positive associations were noted with body weight, hormone replacement therapy (HRT), and oral contraceptive uses [12].

The technique of bone ultrasound measurement is simple, rapid, noninvasive, nonradioactive, inexpensive, and can be implemented with easy-to-use portable devices [17]. It is especially well suited to assess bone quality/strength in isolated communities, where the measurement of bone mineral density (BMD, g/cm^2) by dual-energy X-ray absorptiometry (DXA), the reference method for the diagnosis of osteoporosis according to the World Health Organization [18], cannot be performed. Bone parameters measured by QUS reflect the intrinsic quality and biomechanical properties of bone and provide information complementary to that of BMD on bone strength [19]. Despite its advantages, the QUS method has seldom been used to estimate bone strength/quality in these remote areas inhabited by Inuit.

The main objective of this study was to identify the predictors of calcaneal QUS parameters measured after a follow-up of two years in Greenlandic Inuit women participating in a longitudinal study between 2000 and 2002, among a large number of factors recorded at baseline. As a secondary objective, we aimed to identify the determinant factors of bone parameters at baseline in 2000, using a cross-sectional study design.

2. Methods

2.1. Population. A descriptive cross-sectional study was conducted during September 2000 in Nuuk (Godthab, Greenland, 64°N latitude), home to approximately 14,000 residents, in order to assess bone strength in peri- and postmenopausal Inuit women and identify its determinant factors, with a special focus on exposure to food-chain contaminants. Data collection was previously described by Côté et al. [12]. Inclusion criteria were: being a woman aged between 49 and 64 years and born in Greenland. A random sample of 200 women was drawn from the list of Statistics Greenland, which included 547 women who were potentially eligible. Among the 200 women, 7 died, 11 had moved, and 15 were outside the city at the time of the study (not for medical reasons). Finally, 167 women were invited to participate in the study, at the Primary Health Care Clinic of Queen's Ingrid Hospital in Nuuk. Eight of them refused and six were excluded because of diseases (HIV, mental illness, and influenza). Hence, 153 Inuit women participated in the cross-sectional study [12].

Participants answered a questionnaire to document the most important factors affecting bone health during a face-to-face interview conducted in Danish. The questionnaire was adapted from that of the *Mediterranean Osteoporosis Study* [20]. Subsequently, the women participated in a clinical session that comprised blood sampling, anthropometric measurements, and QUS parameter determination at the right calcaneus. Out of the 153 participants, 148 had enough plasma collected to allow biochemical and toxicological analyses.

Two years later, from August 26 to September 3, 2002, participants at the first QUS measurement were invited for a second measurement using the same technique and instrument as in 2000. From the 153 participants in 2000, 121 completed the study in 2002. Of the 32 nonparticipants in 2002, three had died, five had moved, eleven could not be reached by telephone, seven refused to participate, and six did not show up for their appointment. Among the 121 Inuit women who had the second QUS measurement, 118 had a sufficient quantity of plasma collected to allow all biochemical and toxicological analyses.

2.2. QUS Measurements. SOS (m/s) and BUA (dB/MHz) were measured with the *Achilles Lunar* water-bath ultrasound instrument (Lunar Corporation, Madison, WI, USA) at the right calcaneus of participants. A research nurse performed all QUS measurements. SI, a linear combination of the two QUS parameters, was calculated automatically by the device according to the manufacturer's formula [SI% = (0.67 ∗ BUA) + (0.28 ∗ SOS) − 420].

The instrument was calibrated daily using the acoustic phantom provided by the manufacturer. *In vivo* precision was assessed by repeated measurements conducted in 15 subjects: mean coefficients of variation (CV) were 0.8% for BUA, 0.2% for SOS, and 1.1% for SI measurements at baseline [12]. *In vivo* repeated measures for a 42-year-old woman conducted over a one-year period, prior to beginning the follow up measurements, using the same equipment, yielded CV values of 1.4% for BUA, 0.2% for SOS, and 1.3% for SI.

2.3. Anthropometric Measurements. Weight (kg), height, abdominal circumference, and hip circumference (cm) were measured using standardized techniques by research nurses.

2.4. Laboratory Analyses

2.4.1. Lipids. Omega-3 and omega-6 polyunsaturated fatty acids (PUFA) were measured in erythrocyte membrane phospholipids by gas liquid chromatography using a HP5890 gas chromatograph (Hewlett Packard, Toronto, ON) equipped with a HP8823 capillary column, a 7673A autosampler, and a flame ionization detector (FID). The analyses were performed at the Department of Nutritional Sciences, University of Guelph (Ontario) [12]. Erythrocyte membrane total omega-3 PUFAs and total omega-6 PUFAs contents were calculated and expressed as percentages of all fatty acids in membrane phospholipids. Total omega-3 PUFAs refer to the sum of the following fatty acids: alpha-linolenic acid (C18: 3n-3), eicosapentaenoic acid (C20: 5n-3), docosapentaenoic acid (C22: 5n-3), docosahexaenoic acid (C22: 6n-3), C18: 4n-3, C20: 3n-3, C20: 4n-3. Total omega-6 PUFAs refer to the sum of linoleic acid (C18: 2n-6), arachidonic acid (C20: 4n-6), C18: 3n-6, C20: 2n-6, C20: 3n-6, C22: 2n-6, C22: 4n-6, C22: 5n-6.

Plasma cholesterol and triglycerides concentrations (mmol/L) were determined by standard enzymatic procedures on an AutoAnalyzer II instrument (Technicon Instruments Corporation, Tarrytown, NY).

2.4.2. DL-PCB 156. Concentration of DL-PCB 156 was measured in the plasma of participants using gas chromatography-electron capture detection (GC-ECD). The analyses were performed at the Toxicology Laboratory of the *Institut National de Santé Publique de Québec* (INSPQ, Canada), which is accredited under ISO 17025 by the Standards Council of Canada. The analytical method was described by Côté et al. [12]. CV based on repeated analysis of a standard reference material (SRM 1589, $n = 15$) was 18.5%; the percentage of detection was 100% and the detection limit was 0.02 μg/L [12].

2.5. Questionnaire. A questionnaire was administered to document sociodemographic variables (date and place of birth), lifestyle habits (smoking, yes/no; leisure time physical activity (LPA), inactive/active, yes/no; dairy product consumption (milk, cheese, yogurt) per day and during the last week, yes/no; calcium supplementation during the last month, yes/no; sun exposure over the majority of the body during last year, yes/no), gynaecological history (menopausal status, postmenopausal/nonmenopausal; parity, yes/no; total duration of breastfeeding (months); oral contraceptive use in the past, yes/no; HRT use, yes/no), medical history (major diseases), and personal history of fractures during adulthood (yes/no).

Women were considered postmenopausal if they had no menstrual period for one year before their recruitment in the study or if they had a bilateral oophorectomy for more than six months and/or a level of folliculo-stimulating hormone (FSH) > 40 IU/L.

LPA was documented as the weekly frequency of physical activity during leisure time lasting 20–30 minutes, averaged over the last three months [21]. The LPA variable was dichotomised with the inactive-low activity category corresponding to 0–2 times/week of LPA and the active category to LPA frequency ≥ 3 times/week.

The use of certain drugs during the last year (corticosteroids, heparin, Dilantin, Prednisone, and chemotherapy) and some medical conditions (Cushing's disease, rheumatoid arthritis, bone cancer, gastrectomy, renal or hepatic failure, and thyroid and parathyroid diseases) that are linked to bone loss constitute causes of secondary osteoporosis (CSO) [2]. CSO were deemed present if the participant answered positively to one of the elements listed above.

2.6. Statistical Analyses. Descriptive statistics (mean, standard deviation, minimum, maximum for quantitative variables and numbers, and % per modality for categorical variables) were presented for the participants who participated in QUS measurements in 2000 and 2002. Comparisons of characteristics between participants in both QUS measurements and those who attended only the first measurement were carried out using the Student's t-test for continuous variables. We tested differences between groups for categorical variables using the χ^2 test (if conditions were met) or the Fisher's exact test.

Pearson correlation coefficients were computed to test intercorrelations among QUS parameters. All variables documented at baseline were investigated if they were correlated with QUS parameters measured in 2000. Variables with a P-value ≤0.20 in simple regression were retained and used as "candidate" variables in the predictive models.

Collinearity between "candidate" variables and the predictive models was investigated and redundant variables were removed. Box-Cox procedures were used to resolve problems encountered with the hypotheses of normality and/or homoscedasticity in the multiple linear regression models for the dependent variables SOS and SI, which were subsequently log-transformed.

Firstly, the variables documented in 2000 and related to bone quality were considered for inclusion in predictive models of QUS parameters measured concomitantly. Secondly, the same variables were considered for inclusion in predictive models of QUS parameters measured in 2002. QUS parameters determined at baseline were also considered for inclusion in the latter models. Variables were automatically selected using the stepwise method (P-value =0.10 to enter and P-value =0.15 to exit).

We also calculated differences (Δ) in QUS parameters between the second (2002) and the first (2000) measurements for each participant, according to the following formula: $\Delta QUS = QUS_{year\,2002} - QUS_{year\,2000}$. The percent change in QUS parameters that occurred over the two-year period was calculated as follows: $\Delta QUS\% = (\Delta QUS/QUS_{year\,2000}) * 100$.

A P value of <0.05 in a bilateral situation is considered statistically significant. All statistical analyses were performed using the SAS Version 9.2 software (SAS Institute Inc., Cary, NC, USA).

2.7. Approval of the Research Project. The project was approved by the Commission for Scientific Research in Greenland (Denmark), by the Ethical Committee of the Greenlandic Health Commission (Denmark), and by the Research Ethics Committees of the Hôpital Saint-François d'Assise (CHUQ, Québec, Canada). Participation in the study was voluntary and a consent form was signed by each participant. All information concerning the participants was kept strictly confidential.

3. Results

3.1. Characteristics of the Participants. The characteristics of the 118 participants to both QUS measures are presented in Table 1. At the time of recruitment (year 2000), our participants were between 49 and 64 years old, predominantly postmenopausal, sedentary, smokers, and had had children. Few participants claimed to have used oral contraceptives in the past and among postmenopausal women, few had taken HRT. A limited number of participants had sun exposure during the last year and were taking calcium supplements. All nine fracture cases were wrist fractures; one woman with wrist fracture also reported a vertebral fracture in adulthood. A third of Inuit women (41/118) had a small stature (i.e., <153 cm), a condition that can be associated with osteoporosis [22]. The majority of participants (83/118) had an abdominal circumference ≥ 88 cm, which defines abdominal obesity in women [23], a condition associated with an increased risk of developing serious health problems such as type II diabetes, coronary heart disease, and hypertension. Regarding the body mass index (BMI) [23], only 37/118 participants had normal values (between 18.5 and 24.9 kg/m^2), 3/118 were underweight (<18.5 kg/m^2), 42/118 were overweight (25.0–29.9 kg/m^2), 20/118 were obese (30.0–34.9 kg/m^2), and 16/118 were obese morbid (≥35 kg/m^2). No difference was observed between the characteristics of the 30 women who participated only in the first QUS measurement in 2000 and those of the 118 participants who attended both measurements in 2000 and 2002 (Table 1).

3.2. Changes in QUS Parameters between 2000 and 2002. Mean annual differences (±SD) in QUS parameters were −2.38 m/s (±5.25) for SOS, −0.78 dB/MHz (±3.16) for BUA, and −1.18% (±2.77) for SI. Mean percent changes over the two-year interval between QUS parameter measurements were −0.31% (±0.69) for SOS, −1.35% (±5.95) for BUA, and −2.84% (±7.12) for SI. Results from paired tests indicate that QUS parameter changes that occurred between 2000 and 2002 were statistically significant (for ΔSOS: Student's t-test, $P < 0.0001$; sign test, $P = 0.0004$, for ΔBUA; Student's t-test $P = 0.0088$; sign test, $P = 0.0329$; for SI: Student's t-test and sign test, $P < 0.0001$).

Based on ΔSI values, two thirds of participants (77/118) experienced a decrease over two years (ΔSI between −18 and −1), 11% (13/118) had no change (ΔSI = 0), while 24% (28/118) exhibited improved bone quality (ΔSI between +1 and +29). QUS parameters determined in 2002 were all significantly and positively correlated to the initial measurements performed in 2000 ($\text{SOS (log)}_{\text{year 2000}}$ with $\text{SOS (log)}_{\text{year 2002}}$: $r = 0.89$; $\text{BUA}_{\text{year 2000}}$ with $\text{BUA}_{\text{year 2002}}$: $r = 0.81$; and $\text{SI (log)}_{\text{year 2000}}$ with $\text{SI (log)}_{\text{year 2002}}$: $r = 0.90$, all P values <0.0001).

3.3. Determinants of QUS Parameters Measured in 2000 (Table 2). QUS measurements obtained in 2000 were determined by four or five factors, depending on the QUS parameter. Age was the statistically significant determinant of lower QUS values ($\text{SOS}_{\text{year 2000}}$ (log), $\text{BUA}_{\text{year 2000}}$, and $\text{SI}_{\text{year 2000}}$ (log)). Three factors were statistically significant determinants of higher QUS values: body weight ($\text{SOS}_{\text{year 2000}}$ (log), $\text{BUA}_{\text{year 2000}}$, $\text{SI}_{\text{year 2000}}$ (log)), height ($\text{BUA}_{\text{year 2000}}$ and $\text{SI}_{\text{year 2000}}$ (log)), and past HRT use ($\text{SI}_{\text{year 2000}}$ (log)). Age, body weight, and height explained together 82.4%, 91.6%, and 93.3% of the variance explained for $\text{SOS}_{\text{year 2000}}$ (log), $\text{BUA}_{\text{year 2000}}$, and $\text{SI}_{\text{year 2000}}$ (log), respectively.

3.4. Predictors of QUS Parameters Measured in 2002 (Table 3). Models for QUS measurements obtained in 2002 each comprised five factors. For all parameters, the QUS measurement of 2000 was the main determinant of the value measured in 2002, representing 96.3%, 91.9%, and 95.2% of the variance explained for $\text{SOS (log)}_{\text{year 2002}}$, $\text{BUA}_{\text{year 2002}}$, and $\text{SI (log)}_{\text{year 2002}}$, respectively. Two other factors were statistically significant predictors of higher QUS values: past HRT use ($\text{SOS}_{\text{year 2002}}$ (log), $\text{BUA}_{\text{year 2002}}$ and $\text{SI}_{\text{year 2002}}$ (log)) and the omega-3/omega-6 PUFA content ratio in erythrocyte membranes ($\text{BUA}_{\text{year 2002}}$ and $\text{SI}_{\text{year 2002}}$ (log)). Smoking status was a statistically significant predictor of lower values of all QUS parameters ($\text{SOS}_{\text{year 2002}}$ (log), $\text{BUA}_{\text{year 2002}}$ and $\text{SI}_{\text{year 2002}}$ (log)) and menopausal status of lower $\text{BUA}_{\text{year 2002}}$ values.

4. Discussion

This longitudinal study identifies determinants of bone strength/quality, as measured by QUS parameters, in peri- and postmenopausal Greenlandic Inuit women. We found that after a two-year follow-up, lower QUS measures were predicted by smoking and postmenopausal status, whereas past HRT use and an elevated omega-3/omega-6 PUFA content ratio in erythrocyte membranes is predictive of higher QUS values. Baseline QUS measures, the strongest determinants of QUS measures after a two-year follow-up, were themselves determined by age, past HRT use, body weight, and height.

Most predictors of QUS values identified in the present study were also shown to influence bone quality parameters in other populations. Several studies have reported that QUS parameters measured by ultrasound at the calcaneus decrease significantly with age [12, 24–33]. Height [28, 29] and body weight [12, 27–29, 32–34] were also often found to be positively correlated to QUS parameters measured at the heel. According to Babaroutsi et al. (2005), overweight (BMI ≥ 25 kg/m^2) or obese (BMI ≥ 30 kg/m^2) women display significantly higher BUA values (measured with a SAHARA instrument) than women with normal BMI, regardless of their age group [34]. While obesity seems protective against osteoporosis, results from recent epidemiologic and clinical studies indicate that a high body fat level might constitute a risk factor for osteoporosis and fragility fractures [35]. The body fat mass was not measured in our participants. In our study, almost a third of women were considered obese according to the international criteria of BMI. While BMI is an index used frequently in the general population, the measure of obesity based on BMI is not appropriate among Inuit, due to their higher sitting height [36]. The impact of obesity on metabolic indicators such as plasma lipids and blood pressure in Inuit is lower than in other Euro-Canadian populations [36, 37].

TABLE 1: Characteristics of Inuit women.

2002 measurements ($N = 118$)	Mean ± SD	Range	
SOS (m/s)	1518.43 ± 22.66	1468–1600	
BUA (dB/MHz)	106.41 ± 10.56	80–144	
SI (%)	76.07 ± 12.11	50–124	
2000 measurements	Participation in 2000 and 2002 ($N = 118$)	Nonparticipation in 2002 ($N = 30$)	Comparison
QUS parameters	Mean ± SD Range	Mean ± SD Range	Student's t-test P value[a]
SOS (m/s)	1523.19 ± 23.12 1464–1595	1520.90 ± 37.01 1463–1592	0.7479
BUA (dB/MHz)	107.96 ± 9.61 84–136	108.43 ± 15.08 82–140	0.8703
SI (%)	78.42 ± 11.85 51–117	78.10 ± 19.71 47–116	0.9319
Other factors			
Age (years)	55.25 ± 4.22 49–64	56.13 ± 4.90 49–63	0.3261
Total breastfeeding duration (months)	32.21 ± 40.10 0–216	25.33 ± 29.20 1–108	0.3797
Height (cm)	155.89 ± 6.66 142–171	156.27 ± 6.44 145–171	0.7810
Body weight (kg)	67.62 ± 14.46 37–99	66.50 ± 17.49 36–99	0.7164
Ratio abdominal/hip circumference	0.93 ± 0.07 0.78–1.09	0.94 ± 0.07 0.77–1.10	0.2672
Total cholesterol (mmol/L)	2.60 ± 0.48 1.73–4.67	2.56 ± 0.54 1.38–4.24	0.6783
Total triglycerides (mmol/L)	1.64 ± 1.34 0.44–13.36	1.53 ± 0.84 0.61–3.87	0.5939
Omega-3 PUFA (%)	13.97 ± 4.63 4.78–27.56	13.78 ± 5.03 6.15–25.18	0.8476
Omega-6 PUFA (%)	22.79 ± 4.47 12.44–31.45	22.18 ± 4.92 10.87–29.55	0.5106
Ratio omega-3/omega-6 PUFA	0.68 ± 0.37 0.17–2.21	0.70 ± 0.44 0.21–2.32	0.7657
DL-PCB 156 (μg/L)	0.70 ± 0.35 0.13–2.12 0.62[b]	0.86 ± 0.56 0.22–2.31 0.72[b]	0.1450
	N (%)	N (%)	P value[a]
Menopausal status	118	30	
Postmenopausal	107 (90.7)	26 (86.7)	0.5062[c]
Nonmenopausal	11 (9.3)	4 (13.3)	
Parity	118	30	
Yes	108 (91.5)	30 (100)	0.2139[c]
No	10 (8.5)	0 (0)	
Personal history of fracture	118	30	
Yes	9 (7.6)	4 (13.3)	0.3002[c]
No	109 (92.4)	26 (86.7)	

Table 1: Continued.

Causes of secondary osteoporosis (CSO)	118	30	
Yes	12 (10.2)	3 (10)	1.0000[c]
No	106 (89.8)	27 (90)	
Calcium supplement use	118	30	
Yes	12 (10.2)	1 (3.3)	0.4679[c]
No	106 (89.8)	29 (96.7)	
HRT use	118	30	
Yes	10 (8.5)	3 (10)	0.7272[c]
No	108 (91.5)	27 (90)	
Oral contraceptive use	118	30	
Yes	47 (39.8)	12 (40)	0.9865[d]
No	71 (60.2)	18 (60)	
Leisure physical activity (LPA)	118	30	
Active	12 (10.2)	4 (13.3)	0.7415[c]
Inactive or little activity	106 (89.8)	26 (86.7)	
Smoking status	118	30	
Yes	85 (72)	25 (83.3)	0.2059[d]
No	33 (28)	5 (16.7)	
Sun exposure	118	30	
Yes	25 (21.2)	7 (23.3)	0.7987[d]
No	93 (78.8)	23 (76.7)	
Alcohol intake	118	30	
Yes	73 (61.9)	17 (56.7)	0.6026[d]
No	45 (38.1)	13 (43.3)	
Consumption of dairy products	118	30	
Yes (≥1/jour)	106 (89.8)	27 (90)	1.0000[c]
No (0/jour)	12 (10.2)	3 (10)	

[a]Comparison between the participants ($n = 118$) and the nonparticipants ($n = 30$) to the second QUS measurement (2002); [b]Geometric mean; [c]Fisher's exact test; [d]Chi square test.

Several studies have reported that QUS parameters measured at the calcaneus significantly decrease in women going through menopause [24, 25, 30]. Smoking was also identified as a risk factor for decreased bone quality as determined by ultrasonography at the heel [26, 27, 31, 38, 39]. Current or past HRT use has been positively associated with QUS parameters [12, 26]. Women participating in the *Epidemiological Study on the Prevalence of Osteoporosis*, who took HRT for more than a year, had significantly higher SI values compared to those of nonusers, and differences remained significant even 20 years after menopause [27]. HRT use for more than 3 years was associated with higher QUS values compared to those measured in nonusers [40]. In the *EPIC-Norfolk* cohort, BUA values (measured with a CUBA instrument) in women with past HRT use exceeded those of nonusers by an average of 5 dB/MHz [39].

Results of our predictive modelling approach corroborate the positive association previously reported in an explanatory study between increased omega-3/omega-6 PUFA content ratio in erythrocyte membranes and BUA values in Greenlandic Inuit women [16]. The content of omega-3 PUFA in erythrocyte membranes reflects dietary omega-3 PUFA intake. EPA and DHA content of erythrocyte membranes increased with the frequency of 3 or more fish meals per week among the Inuit women of Nuuk ($P = 0.0018$) [16]. Results from *in vitro* studies, laboratory animal experiments, and human studies suggest a beneficial effect of omega-3 PUFAs and low omega-6/omega-3 PUFA ratio on bone health and osteoporosis [41–43].

Côté et al. previously reported that the plasma concentration of DL-PCB 156 was negatively associated with calcaneal QUS parameters in 153 Inuit women from Nuuk [12]. In the current cross-sectional and longitudinal study, DL-PCB 156 concentration measured at baseline was not a determinant of QUS parameters values measured concomitantly or after a two-year follow-up. Also in contrast to the previous results [12], past oral contraceptive use was not found to be a significant predictive factor of QUS parameters. Côté et al.'s study was explanatory and focused exclusively on organochlorine compounds as the main exposure variable; only four adjustment factors (age, body weight, oral contraceptive, and HRT use) were considered in the multivariate models.

Some determinant factors were associated with either BUA or SOS, but not with both parameters. Height was

Table 2: Determinants of QUS parameters at the first measurement (2000).

Model[a]			
$N = 118$			
SOS $(\log)_{\text{year 2000}}$ (m/s)[b]			
$R^2 = 0.2709$			
Variables	R^2 partial	β coefficient (SE)	P value
Intercept	—	7.34480 (0.04531)	<0.0001
Height (cm)	0.1207	0.00035 (0.00022)	0.1077
Age (years)	0.0835	−0.00093 (0.00030)	0.0025
HRT use (Yes/No)	0.0281	0.00862 (0.00456)	0.0610
Weight (kg)	0.0190	0.00027 (0.00011)	0.0172
Ratio waist circumference/hip circumference	0.0196	−0.04157 (0.02396)	0.0856
$\text{BUA}_{\text{year 2000}}$ (dB/MHz)[b]			
$R^2 = 0.4029$			
Variables	R^2 partial	β coefficient (SE)	P value
Intercept	—	48.71032 (20.93768)	0.0218
Height (cm)	0.2147	0.41009 (0.11485)	0.0005
Weight (kg)	0.1234	0.24673 (0.05054)	<0.0001
Age (years)	0.0309	−0.40096 (0.17109)	0.0209
Calcium supplements use (Yes/No)	0.0185	4.03632 (2.34922)	0.0885
HRT use (Yes/No)	0.0155	4.45645 (2.61774)	0.0915
SI $(\log)_{\text{year 2000}}$ (%)[b]			
$R^2 = 0.3657$			
Variables	R^2 partial	β coefficient (SE)	P value
Intercept	—	3.56182 (0.33487)	<0.0001
Height (cm)	0.2065	0.00664 (0.00184)	0.0005
Weight (kg)	0.0734	0.00311 (0.00082)	0.0002
Age (years)	0.0614	−0.00840 (0.00275)	0.0028
HRT use (Yes/No)	0.0243	0.08752 (0.04208)	0.0398

[a]Automatic selection of variables by the stepwise method (entry P value of 0.10 and exit P value of 0.15).
"Candidate" variables in the predictive model were age, height, body weight, waist circumference/hip circumference ratio, ratio omega-3/omega-6 PUFA (or % omega-6 PUFA), DL-PCB 156, total breastfeeding duration, menopausal status, oral contraceptive use, HRT use, smoking status, calcium supplement use, sun exposure, and consumption of dairy products ("candidate" variables were measured at baseline (year 2000) and all these variables in simple linear regression for $\text{QUS}_{\text{year 2000}}$ models had a P value ≤ 0.20).
[b]The same determinants were identified in a predictive model that comprised a greater number of "candidate" variables, for example, variables listed in note [a] plus eight variables with a P value >0.20 in simple regression models. This model included only 101 participants for whom dataset was complete. "Candidate" variables in this predictive model were age, height, body weight, waist circumference/hip circumference ratio, % omega-6 PUFA, DL-PCB 156, total breastfeeding duration, menopausal status, oral contraceptive use, HRT use, smoking status, calcium supplement use, sun exposure, consumption of dairy products, and total cholesterol, total triglycerides, % omega-3 PUFA, personal history of fracture, LPA, CSO, parity, and alcohol intake. All "candidate" variables were measured at baseline (year 2000).

a statistically significant determinant of BUA but not SOS at baseline (year 2000). Omega-3/omega-6 PUFA ratio and menopausal status were determinants of BUA but not SOS at follow-up (year 2002). SOS is the ratio of propagation distance to the pulse transit time across bone. BUA is the rate of attenuation in the acoustic energy across a broad range of frequency; this attenuation is due to the absorption and scattering of ultrasound in the bone, marrow, and soft tissue. Although both SOS and BUA parameters provide information on bone strength, they do not reflect exactly the same bone properties (microarchitectural parameters, bone geometry and composition, or elastic properties) [19, 44]. This may explain the differences observed among the identified predictors. SI, a composite parameter that combines BUA and SOS, appears more useful than the individual parameters for a global evaluation of bone strength determinants.

QUS can evaluate quantitative factors known to be associated with bone strength that are not assessed by DXA, such as cortical thickness, microarchitecture (bone geometry, trabecular orientations), material properties (i.e., bone size, bone mineral content, degree of mineralization, and porosity), and bone elasticity [19, 44]. Bone strength and elasticity determine bone resistance to fractures. Recent studies reported that bone parameters measured by QUS at the calcaneus can predict fractures as effectively as DXA in postmenopausal women and men aged 65 years and older [18, 45]. Values of QUS parameters are generally lower in osteoporotic patients than in healthy subjects [46]. However, it remains unclear

TABLE 3: Predictors of QUS parameters at the second measurement (2002).

Model[a]			
$N = 118$			
SOS $(\log)_{\text{year 2002}}$ (m/s)[b] $R^2 = 0.8306$			
Variables	R^2 partial	β coefficient (SE)	P value
Intercept	—	1.19773 (0.32028)	0.0003
SOS $(\log)_{\text{year 2000}}$ (m/s)	0.7997	0.84241 (0.04380)	<0.0001
Smoking status (Yes/No)	0.0108	−0.00410 (0.00132)	0.0024
HRT use (Yes/No)	0.0102	0.00609 (0.00219)	0.0063
Height (cm)	0.0052	−0.00019 (0.00009)	0.0520
Age (years)	0.0047	−0.00027 (0.00015)	0.0805
$\text{BUA}_{\text{year 2002}}$ (dB/MHz)[c] $R^2 = 0.7092$			
Variables	R^2 partial	β coefficient (SE)	P value
Intercept	—	19.77795 (7.15003)	0.0066
$\text{BUA}_{\text{year 2000}}$ (dB/MHz)	0.6517	0.82784 (0.05972)	<0.0001
Smoking status (Yes/No)	0.0178	−3.53459 (1.21960)	0.0045
Ratio omega-3/omega-6 PUFA	0.0199	4.29757 (1.45547)	0.0038
HRT use (Yes/No)	0.0090	4.28491 (2.01686)	0.0358
Menopausal status (Yes/No)	0.0108	−3.83486 (1.87776)	0.0435
SI $(\log)_{\text{year 2002}}$ (%)[d] $R^2 = 0.8410$			
Variables	R^2 partial	β coefficient (SE)	P value
Intercept	—	0.75016 (0.23022)	0.0015
SI $(\log)_{\text{year 2000}}$ (%)	0.8005	0.85902 (0.04289)	<0.0001
Smoking status (Yes/No)	0.0140	−0.05410 (0.01377)	0.0001
Ratio omega-3/omega-6 PUFA	0.0119	0.05795 (0.01677)	0.0008
HRT use (Yes/No)	0.0092	0.05307 (0.02183)	0.0166
Age (years)	0.0055	−0.00313 (0.00160)	0.0523

[a]Automatic selection of variables by the stepwise method (entry P value of 0.10 and exit P value of 0.15).
"Candidate" variables in the predictive model were $\text{QUS}_{\text{year 2000}}$, age, height, body weight, waist circumference/hip circumference ratio, ratio omega-3/omega-6 PUFA, DL-PCB 156, total breastfeeding duration, menopausal status, oral contraceptive use, HRT use, smoking status, calcium supplement use, sun exposure, and consumption of dairy products ("candidate" variables were measured at baseline, year 2000).

[b]The same predictive variables were identified in a predictive model that comprised a greater number of "candidate" variables: SOS $(\log)_{\text{year 2000}}$, age, height, body weight, waist circumference/hip circumference ratio, % omega-6 PUFA, DL-PCB 156, total breastfeeding duration, menopausal status, oral contraceptive use, HRT use, smoking status, calcium supplement use, sun exposure, consumption of dairy products, and total cholesterol, total triglycerides, % omega-3 PUFA, personal history of fracture, LPA, CSO, parity, and alcohol intake. All "candidate" variables were measured at baseline (year 2000). This model included only 101 participants for whom dataset was complete.

[c]The same predictive variables were identified when all "candidate" variables were included in the predictive model ($\text{BUA}_{\text{year 2000}}$ and the other variables listed in note[b]; $n = 101$).
When % omega-3 PUFA and % omega-6 PUFA were included as "candidate" variables instead of the omega-3/omega-6 PUFA ratio, the % omega-3 PUFA was significant ($P = 0.0049$; R^2 partial = 0.0202). The model ($R^2 = 0.7080$) was $\text{BUA}_{\text{year 2002}} = 18.50058 + 0.82080\text{BUA}_{\text{year 2000}} - 3.42455$ smoking status + 0.33554% omega-3 PUFA + 4.17829HRT use − 3.61551 menopausal status.

[d]The same predictive variables were identified when all "candidate" variables for the predictive model [SI $(\log)_{\text{year 2000}}$ and the other variables given in note[b]] were used ($n = 101$).
When % omega-3 PUFA and % omega-6 PUFA were included as "candidate" variables instead of the omega-3/omega-6 PUFA ratio, the % omega-3 PUFA was significant ($P = 0.0013$; R^2 partial = 0.0113). The model ($R^2 = 0.8397$) was SI $(\log)_{\text{year 2002}} = 0.75160 + 0.85030$SI $(\log)_{\text{year 2000}} - 0.05201$ smoking status + 0.00441% omega-3 PUFA + 0.05289HRT use − 0.00290 age.

as to what elements evaluated by QUS truly correlate with measures of bone strength; a fundamental understanding is still lacking [47]. Differences exist also between the various QUS devices and skeletal sites measured [18].

4.1. Considerations Regarding Our Study. The main advantage of our study is its longitudinal design with repeated measures of QUS parameters two years apart. Causal inference is supported by the fact that exposure factors were measured in 2000, prior to QUS parameter measurements in 2002. In addition, the type of sampling and recruitment allows for generalising our results to the population of Inuit women aged 49 to 64 years living in Nuuk (Greenland). Our study also benefits from the inclusion of a relatively large number of factors known to be associated with bone strength.

Measurement biases in QUS parameters are relatively unlikely. None of the participants had suffered a fracture and none showed oedema of the foot. The temperature of the water bath was constantly monitored and that of the foot verified prior to conducting measurements, because it is known that the temperature of the skin and soft tissue may affect SOS values [18]. Furthermore, data collection in the field (ultrasound measurements, anthropometric measurements) and blood sampling were performed by research nurses using standardized techniques. All laboratory analyses were carried out using standardized methods.

However, our study has some limitations. From the outset, the number of participants of the first QUS measure was low. The percentage of participants lost to follow-up in 2002 was important (20%), which might lead to a selection bias. However, being lost to follow-up was neither related to bone fragility nor to exposures. Women who did not participate in the second bone measurement in 2002 were not different from those who participated in both measures for all factors investigated.

Some potential predictors of bone quality documented by questionnaires may not have been properly assessed. For example, regarding exposure to sunlight as a source of vitamin D, only one question was asked to inquire about any occurrence of whole-body exposure during the last year. The frequency of sun bathing per week, the time of day, or the season during which exposure occurred [48] were not assessed, which may have led to exposure misclassification. The assessment of LPA considered only the frequency of activities; no information was collected on the type of activity performed or its intensity. COS comprised several different diseases and medications [2], without the possibility of distinguishing between different categories because the numbers were too small in each of them. Finally, questions on dietary supplementation covered only calcium and not vitamin D supplements.

In conclusion, even over a short period of two years, significant decreases in QUS parameters were observed in this group of mostly postmenopausal Inuit women. QUS parameters measured two years apart were predicted by a number of modifiable factors, including dietary and lifestyle habits. Reducing smoking prevalence and promoting the traditional diet rich in omega-3 PUFA may improve bone strength of women in this population.

Conflict of Interests

The authors declare that there is no conflict of interests regarding the publication of this paper.

Acknowledgments

The authors would like to thank the Inuit women of Nuuk who participated in this research project and the medical and health care professionals from the Center of Primary Health Care Queen's Ingrid Hospital for their assistance in collecting data. This study was funded by the Commission for Scientific Research in Greenland and by Helsefonden from Denmark. ACP is the recipient of a Doctoral Training Award from the Fonds de Recherche du Québec—Santé and a doctoral scholarship from Nasivvik—Centre for Inuit Health and Changing Environments.

References

[1] S. G. Donaldson, J. Van Oostdam, C. Tikhonov et al., "Environmental contaminants and human health in the Canadian Arctic," *Science of the Total Environment*, vol. 408, no. 22, pp. 5165–5234, 2010.

[2] The Journal of The North American, "Menopause Society, Management of osteoporosis in postmenopausal women: 2010 Position Statement of the North American Menopause Society," *Menopause*, vol. 17, no. 1, pp. 25–54, 2010.

[3] R. B. Mazess and W. Mather, "Bone mineral content of North Alaskan Eskimos," *American Journal of Clinical Nutrition*, vol. 27, no. 9, pp. 916–925, 1974.

[4] R. B. Mazess and W. E. Mather, "Bone mineral content in Canadian Eskimos," *Human Biology*, vol. 47, no. 1, pp. 45–63, 1975.

[5] I. G. Pawson, "Radiographic determination of excessive bone loss in Alaskan Eskimos," *Human Biology*, vol. 46, no. 3, pp. 369–380, 1974.

[6] D. D. Thompson and M. Gunness-Hey, "Bone mineral-osteon analysis of Yupik-Inuping skeletons," *American Journal of Physical Anthropology*, vol. 55, no. 1, pp. 1–7, 1981.

[7] D. D. Thompson, "Age changes in bone mineralization, cortical thickness, and haversian canal area," *Calcified Tissue International*, vol. 31, no. 1, pp. 5–11, 1980.

[8] D. D. Thompson, E. M. Salter, and W. S. Laughlin, "Bone core analysis of Baffin Island skeletons," *Arctic Anthropology*, vol. 18, no. 1, pp. 87–96, 1981.

[9] A. B. Harper, W. S. Laughlin, and R. B. Mazess, "Bone mineral content in St. Lawrence Island Eskimos," *Human Biology*, vol. 56, no. 1, pp. 63–78, 1984.

[10] M. F. Ericksen, "Patterns of microscopic bone remodeling in three aboriginal American populations," in *Early Native Americans: Prehistoric Demography, Economy, and Technology*, D. L. Browman, Ed., pp. 239–270, Mouton Publishers, The Hague, The Netherlands, 1980.

[11] E. A. Richman, D. J. Ortner, and F. P. Schulter-Ellis, "Differences in intracortical bone remodeling in three aboriginal American populations: possible dietary factors," *Calcified Tissue International*, vol. 28, no. 3, pp. 209–214, 1979.

[12] S. Côté, P. Ayotte, S. Dodin et al., "Plasma organochlorine concentrations and bone ultrasound measurements: a cross-sectional study in peri-and postmenopausal Inuit women from Greenland," *Environmental Health*, vol. 5, article 33, 2006.

[13] R. B. Martin, D. B. Burr, and M. B. Schaffler, "Effects of age and sex on the amount and distribution of mineral in Eskimo tibiae," *American Journal of Physical Anthropology*, vol. 67, no. 4, pp. 371–380, 1985.

[14] J. J. Filner, K. D. Krohn, J. A. Lapidus, and T. M. Becker, "Risk factors for osteoporosis in Alaska Native women: a cross-sectional survey," *Alaska Medicine*, vol. 44, no. 1, pp. 8–21, 2002.

[15] L. Rejnmark, M. E. Jorgensen, M. B. Pedersen et al., "Vitamin D insufficiency in greenlanders on a westernized fare: ethnic differences in calcitropic hormones between greenlanders and danes," *Calcified Tissue International*, vol. 74, no. 3, pp. 255–263, 2004.

[16] A. C. Paunescu, P. Ayotte, E. Dewailly et al., "Polyunsaturated fatty acids and calcaneal ultrasound parameters among Inuit women from Nuuk (Greenland): a longitudinal study," *International Journal of Circumpolar Health*, vol. 72, Article ID 20988, 2013.

[17] P. Laugier, "Quantitative ultrasound instrumentation for bone in vivo characterization," in *Bone Quantitative Ultrasound, Springer Science+Business Media B.V*, P. Laugier and G. Haïat, Eds., Chapter 3, pp. 47–71, 2011.

[18] M. A. Krieg, R. Barkmann, S. Gonnelli et al., "Quantitative ultrasound in the management of osteoporosis: the 2007 ISCD Official Positions," *Journal of Clinical Densitometry*, vol. 11, no. 1, pp. 163–187, 2008.

[19] F. Padilla and P. Laugier, "Recent developments in trabecular bone characterization using ultrasound," *Current Osteoporosis Reports*, vol. 3, no. 2, pp. 64–69, 2005.

[20] J. Dequeker, J. Ranstam, J. Valsson, B. Sigurgevisson, and E. Allander, "The Mediterranean Osteoporosis (MEDOS) Study questionnaire," *Clinical Rheumatology*, vol. 10, no. 1, pp. 54–72, 1991.

[21] G. Godin and R. J. Shephard, "A simple method to assess exercise behavior in the community," *Canadian Journal of Applied Sport Sciences*, vol. 10, no. 3, pp. 141–146, 1985.

[22] J. L. Newton, D. E. J. Jones, K. Wilton, J. Pairman, S. W. Parry, and R. M. Francis, "Calcaneal bone mineral density in older patients who have fallen," *QJM—Monthly Journal of the Association of Physicians*, vol. 99, no. 4, pp. 231–236, 2006.

[23] Santé Canada, "Lignes directrices canadiennes pour la classification du poids chez les adultes," 2013, http://www.hc-sc.gc.ca/fn-an/nutrition/weights-poids/guide-ld-adult/index-fra.php.

[24] V. T. T. Hien, N. C. Khan, N. T. Lam et al., "Determining the prevalence of osteoporosis and related factors using quantitative ultrasound in Vietnamese adult women," *American Journal of Epidemiology*, vol. 161, no. 9, pp. 824–830, 2005.

[25] H. F. Saadi, R. L. Reed, A. O. Carter, E. V. Dunn, H. S. Qazaq, and A. R. Al-Suhaili, "Quantitative ultrasound of the calcaneus in Arabian women: relation to anthropometric and lifestyle factors," *Maturitas*, vol. 44, no. 3, pp. 215–223, 2003.

[26] C. Blanchet, Y. Giguère, D. Prud'homme et al., "Leisure physical activity is associated with quantitative ultrasound measurements independently of bone mineral density in postmenopausal women," *Calcified Tissue International*, vol. 73, no. 4, pp. 339–349, 2003.

[27] S. Adami, S. Giannini, R. Giorgino et al., "The effect of age, weight, and lifestyle factors on calcaneal quantitative ultrasound: the ESOPO study," *Osteoporosis International*, vol. 14, no. 3, pp. 198–207, 2003.

[28] C. Heldan de Moura Castro, M. Medeiros Pinheiro, and V. Lúcia Szejnfeld, "Quantitative ultrasound of the calcaneus in Brazilian Caucasian women: normative data are similar to the manufacturer's normal range," *Osteoporosis International*, vol. 11, no. 11, pp. 923–928, 2000.

[29] W. Liu, C. L. Xu, Z. Q. Zhu, S. M. Han, S. Y. Zu, and G. J. Zhu, "Assessment of low quantitative ultrasound values of calcaneus in chinese mainland women," *Journal of Clinical Densitometry*, vol. 9, no. 3, pp. 351–357, 2006.

[30] J. Yamaguchi, G. Truman, and I. D. Cameron, "Lifestyle factors affecting bone ultrasonometry of the calcaneus in Japanese women," *Calcified Tissue International*, vol. 66, no. 1, pp. 43–46, 2000.

[31] J.-D. Lin, J.-F. Chen, H.-Y. Chang, and C. Ho, "Evaluation of bone mineral density by quantitative ultrasound of bone in 16 862 subjects during routine health examination," *British Journal of Radiology*, vol. 74, no. 883, pp. 602–606, 2001.

[32] B. Durmaz, S. Öncel, Y. Kirazli et al., "Quantitative calcaneal ultrasonometry: normative data and age-related changes for stiffness index in the Turkish population," *Journal of Clinical Densitometry*, vol. 9, no. 2, pp. 217–221, 2006.

[33] S. Maggi, M. Noale, S. Gonnelli et al., "Quantitative ultrasound calcaneous measurements: normative data for the Italian population. The ESOPO Study," *Journal of Clinical Densitometry*, vol. 10, no. 3, pp. 340–346, 2007.

[34] E. Babaroutsi, F. Magkos, Y. Manios, and L. S. Sidossis, "Lifestyle factors affecting heel ultrasound in Greek females across different life stages," *Osteoporosis International*, vol. 16, no. 5, pp. 552–561, 2005.

[35] S. Migliaccio, E. A. Greco, R. Fornari, L. M. Donini, and A. Lenzi, "Is obesity in women protective against osteoporosis?" *Diabetes, Metabolic Syndrome and Obesity*, vol. 4, pp. 273–282, 2011.

[36] T. K. Young, "Are the circumpolar inuit becoming obese?" *American Journal of Human Biology*, vol. 19, no. 2, pp. 181–189, 2007.

[37] T. K. Young, P. Bjerregaard, E. Dewailly, P. M. Risica, M. E. Jørgensen, and S. E. O. Ebbesson, "Prevalence of obesity and its metabolic correlates among the circumpolar inuit in 3 countries," *American Journal of Public Health*, vol. 97, no. 4, pp. 691–695, 2007.

[38] C. M. Bernaards, J. W. R. Twisk, J. Snel, W. Van Mechelen, P. Lips, and H. C. G. Kemper, "Smoking and quantitative ultrasound parameters in the calcaneus in 36-year-old men and women," *Osteoporosis International*, vol. 15, no. 9, pp. 735–741, 2004.

[39] A. Welch, J. Camus, N. Dalzell, S. Oakes, J. Reeve, and K. T. Khaw, "Broadband ultrasound attenuation (BUA) of the heel bone and its correlates in men and women in the EPIC-Norfolk cohort: a cross-sectional population-based study," *Osteoporosis International*, vol. 15, no. 3, pp. 217–225, 2004.

[40] P. Hadji, O. Hars, M. Schüler et al., "Assessment by quantitative ultrasonometry of the effects of hormone replacement therapy on bone mass," *American Journal of Obstetrics & Gynecology*, vol. 182, no. 3, pp. 529–534, 2000.

[41] P. Salari, A. Rezaie, B. Larijani, and M. Abdollahi, "A systematic review of the impact of n-3 fatty acids in bone health and osteoporosis," *Medical Science Monitor*, vol. 14, no. 3, pp. RA37–RA44, 2008.

[42] P. Albertazzi and K. Coupland, "Polyunsaturated fatty acids. Is there a role in postmenopausal osteoporosis prevention," *Maturitas*, vol. 42, no. 1, pp. 13–22, 2002.

[43] M. Maggio, A. Artoni, F. Lauretani et al., "The impact of omega-3 fatty acids on osteoporosis," *Current Pharmaceutical Design*, vol. 15, no. 36, pp. 4157–4164, 2009.

[44] N. Malavolta, R. Mule, and M. Frigato, "Quantitative ultrasound assessment of bone," *Aging Clinical and Experimental Research*, vol. 16, no. 3, pp. 23–28, 2004.

[45] A. Moayyeri, J. E. Adams, R. A. Adler et al., "Quantitative ultrasound of the heel and fracture risk assessment: an updated meta-analysis," *Osteoporosis International*, vol. 23, no. 1, pp. 143–153, 2012.

[46] R. D. Danese and A. A. Licata, "Ultrasound of the skeleton: review of its clinical applications and pitfalls," *Current Rheumatology Reports*, vol. 3, no. 3, pp. 245–248, 2001.

[47] C. M. Langton and C. F. Njeh, "The measurement of broadband ultrasonic attenuation in cancellous bone—a review of the science and technology," *IEEE Transactions on Ultrasonics, Ferroelectrics, and Frequency Control*, vol. 55, no. 7, pp. 1546–1554, 2008.

[48] M. F. Holick, "Sunlight and vitamin D for bone health and prevention of autoimmune diseases, cancers, and cardiovascular disease," *The American Journal of Clinical Nutrition*, vol. 80, no. 6, pp. 1678–1688, 2004.

15

Do Demographic Profiles of Listed and Unlisted Households Differ? Results of a Nationwide Telephone Survey

Renee N. Carey,[1,2] Alison Reid,[1] Susan Peters,[1] and Lin Fritschi[1]

[1] *Harry Perkins Institute of Medical Research, The University of Western Australia, Perth, WA 6009, Australia*
[2] *Sir Charles Gairdner Hospital, B Block, Hospital Avenue, Nedlands, WA 6009, Australia*

Correspondence should be addressed to Lin Fritschi; lin.fritschi@uwa.edu.au

Academic Editor: Susana Sans Menendez

A growing number of households are not reachable through traditional directory-based samples, which can have important implications for the representativeness of telephone surveys. The current study aims to investigate the demographic differences between households which have their telephone numbers listed or not listed in the Australian White Pages telephone directory. A total of 5,023 eligible Australian residents who were currently in paid employment participated in this study. Each respondent's telephone number was individually matched to the residential White Pages to determine its listed status, and demographic variables were compared between those with a listed and unlisted telephone number. Those with an unlisted number were significantly more likely to be younger, to have been born in a country outside of Australia, and to live in a lower socioeconomic area than those who were listed in the White Pages. These demographic differences should be considered when undertaking telephone surveys using a White Pages sample.

1. Introduction

Those wishing to gather information from large groups of individuals have long turned to the telephone as a means of reaching a representative sample of the population. Telephone surveys have the advantage of cost efficiency and timeliness [1, 2] and generally achieve higher response rates than mail surveys [3]. The traditional sampling frame for such surveys is the telephone directory. However, although approximately 85% of Australians have a fixed line home telephone [4], a growing number of households are not reachable through traditional directory-based samples, with an estimated 18% of Queensland households in 2004 [5] and 31% of South Australian households in 2008 not having a fixed line or mobile telephone number listed in the White Pages telephone directory [1]. This may largely be due to the fact that many people choose to only have a mobile telephone, and these numbers are only listed in the Australian directory if the owner requests it.

Excluding unlisted numbers from the sampling frame can have important implications for the representativeness of the final sample [6] and may result in certain subgroups of the population being omitted [7]. For example, people living in unlisted households have generally been reported to be younger, to live in metropolitan areas, and to reside in lower socioeconomic status areas than those in households with a telephone directory listing [1, 6, 8, 9]. In addition, studies conducted in South Australia and New South Wales have shown that those with an unlisted residential telephone number are more likely to have been born outside of Australia and to speak a language other than English [1, 10]. Important health and lifestyle differences have also been found, with those living in unlisted households more likely to be current smokers and less likely to report high blood pressure or cholesterol levels [11].

The literature is, however, less consistent with regard to educational attainment. A South Australian study, for example, found that those in unlisted households were more likely to have achieved a higher educational level than those living in listed households [1], while in New South Wales no significant difference between listed and unlisted households was observed in terms of educational attainment [10]. International studies have also reported inconsistent results in this regard, with unlisted Chicago residents being more likely to have a lower educational level [6] and those living in unlisted households in Germany being more likely to have received a tertiary education than those with a listed number [9].

It is possible that differences in the characteristics of listed and unlisted households vary by country, and so local information is vital in order to ensure that researchers are not obtaining a biased sample. Although previous Australian studies have been published in this area [1, 8, 10, 11], these have been limited to two states. One aim of the current study is therefore to investigate whether the proportion of listed and unlisted households differs between states, in an attempt to explore whether these earlier findings may be applicable to Australia as a whole. In addition, this study aims to investigate differences in terms of other demographic variables, including age, country of birth, and socioeconomic status, and to further explore the role of educational level in light of past inconsistent findings.

2. Materials and Methods

This study was conducted as part of the Australian Work Exposures Study (AWES), a nationwide telephone survey investigating the prevalence of occupational exposure to carcinogens in Australia. Ethics approval for this study was received from the University of Western Australia's Human Research Ethics Committee.

The sample for this study was randomly selected from a list of approximately 6 million Australian households supplied by a commercial survey sampling firm. This list consisted of household telephone numbers and address details which had been sourced from various public domain data sources. Both landline and mobile telephone numbers were available but we excluded mobile numbers from this paper because only 5% of the numbers were mobiles; mobile numbers tend to be an individual rather than a household sampling frame, and there are different processes for listing mobiles in the directory. Each telephone number was individually matched to the residential White Pages to determine its listed status. Where a number could not be matched, it was assigned to the unlisted group.

Telephone interviews were conducted with Australian residents aged between 18 and 65 who were currently in paid employment. The sample was stratified to approximate the distribution of the Australian work force by state and territory according to the Australian Bureau of Statistics Labour Force Statistics from March 2011 [12]. In addition, an attempt was made to recruit respondents in the gender ratio of two males to every female via the use of a modified interview request, whereby the interviewer asked to speak to a male in six out of seven telephone calls. If there was more than one person in the household of the required gender, the interviewer asked for the person who was next to have a birthday. Up to ten call attempts to each household were made before attempts at contact were terminated.

All interviews were conducted by trained interviewers, who gave a brief description of the study and obtained oral informed consent from the respondent. Demographic information collected from each respondent included age, gender, postcode of residence, country of birth, length of residence in Australia (if relevant), language most commonly spoken at home, and education level. Socioeconomic status (SES) and remoteness were determined by applying the Australian Bureau of Statistics Socio-Economic Indexes for Areas Index of Relative Socio-Economic Disadvantage (SEIFA IRSD; [13]) and Australian Standard Geographical Classification Accessibility/Remoteness Index of Australia (ARIA+; [14]) to each postcode of residence. The IRSD scores were grouped into quintiles for analysis, with the lowest quintile comprising the most disadvantaged areas.

Odds ratios (ORs) and 95% confidence intervals (CIs) were estimated using logistic regression in order to explore which demographic variables were associated with having an unlisted telephone number. Univariate analyses were carried out for each variable and then all variables were entered simultaneously to adjust for confounding. All analyses were conducted using Stata version 12 [15].

3. Results

Of the 6,895 eligible households contacted, interviews were conducted with 5,023 respondents, resulting in a cooperation rate (completed interviews/eligible households) of 72.8%. After omitting mobile telephone numbers we were left with a sample size of 805 unlisted and 3972 listed fixed line numbers. When the demographic characteristics of listed and unlisted households were compared, respondents from unlisted households were significantly more likely to be aged under 35 and less likely to be aged over 50. They were also more likely to have been born in a country other than Australia and to live in a major city (Table 1). Those with an unlisted number were also more likely to live in New South Wales and Western Australia as compared to Victoria.

In addition, although socioeconomic status was not associated with having an unlisted telephone number in the unadjusted analysis, when adjusted for all other demographic variables in the model, the relationship between having an unlisted number and living in a low socioeconomic status area became statistically significant. Similar results emerged for state, whereby living in Queensland was associated with having an unlisted telephone number in the adjusted analysis only.

In an attempt to further explore the role of country of birth, length of residence in Australia was also investigated. In multivariate analyses, adjusting for age, those residing in Australia for less than 10 years ($n = 150$) were 2.48 times (95% CI 1.66–3.69) more likely to have an unlisted number (29.7% of unlisted versus 11.4% of listed) than those who had resided in Australia for 10 or more years ($n = 830$; 70.3% of unlisted versus 88.6% of listed).

Table 1: Odds ratios (OR) and 95% confidence intervals (CI) for association between demographic characteristics and having an unlisted telephone number.

Demographic characteristic	Unlisted *n*	Unlisted %	Listed *n*	Listed %	Unadjusted OR	Unadjusted 95% CI	Adjusted[a] OR	Adjusted[a] 95% CI
Gender								
Male	458	56.9	2165	54.5	1.00		1.00	
Female	347	43.1	1807	45.5	0.91	0.78–1.06	0.89	0.76–1.04
Age								
18–34	179	22.4	508	12.9	1.59	1.30–1.94	1.61	1.31–1.97
35–50	408	51.1	1840	46.7	1.00		1.00	
51–65	211	26.4	1589	40.4	0.60	0.50–0.72	0.62	0.52–0.74
Country of birth								
Australia	593	73.8	3194	80.5	1.00		1.00	
Other	210	26.2	774	19.5	1.46	1.23–1.74	1.38	1.14–1.68
Main language								
English	780	97.0	3902	98.2	1.00		1.00	
Other	24	3.0	70	1.8	1.72	1.07–2.74	1.00	0.60–1.66
Highest education								
High school or less	286	35.6	1473	37.2	1.00		1.00	
Trade certificate/diploma	195	24.2	1126	28.5	0.89	0.73–1.09	0.91	0.75–1.12
Bachelor degree or higher	323	40.2	1358	34.3	1.23	1.03–1.46	1.17	0.97–1.41
Socioeconomic status[b]								
Highest quintile	228	28.3	1102	27.7	1.00		1.00	
4th quintile	207	25.7	998	25.1	1.00	0.82–1.23	1.05	0.85–1.31
3rd quintile	165	20.5	798	20.1	1.00	0.80–1.25	1.22	0.96–1.55
2nd quintile	110	13.7	698	17.6	0.76	0.60–0.97	1.00	0.76–1.30
Lowest quintile	95	11.8	376	9.5	1.22	0.94–1.59	1.44	1.07–1.94
Remoteness[c]								
Major city	553	68.7	2371	59.7	1.00		1.00	
Inner regional	173	21.5	1127	28.4	0.66	0.55–0.79	0.68	0.56–0.84
Outer regional	69	8.6	409	10.3	0.72	0.55–0.95	0.64	0.47–0.87
Remote/very remote	10	1.2	65	1.6	0.66	0.34–1.29	0.56	0.27–1.17
State								
Victoria	173	21.5	677	17.1	1.00		1.00	
New South Wales	189	23.5	1002	25.2	0.74	0.59–0.93	0.72	0.57–0.92
Queensland	93	11.5	437	11.0	0.83	0.63–1.10	0.75	0.56–1.00
Western Australia	241	29.9	1430	36.0	0.66	0.53–0.82	0.63	0.50–0.78
South Australia	27	3.4	83	2.1	1.27	0.80–2.03	1.01	0.62–1.65
Australian Capital Territory	17	2.1	72	1.8	0.92	0.53–1.61	1.08	0.60–1.93
Tasmania	11	1.4	41	1.0	1.05	0.53–2.09	1.61	0.76–3.43
Northern Territory	54	6.7	230	5.8	0.92	0.65–1.29	0.80	0.56–1.14

[a]Mutually adjusted analysis.
[b]Based on Socio-Economic Indexes For Areas Index of Relative Socio-Economic Disadvantage (SEIFA IRSD); highest quintile comprises least disadvantaged.
[c]Based on Accessibility/Remoteness Index of Australia (ARIA+).

4. Discussion

As traditional directory-based telephone surveys are likely to exclude those whose telephone numbers are not listed in the White Pages directories, it is important to understand how these individuals may differ from those with listed numbers. This study investigated the demographic differences between listed and unlisted households in the Australian working population, updating previous research conducted in two Australian states. In addition, this study further explored differences in terms of educational attainment, as past research has produced inconsistent findings in this regard.

In line with previous research, age and country of birth were significantly associated with having an unlisted telephone number [1, 6, 8, 10]. Specifically, respondents aged between 18 and 34 were more likely than those aged between 35 and 50 to have an unlisted number, while those aged over 50 were significantly less likely to live in an unlisted household. In addition, foreign-born respondents were 1.4 times more likely than Australian-born respondents to live in a household which was not listed in the White Pages. Education was not significantly associated with having an unlisted number. This is consistent with previous research conducted in New South Wales [10] but not with a South Australian study which found that those with an unlisted number were more likely to have attained a higher educational level [1].

After adjusting for all other demographic variables, living in a low socioeconomic status area was also found to be significantly associated with having an unlisted telephone number, in line with past research [1]. Similarly, living in a major city was significantly associated with having an unlisted number, consistent with previous studies [1, 9]. Differences in the proportion of unlisted households were also found between the states, with those in New South Wales, Queensland, and Western Australia more likely to have an unlisted number than those in Victoria. Previous Australian studies have not looked at differences between states in terms of their listed status, although studies in the US have found differences in the proportion of unlisted households across districts [6].

The results of this study show that an unrepresentative sample may be obtained if recruitment is limited to those with listed telephone numbers only. Young people are less likely to have a listed telephone number and young men in particular are a subset of the population from whom recruitment and participation in research is already difficult [16]. Similarly, people born outside of Australia, and particularly those arriving in recent years, are less likely to have a listed telephone number. Australia is a nation of migrants with one in four being born overseas [17, 18]. People from ethnic minority groups are as likely to participate in scientific research as those from majority populations [19, 20], and therefore a sampling frame as wide as possible should be utilised.

The current results may be biased due to the potential nonrepresentativeness of the original sample, as well as those who agreed to participate. This is a limitation of using commercial samples, as the original sampling frame is somewhat unknown. However, the sample does reflect the distribution of listed and unlisted households in the general population, with a similar proportion of unlisted households found in this study (18%) as has been found in past research [10]. In addition, the cooperation rate observed in this study (72.8%) is very acceptable for a telephone survey, particularly in the context of declining response rates in epidemiological studies as a whole [21]. Further, this study aimed only to gain a representative sample of the working population, and so, generalisation of these results to the wider population may be inappropriate. This study may also be limited by the small numbers observed in some remoteness and state groups, meaning that results pertaining to these variables may need to be interpreted with caution. Additionally, the socioeconomic status measure we used was an ecological measure, rather than individual level, and this may be a potential source of bias in our results [22].

5. Conclusions

The current study has shown important demographic differences between listed and unlisted households, supporting previous state-based findings on a national level. However, differences between states have also been found, indicating that these previous state-based studies may not be entirely generalisable to the Australian population as a whole. In conclusion, our results suggest that care should be taken when generalising findings from studies which exclude unlisted households, especially where the variables under study are thought to be associated with demographic variables such as age and country of birth [10].

Conflict of Interests

The authors declare that there is no conflict of interests regarding the publication of this paper.

Acknowledgments

This study was funded by the National Health and Medical Research Council (NHMRC), Project Grant no. 1003563, and the Cancer Council Western Australia. Professor Lin Fritschi is supported by NHMRC and the Cancer Council Western Australia fellowships. The authors acknowledge the coinvestigators in this study: Associate Professor Deborah Glass, Associate Professor Tim Driscoll, and Dr. Geza Benke. The authors also thank Vicki Graham and Theresa Wilkes at the Survey Research Centre, Edith Cowan University, Western Australia, for their assistance in the data collection for this paper.

References

[1] E. D. Grande and A. W. Taylor, "Sampling and coverage issues of telephone surveys used for collecting health information in Australia: results from a face-to-face survey from 1999 to 2008," *BMC Medical Research Methodology*, vol. 10, article 77, 2010.

[2] C. Rissel, L. Jorm, and J. Ward, "Representativeness of three survey methods in ethnic health research," *Asia-Pacific Journal of Public Health*, vol. 10, no. 2, pp. 100–105, 1998.

[3] J. J. Hox and E. D. De Leeuw, "A comparison of nonresponse in mail, telephone, and face-to-face surveys—applying multilevel modeling to meta-analysis," *Quality & Quantity*, vol. 28, no. 4, pp. 329–344, 1994.

[4] Australian Communications and Media Authority, "Communications report 2010-11," Tech. Rep., Commonwealth of Australia, Melbourne, Australia, 2011.

[5] Australian Bureau of Statistics, *Household Telephone Connections: Queensland*, Australian Bureau of Statistics, Canberra, Australia, 2004.

[6] S. R. Orden, A. R. Dyer, K. Liu et al., "Random digit dialing in Chicago CARDIA: comparison of individuals with unlisted and listed telephone numbers," *American Journal of Epidemiology*, vol. 135, no. 6, pp. 697–709, 1992.

[7] A. W. Taylor, D. H. Wilson, and M. Wakefield, "Differences in health estimates using telephone and door-to-door survey methods—a hypothetical exercise," *Australian and New Zealand Journal of Public Health*, vol. 22, no. 2, pp. 223–226, 1998.

[8] E. Dal Grande, A. Taylor, and D. Wilson, "Is there a difference in health estimates between people with listed and unlisted telephone numbers?" *Australian and New Zealand Journal of Public Health*, vol. 29, no. 5, pp. 448–456, 2005.

[9] E. von der Lippe, P. Schmich, and C. Lange, "Advance letters as a way of reducing non-response in a National Health Telephone Survey: differences between listed and unlisted numbers," *Survey Research Methods*, vol. 5, no. 3, pp. 103–116, 2011.

[10] W. Smith, P. Mitchell, K. Attebo, and S. Leeder, "Selection bias from sampling frames: telephone directory and electoral roll compared with door-to-door population census: results from the Blue Mountains Eye Study," *Australian and New Zealand Journal of Public Health*, vol. 21, no. 2, pp. 127–133, 1997.

[11] D. H. Wilson, G. J. Starr, A. W. Taylor, and E. Dal Grande, "Random digit dialling and electronic white pages samples compared: demographic profiles and health estimates," *Australian and New Zealand Journal of Public Health*, vol. 23, no. 6, pp. 627–633, 1999.

[12] Australian Bureau of Statistics, *Labour Force Australia*, Australian Bureau of Statistics, Canberra, Australia, 2011.

[13] Australian Bureau of Statistics, *Socio-Economic Indexes For Areas 2006*, Australian Bureau of Statistics, Canberra, Australia, 2008.

[14] Australian Bureau of Statistics, *Australian Standard Geographical Classification*, Australian Bureau of Statistics, Canberra, Australia, 2011.

[15] StataCorp, "Stata Statistical Software: release 12," Tech. Rep., StataCorp LP, Lakeway, Tex, USA, 2011.

[16] Australian Bureau of Statistics, "Census of population and housing: details of undercount 2011," Tech. Rep., Australian Bureau of Statistics, Canberra, Australia, 2012.

[17] S.-E. Khoo, "Ethnic disparities in social and economic wellbeing of the immigrant aged in Australia," *Journal of Population Research*, vol. 29, no. 2, pp. 119–140, 2012.

[18] "Fact sheet 4—more than 60 years of post-war migration," Department of Immigration and Citizenship, 2009, http://www.immi.gov.au/media/fact-sheets/04fifty.htm.

[19] D. Wendler, R. Kington, J. Madans et al., "Are racial and ethnic minorities less willing to participate in health research?" *PLoS Medicine*, vol. 3, no. 2, pp. 201–210, 2006.

[20] S. Mason, M. Hussain-Gambles, B. Leese, K. Atkin, and J. Brown, "Representation of South Asian people in randomised clinical trials: analysis of trials' data," *British Medical Journal*, vol. 326, no. 7401, pp. 1244–1245, 2003.

[21] S. Galea and M. Tracy, "Participation Rates in Epidemiologic Studies," *Annals of Epidemiology*, vol. 17, no. 9, pp. 643–653, 2007.

[22] H. Gravelle, "How much of the relation between population mortality and unequal distribution of income is a statistical artefact?" *British Medical Journal*, vol. 316, no. 7128, pp. 382–385, 1998.

16

Assessment of the Knowledge of Poultry Farmers and Live Poultry Sellers to Preventive and Control Measures on Bird Flu, Benin City, Nigeria

V. Y. Adam,[1] A. M. Qasim,[1,2] and M. O. Kazeem[3]

[1] *Department of Community Health, University of Benin, Benin City, Nigeria*
[2] *National Veterinary Research Institute, Livestock Investigation Department, Poultry Division, Vom, Nigeria*
[3] *Department of Microbiology, University of Ilorin, Ilorin, Nigeria*

Correspondence should be addressed to A. M. Qasim; abdullahifirm@yahoo.com

Academic Editor: M. L. Wilson

Investigated was the knowledge of preventive measures of avian influenza from farmers, live chicken sellers, and poultry veterinarian in Benin City, Edo State, Nigeria. A cross-sectional descriptive study using standardized questionnaire was conducted. Respondents included 236 poultry farmers, live chicken sellers (LCS), and veterinarian aged 12–70 years in contact with birds through husbandry. The study duration was from October 2010 to May 2011. Participants knowledge on transmission sources showed low understanding with highest being from bird-bird (57.3%). The medium most commonly utilized was electronic media (82.5%) as information source. Respondents thought that vaccination of birds (80.6%) would prevent infection. Farmers' education on bird flu needs to be improved through veterinary public health and health promotion approach. Nonpharmaceutical preventive measures such as hand washing freely and avoidance of eye, nose, and mouth touching must be improved.

1. Introduction

During an outbreak of avian influenza among poultry, there is a possible risk to people who have contact with infected birds or surfaces that have been contaminated with secretions or excretions from infected birds [1]. Avian influenza (AI) is a disease peculiar to avian species; it has been reported recently to have caused diseases in human through close contact with infected chicken [1]. The recent emergence of highly pathogenic avian influenza virus (HPAI) strains in poultry and their subsequent transmission to humans in Southeast Asia have raised concerns about the potential pandemic spread of lethal disease [2]. The small numbers of the human deaths associated with the highly pathogenic avian influenza virus (HPAIV) H5N1 appeared to be from direct exposure to infected birds on farms and in markets [2].

So far outbreaks have receded globally. Sporadic cases do occur in farms, signaling endemicity. Nigeria is surrounded by four countries with long porous borders with high risk of introduction of diseases of animal (zoonotic), fish, and plant during trade and movement [3]. Approximately 1.5 million birds have died or been depopulated as a result of avian influenza infection among poultry in Nigeria. In addition, one human fatal case was reported in the country [4]. There were four recorded outbreaks in Edo State from 2006 to 2008, three of which occurred in farms in Benin City. During this period the live poultry markets did not report cases of bird flu (Federal Livestock Department, Benin City, unpublished). This study was conducted to assess the knowledge of poultry farmers and live poultry sellers on the preventive measures against bird flu in Benin City, Nigeria.

2. Materials and Method

Benin City, the study area is southern Nigeria, is comprised of a population of 3,497,502 people based on the 2006 census [5]. Benin City has the largest concentration (>95%) of poultry farms in Edo State. It remained a major transit route for poultry distribution to the South-South zone and parts of Southeast Zone, Nigeria from the hatcheries in Ibadan, Oyo state, Southwest Nigeria. Large numbers of day old chick broiler, cockerel, and pullets, turkey poult, and also points of lay (18–21 week old) pullets are transported on road to and through Benin City. Also indigenous chicken, Japanese quail, pigeons, guinea fowl, water birds, and other wild birds are transported from the northern Nigeria to and through Benin City [6]. Poultry eggs from commercial farms are transported from Benin City to the northern zones, Nigeria.

Farmers were identified by list of members of Poultry Association of Nigeria (PAN), Edo State. Out of the 91 listed members, 76 were members who located their farms in Benin City. These populations represent farmers with the low and high density flock sizes and were given questionnaire at their weekly poultry association meeting. Those farmers (163) who are not registered members of PAN were also reached through visitation to a total of 15 farms, 9 veterinary drug, and 5 feed stores and the live animal markets (LAM). Data were collected by self-administered questionnaire to the participants, who fill in and returned to designated Veterinary stores along Murtala Mohammad Way, Benin City.

The questionnaire was also administered to 48 live chicken sellers (LCS) who are mostly illiterate by interview at the five LAM, such as Oba market, Oliha market, Third circular junction market, Aduwawa market, and New Benin market. The questionnaire comprises questions on the demographic characteristics of participants and 46 questions on the knowledge of bird flu which included sources of information, transmission, and the practice of prevention and control measures at farms and markets. In this study, the disease was identified as "bird flu" because this was the term most commonly used in the media in Nigeria at the time of the 2006-2007 epidemic and was accepted by the public. The study period covered October 2010–May 2011. Research assistants (6 veterinary doctors and 7 animal health technologists) who are poultry veterinarian and assistants, respectively, were trained for 2 days. Verbal informed consent was obtained from the participants. Respondents' confidentiality was assured and that the research had no harm to the respondents. Analysis was conducted by using SPSS 15.0 statistical software to generate frequency distributions.

3. Result

In this study, 236 (77.9%) respondents participated in the research and 39 respondents declined participation with reasons such as there is no need, no monetary benefit, and outright rejection. Twenty farmers did not return their questionnaire.

The 236 respondents involved in the research included 56.8% males and 43.2% females. The age groupings were 21–40 years (47.5%) as the highest, 41–60 years (41.5%), 0–20 years (5.9%), and ≥61 years (5.1%). More married people (69.1%) were engaged than single (29.2%) population in poultry farming. Most participants attended secondary and tertiary education (72.0%) and primary (22.9%) and 3.0% had no formal education. The others occupational group owns more poultry farms 40.4%; poultry farmers accounted for 29.2% and LPS are 23.3% while veterinarian 3.8% and pork sellers 0.8%, respectively.

Table 1: Awareness on information sources concerning bird flu by poultry farmers and live poultry sellers in Benin City.

Information sources variable	Frequency (%), n = 234		
	Yes	No	Total
Heard about bird flu	229 (97.9)	5 (2.1)	234 (100.0)
Through television	193 (82.5)	41 (17.5)	234 (100.0)
Radio	135 (57.7)	99 (42.3)	234 (100.0)
Newspaper	92 (39.3)	142 (60.7)	234 (100.0)
Colleagues	95 (40.6)	139 (59.4)	234 (100.0)
Health worker	47 (20.1)	187 (79.9)	234 (100.0)
Place of worship	10 (4.3)	224 (95.7)	234 (100.0)
Seminar/workshop	52 (22.2)	182 (77.8)	234 (100.0)
Others	9 (3.8)	225 (96.2)	234 (100.0)

Multiple response, n: number of respondents, %: percentage, others: media such as internet and school.

Table 2: Awareness of the sources of transmission of bird flu by poultry farmers and live poultry sellers in Benin City.

Variable	Frequency (%), n = 234		
	Yes	No	Total
Bird—bird	134 (57.3)	100 (42.7)	234 (100.0)
Bird—man	118 (50.4)	116 (49.6)	234 (100.0)
Man—bird	22 (9.4)	112 (90.6)	234 (100.0)
Man—man	34 (14.5)	200 (85.5)	234 (100.0)
Pig—man	25 (10.7)	209 (89.3)	234 (100.0)
Bird—pig	32 (13.7)	202 (86.3)	234 (100.0)
Bird feces	71 (30.3)	163 (69.7)	234 (100.0)
Handling of eggs	62 (26.5)	172 (73.5)	234 (100.0)
Vehicles	40 (17.1)	194 (82.9)	234 (100.0)
Slaughter surfaces	68 (29.1)	166 (70.9)	234 (100.0)

Multiple response, %: percentage.

Information sources through which farmers heard about bird flu were radio (57.7%), newspaper (39.3%), colleagues (40.6%), and seminar/workshop (22.2%); the medium most commonly utilized was electronic media (82.5%) (Table 1).

Farmers knowledge of sources of bird flu transmission revealed bird-bird 57.3%, bird-man 50.4%, man-bird 9.4%, slaughter surfaces 29.1%, bird feces 30.3%, vehicles 17.1%, and handling of eggs 26.5% (Table 2).

Respondents awareness of transmission through contacts showed low to high levels with 39.7% indicating that avian influenza can infect only chicken and 67.9% showing that bird flu can infect man. Transmission through contact with infected birds 73.9% and close contact with infected person 56.8% were revealed. Respondents 41.5% indicated that many birds died and 37.2% reported to veterinary authority. Visitation to farms showed 67.5%, 66.2%, and 71.4% (Table 3).

Respondents (80.6%) believed that vaccination of bird will prevent bird flu and 86.6% are aware that bird flu can be prevented; 86.2% cover their mouth when coughing and sneezing; fewer respondents (23.7%) indicated using face mask while working in the pen and training of workers on

TABLE 3: Awareness of bird flu transmission through contact and reporting to veterinary authority.

Variable	Frequency (%), n = 234		
	Yes	No	Total
Bird flu infects only chicken	93 (39.7)	141 (60.3)	234 (100.0)
Bird flu can infect man	159 (67.9)	75 (32.1)	234 (100.0)
By touching infected chicken	120 (51.3)	114 (48.7)	234 (100.0)
Contact with infected birds	173 (73.9)	61 (26.1)	234 (100.0)
Close contact with infected person	133 (56.8)	101 (43.2)	234 (100.0)
Have many birds died at once	97 (41.5)	137 (58.4)	234 (100.0)
Report to Vet. authority	87 (37.2)	147 (62.8)	234 (100.0)
Wild birds fly into farms	122 (52.1)	112 (47.9)	234 (100.0)
Visit to other farms	158 (67.5)	76 (32.5)	234 (100.0)
Other farmers' visit	155 (66.2)	79 (33.8)	234 (100.0)
Chicken sellers' visit	167 (71.4)	67 (28.6)	234 (100.0)

n: respondents awareness, %: percentage, multiple response.

prevention measures showed 31.9%; 59.1% wash hands with antiseptics after touching birds (Table 4).

An 88.4% respondents believe public health information and communication awareness were helpful in controlling bird flu, 35.3% of respondents indicated staying at home to avoid public places; 21.6% and 37.9% respondents were aware that wearing face mask and wearing hand gloves while handling sick birds could prevent bird flu transmission while 47.8% are aware that disinfection of equipments and contact surfaces could prevent bird flu as shown in Table 5.

4. Discussion

In this study, demographically, the number of males was greater than females who participated. This could be partly because (1) there are more males owning poultry farms than female in the study area, (2) intrinsically because of poultry farming being modernized with the improved breed stocked, a modernized management system, and highly capital intensive to which men are more likely to venture than women [6], and (3) modern poultry farming is more profitable than village chicken rearing by women. And men would choose modern poultry farming as an occupation rather than the traditional chicken rearing.

Most respondents are in the age groups of 21–40 years and 41–60 years, which when linked to most farms being located at home (69.4%) makes this finding of public health significance. And more, 66.9% of respondents are married. Thus population of high socioeconomic importance is involved in poultry farming and sales, which could be a risk factor for bird flu in humans, this findings is corroborated by earlier work [7]. This finding implied that avian influenza is associated with a very high socioeconomic burden.

Participants' awareness of bird flu (Table 1) is higher than the study carried out in Lagelu, Oyo state, Nigeria (92.9%), 2008 [8], with the electronic media being the source from which most farmers heard about bird flu (Table 1). This awareness level reflects in the educational status in which 72.0% respondents had attended secondary and tertiary schools. In a resource limited country like Nigeria, where electrical power is individually generated by a few that could own power generator, information dissemination would be hampered as only few farmers may access the information timely (outbreak and control measure news). Respondents also utilized radio as an important information source. Other sources were poorly utilized in knowing about bird flu. Extremely few respondents attended seminars on bird flu or there were just few seminars at the time of epidemic and subsequently. The findings suggested that mass communication with electronic and radio media would be the most effective media of information dissemination to the farmers and the populace.

Respondents' knowledge of bird flu transmission among birds and from bird to man is moderate (Table 2). Abysmally low understanding of transmission routes from man to bird, pig to bird, and vehicles and slaughter surfaces to birds and human was an important finding which suggested a knowledge gap by the respondents. Findings as such give an impression that farmers in this investigation have low knowledge of bird flu with increased possibility of ease of pathogen spread in farms which agreed with the study [9].

Respondents' knowledge of transmission from infected birds to man is higher than transmission from infected man (Table 3), which suggests increased awareness; this finding is higher than the study in turkey [10]. Infected birds is at the center of reported human cases that have resulted in mortality; rare cases of human to human transmission though have been reported [9, 11] but not in Benin City (Nigeria) the study area (personal communication). Awareness of the transmission of bird flu through contact with infected chickens, by touching infected chicken, is high; as well 67.9% respondents are aware of the zoonotic nature of the disease. Many respondents had experienced high mortality but only 37.2% reported such mortality to the veterinarian. Importantly, it implied poor level of awareness on the significance of disease reporting. This is supported by earlier finding of more respondents that got bird flu information from colleagues than from veterinarian (Table 1).

The LPS, an important stakeholder in poultry trade, practiced non consultation of the veterinarian for treatment of morbidity and mortality of poultry in the live animal markets, which is an important finding. This constituted a great risk to public health safety and contributed immensely perhaps to under diagnosis and reporting of avian influenza in Nigeria. The finding of increased interfarm visitation by respondents also showed poor understanding of the epidemiology of the disease, particularly the role of human, poultry, and poultry by-products movements and trade in pathogen spread and persistence in farms (Figures 2 and 3). This could suggest low awareness of biosecurity measures, increased risk of pathogen spread among farms, and a less organized poultry farming and trade. There is a moderate level of awareness of transmission through touching infected chicken (Table 3). This reflected the low usage of coverall, hand gloves, and face

TABLE 4: Public health preventive measures that prevent zoonotic transmission of bird flu.

Variable	Frequency (%), n = 232		
	Yes	No	Total
Hand washing with antiseptic			
Before entering pen	104 (44.8)	128 (55.2)	232 (100.0)
Coming out of pen	132 (56.9)	100 (43.1)	232 (100.0)
Disinfection of clothing			
On entering pen	62 (26.7)	170 (73.3)	232 (100.0)
On leaving farm	82 (35.3)	150 (64.7)	232 (100.0)
Hand washing with antiseptic after touching birds	137 (59.1)	95 (40.9)	232 (100.0)
Covering of mouth on coughing/sneezing	200 (86.2)	32 (13.8)	232 (100.0)
Use of face mask while in the pen	55 (23.7)	177 (76.3)	232 (100.0)
Can bird flu be prevented	201 (86.6)	31 (13.4)	232 (100.0)
Vaccination of birds	187 (80.6)	45 (19.4)	232 (100.0)
Vaccination of humans	109 (47.0)	123 (53.0)	232 (100.0)
Training of workers on prevention	74 (31.9)	158 (68.1)	232 (100.0)

Multiple response, n: number of respondents, %: percentage.

TABLE 5: Control measures involving pharmaceutical and nonpharmaceutical methods.

Variable	Frequency (%), n = 232		
	Yes	No	Total
Use of antiviral drugs	107 (46.1)	125 (53.9)	232 (100.0)
Use of unorthodox drugs	68 (29.3)	164 (70.7)	232 (100.0)
Public health information and communication awareness	205 (88.4)	27 (11.6)	232 (100.0)
Isolation of sick person	137 (59.1)	95 (40.9)	232 (100.0)
Staying at home to avoid public places	82 (35.3)	150 (64.7)	232 (100.0)
Wearing protective clothing in public places	96 (41.4)	136 (58.6)	232 (100.0)
Wearing face mask while handling sick birds	50 (21.6)	182 (78.4)	232 (100.0)
Wearing hand gloves while handling sick birds	88 (37.9)	144 (62.1)	232 (100.0)
Disinfection of equipments and contact surfaces	111 (47.8)	121 (52.2)	232 (100.0)

n: number of respondents, %: percentage.

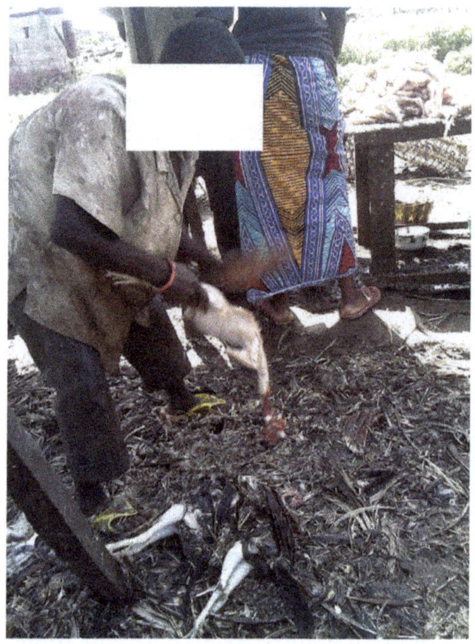

FIGURE 1: Worker dressing live chicken after slaughtering without personnel protective equipments (PPE), unhygienic processing that increases risk of viral transmission at the live poultry market.

masks in the farms and markets as observed from the study (Figure 1), which agreed with the findings in turkey [12].

Awareness on practices (Table 4) that prevent zoonotic transmission and contagious spread among humans is low to moderate. The reasons are the following: (a) since the 2006–2008 epidemic avian influenza in poultry farms recorded no reported human cases, it could have caused farmers to quickly relax the practice of these measures; (b) due to few reported bird flu cases in farms, as such awareness of these measures perhaps must have been forgotten because usage might have stopped shortly after the epidemic recession; (c) human disease is rare, so a case definition for identification has not been established.

More respondents 86.6% of the respondents believed bird flu is preventable (Table 4) is higher than the 78.6% findings of an earlier study in Oyo, Nigeria [8]; this could perhaps be due to the practice of vaccination of birds against diseases like Newcastle disease, fowl typhoid, and infectious bursal disease that had resulted in the control of those diseases in farms. Disinfection of clothing in farms, hand washing with antiseptics before entering pens, and face mask use

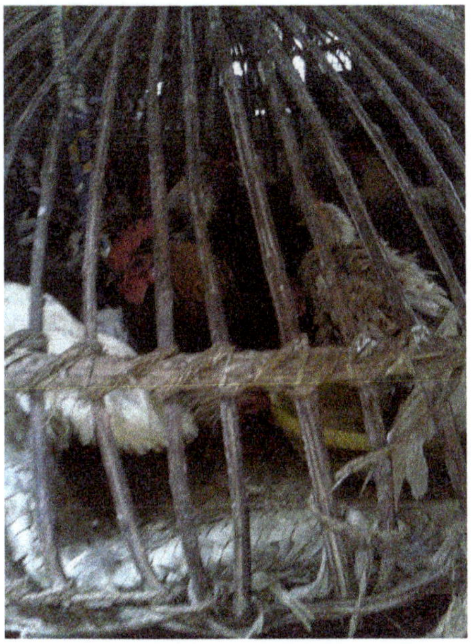

FIGURE 2: Cone shaped basket containing duck, chicken, and guinea fowl at the live poultry market.

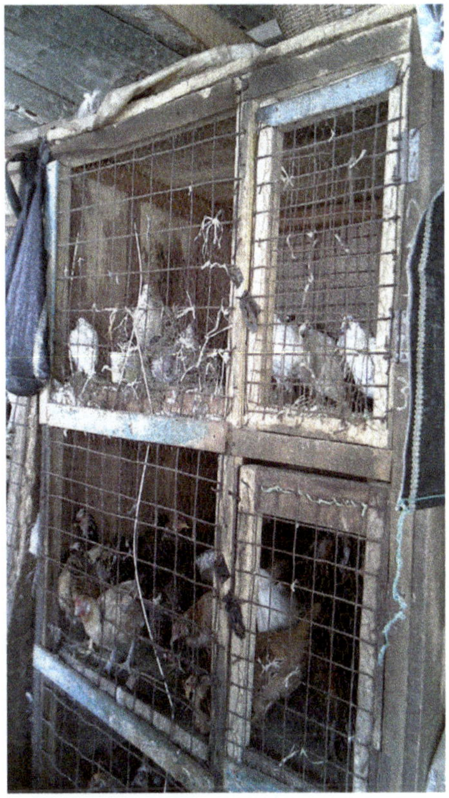

FIGURE 3: Wooden cage containing live pigeon and chicken in a multianimal live poultry market transported from the northern states, Nigeria, to Benin City (southern Nigeria).

(Table 4) as found indicated poor awareness which could imply low hygienic practices and poor understanding of disease dynamics in farms. These observations coupled with the increased interfarm visitation would mean that in the study area, increased movements and contacts among human and farms would greatly enhance bird flu transmission and ensure epidemics. High response to hand washing with antiseptics on leaving pens showed good awareness and invariably limiting the pathogen spread. The behavior could mean washing with clean water and bathing at the close of work only, especially in the commercial farms as witnessed by this author. Higher response to vaccination of birds with avian influenza vaccine indicated increased awareness and possibly acceptance of vaccination in farms; it could also mean ongoing vaccination of birds in the study area.

Public health information and communication awareness though helpful in educating the public on the disease, participants showed low usage of such information in this current study (Table 5). It could mean that they are poorly understood which corroborates findings elsewhere [8, 12]. Respondents' awareness of antiviral and unorthodox drugs use is low, suggesting that human bird flu is unknown to the respondents. This perhaps would best explain the poor awareness of the nonpharmaceutical measures such as isolation of sick persons, staying at home to avoid public places, wearing face masks and hand gloves when handling sick birds. Wearing face masks and hand gloves responses could be as a result of non provision to the farm workers and poor acceptance as witnessed in farms by the author. These findings as corroborated by [9] implied increased and rapid possible zoonotic and epidemic transmission should there be an incidence of the HPAI (H5N1) V in this investigated area. In case of increased viral fitness for zoonotic transmission, large population could be quickly affected with a resultant increased mortality due to lack of disease identification, inadequate diagnostic capacity, lack of vaccine and non to existent but poorly equipped health care facility [9, 13, 14].

Limitations. Due to self reporting, the data could not be validated independently. Refusal of some farmers to participate in the study is a potential bias. Increase in the participants on the tertiary education category did not give a true representation which could influence information education communication program.

5. Conclusion

There is an increased need to improve the awareness of these occupational groups on this important disease towards behavioral and attitudinal change to ensure compliance on the preventive measures. This is so because new farms and farmers have emerged since the recession of avian influenza that are might be insufficiently aware of disease dynamics and prevention. Governmental incentives to cushion the effect of severe bird mortality in farms will greatly enhance behavioral practices to protect farmers and improve disease reporting. An important finding is the poor awareness of avian influenza in humans which reflects poor understanding of pharmaceutical and nonpharmaceutical measures that could control zoonotic spread. Intersectoral collaboration of the veterinary and medical disciplines are required for case identification through occupational relationship to medical management. The poultry farms and LAM remain important as foci for epidemiological surveillance.

This study will greatly contribute to the understanding of the disease epidemiology in Nigeria. It is helpful in designing appropriate planning towards mitigating socioeconomic consequences associated with avian influenza.

Consent

Informed consent of individual participant was gotten.

Conflict of Interests

The authors declare that they have no conflict of interests.

Acknowledgments

Researchers privately funded the study. The authors are sincerely grateful to Dr. Ugochuwkwu, management and staff of Dominion Veterinary Consult, Faith Animal Concept, Jappar Nigeria Ltd., animal doctor, Poultry Association of Nigeria, Benin City, Edo State, for their assistance in data collection. Management of NVRI, Vom, are appreciated for their cooperation.

References

[1] R. A. Ocholi, I. L. Oyetunde, P. Kumbish et al., "Epidemiology of an outbreak of highly pathogenic avian influenza caused by the virus subtype H5N1 in Nigeria in 2006," *Vom Journal of Veterinary Science*, vol. 3, no. 1, p. 12, 2006.

[2] W. Gao, A. C. Soloff, X. Lu et al., "Protection of mice and poultry from lethal H5N1 avian influenza virus through adenovirus-based immunization," *Journal of Virology*, vol. 80, no. 4, pp. 1959–1964, 2006.

[3] M. E. Quiñones-Mateu and E. J. Arts, "Virus fitness: concept, quantification, and application to HIV population dynamics," *Current Topics in Microbiology and Immunology*, vol. 299, pp. 83–140, 2006.

[4] S. U. Schnitzler and P. Schnitzler, "An update on swine-origin influenza virus A/H1N1: a review," *Virus Genes*, vol. 39, no. 3, pp. 279–292, 2009.

[5] Nigerian Bureau of Statistics (NBS), "Federal Republic of Nigeria 2006 population census. Official Gazatte (FGP 71/52007/2, 500(OL24)," 2011, http://www.nigerianstat.gov.ng/.

[6] M. M. Kazeem, *Assessment of the knowledge, attitude and practice of control measures to avert avian influenza (bird flu) among poultry farmers in Benin City, Edo State, Nigeria [MPH thesis]*, 2011.

[7] M. E. Thomas, A. Bouma, H. M. Ekker, A. J. M. Fonken, J. A. Stegeman, and M. Nielen, "Risk factors for the introduction of high pathogenicity Avian Influenza virus into poultry farms during the epidemic in the Netherlands in 2003," *Preventive Veterinary Medicine*, vol. 69, no. 1-2, pp. 1–11, 2005.

[8] A. A. Fatiregun and M. M. Saani, "Knowledge, attitudes and compliance of poultry workers with preventive measures for avian influenza in Lagelu, Oyo State, Nigeria," *Journal of Infection in Developing Countries*, vol. 2, no. 2, pp. 130–134, 2008.

[9] J. Beigel, J. Bion, J. D. Chiche, Z. Gao, and F. Hayden, "WHO Clinical management of infection with avian influenza A, (H5N1) virus," Updated advice, 2007.

[10] B. S. Kuckkaya and T. Erbaydar, "Behaviors and experiences of poultry owners in Dogubayazit whose poultry were culled during the avian influenza epidemic," *European Journal of Public Health*, vol. 22, no. 2, pp. 174–177, 2012.

[11] A. Kandeel, S. Manoncourt, E. A. el Kareem et al., "Zoonotic transmission of avian influenza virus (H5N1), Egypt, 2006–2009," *Emerging Infectious Diseases*, vol. 16, no. 7, pp. 1101–1107, 2010.

[12] J. T. Lau, J. H. Kim, H. Y. Tsui, and S. Griffiths, "Perception related bird-to human avian influenza, Influenza vaccination and use of face mask," *Infection*, vol. 36, no. 5, pp. 434–443, 2008.

[13] M. M. Kazeem and M. O. Kazeem, "How prepared are we for the pandemic influenza in Nigeria," in *Proceedings of the Nigerian Veterinary Medical Association Congress*, pp. 69–72, 2010.

[14] WHO, "Vaccine research and development: current status," 2005, http://www.who.int/csr/disease/avian_influenza/.

17

The Mississippi Delta Cardiovascular Health Examination Survey: Study Design and Methods

Vanessa L. Short,[1] Tameka Ivory-Walls,[2] Larry Smith,[3] and Fleetwood Loustalot[4]

[1] *Mississippi State Department of Health, 570 East Woodrow Wilson, Osborne-429B, Jackson, MS 39215, USA*
[2] *Office of Preventive Health, Mississippi State Department of Health, 522 West Park Avenue, Suite P, Greenwood, MS 38930, USA*
[3] *Office of Preventive Health, Mississippi State Department of Health, 570 East Woodrow Wilson, Osborne-429B, Jackson, MS 39215, USA*
[4] *Division for Heart Disease and Stroke Prevention, Centers for Disease Control and Prevention, 1600 Clifton Road, Atlanta, GA 30333, USA*

Correspondence should be addressed to Vanessa L. Short; vanessa.short@msdh.state.ms.us

Academic Editor: Jaume Marrugat

Assessment of cardiovascular disease (CVD) morbidity and mortality in subnational areas is limited. A model for regional CVD surveillance is needed, particularly among vulnerable populations underrepresented in current monitoring systems. The Mississippi Delta Cardiovascular Health Examination Survey (CHES) is a population-based, cross-sectional study on a representative sample of adults living in the 18-county Mississippi Delta region, a rural, impoverished area with high rates of poor health outcomes and marked health disparities. The primary objectives of Delta CHES are to (1) determine the prevalence and distribution of CVD and CVD risk factors using self-reported and directly measured health metrics and (2) to assess environmental perceptions and existing policies that support or deter healthy choices. An address-based sampling frame is used for household enumeration and participant recruitment and an in-home data collection model is used to collect survey data, anthropometric measures, and blood samples from participants. Data from all sources will be merged into one analytic dataset and sample weights developed to ensure data are representative of the Mississippi Delta region adult population. Information gathered will be used to assess the burden of CVD and guide the development, implementation, and evaluation of cardiovascular health promotion and risk factor control strategies.

1. Introduction

Cardiovascular disease (CVD) is the leading cause of mortality in the United States [1], accounting for over 25% of all deaths [1]. CVD data collected by surveillance systems allow for the appropriate allocation of limited resources and focused programmatic planning and intervention. National surveillance systems track CVD and its related risk factors using a collection of representative surveys (e.g., National Health and Nutrition Examination Survey (NHANES)). However, equivalent regional or local level surveillance of CVD is not currently available, and coordination of CVD surveillance is lacking [2]. Development of a replicable, scalable, and flexible model for local level surveillance is needed, particularly among vulnerable populations potentially underrepresented in current systems.

The 18-county Mississippi Delta region consistently ranks among the most disadvantaged areas in the nation, with approximately one-quarter of its population living below the federal poverty level (Table 1) [3]. Residents of the Mississippi Delta region experience age-adjusted rates of death due to major CVDs that are considerably higher than Mississippi and national rates and marked racial health disparities exist (Table 2).

States and localities benefit from reliable, timely, and accurate health information. The Behavioral Risk Factor Surveillance System (BRFSS) is frequently used to track a broad range of health indicators and direct programmatic

Table 1: Sociodemographic characteristics of the Mississippi Delta region, Mississippi, and the United States.

Delta county	Population size[a]	% total Delta population	% non-Hispanic black[a]	% non-Hispanic white[a]	% other[a]	Median household income[b]	% persons below FPL[b]	Urban-rural classification[c,d]
Bolivar	33,771	6.1	64.2	34.4	1.4	$28,984	33.9	Micropolitan
Carroll	10,373	1.9	33.0	65.5	1.4	$34,436	18.8	Micropolitan
Coahoma	25,913	4.7	75.1	23.7	1.3	$25,719	38.7	Micropolitan
Desoto	164,053	29.6	22.8	74.1	3.1	$58,979	10.4	Large fringe metro
Holmes	18,818	3.4	82.6	16.4	1.0	$22,536	41.2	Noncore
Humphreys	9,312	1.7	74.4	24.3	1.4	$24,205	42.2	Noncore
Issaquena	1,392	0.3	64.2	35.1	0.7	$27,124	43.3	Noncore
Leflore	31,861	5.8	72.5	25.8	1.7	$26,037	37.2	Micropolitan
Panola	34,602	6.2	48.9	49.7	1.4	$32,377	27.9	Noncore
Quitman	8,134	1.5	69.4	29.2	1.4	$25,507	36.9	Noncore
Sharkey	4,892	0.9	70.8	28.3	0.9	$24,987	37.9	Noncore
Sunflower	29,296	5.3	72.4	26.4	1.2	$26,921	39.2	Micropolitan
Tallahatchie	15,318	2.8	56.7	41.1	2.2	$27,352	34.8	Noncore
Tate	28,719	5.2	30.6	67.7	1.7	$41,465	18.2	Large fringe metro
Tunica	10,628	1.9	72.8	25.3	1.9	$29,808	28.1	Large fringe metro
Warren	48,346	8.7	46.9	51.0	2.1	$37,578	23.3	Micropolitan
Washington	50,406	9.1	71.0	27.5	1.5	$25,559	42.2	Micropolitan
Yazoo	27,886	5.0	57.1	41.2	1.7	$28,474	39.0	Micropolitan
Delta Region	553,720		49.7	48.3	2.0	$30,447	25.5	
Mississippi	2,978,512		37.3	60.0	2.6	$36,992	21.7	
United States	311,591,917		13.1	78.1	8.8	$50,046	15.3	

FPL: Federal Poverty Level. [a]Data source: U.S. Census Bureau—2011 Census of Population. [b]Data source: U.S. Census Small Area Income and Poverty Estimates for State and Counties. [c]Data Source: 2006 National Center for Health Statistics Urban-Rural Classification Scheme for Counties. [d]Categories and classification rules: large central metro: central counties of MSAs of 1 million or more population; large fringe metro: counties in MSA of 1 million or more population that do not qualify as large central; medium metro: counties within MSAs of 250,000–999,999 population; small metro: counties within MSAS of 50,000 to 249,999 population; micropolitan: counties in micropolitan statistical area; noncore: counties not in micropolitan statistical area [4].

planning at the state level. The methodology of the BRFSS allows for a large annual sample size and comparisons across states and large metropolitan areas. However, the BRFSS has limitations, including the use of random-digit-dialing to select participants and reliance on self-reported data. Moreover, telephone-based surveillance systems have noncoverage biases and comparisons between self-reported and measured health metrics have found inconsistencies, with significant over- and underestimation of CVD risk factors among population subgroups [5–9].

To further develop a model for CVD surveillance at the regional level and to examine the CVD risk factors in an area with significant health needs, the Mississippi State Department of Health (MSDH), with support from the Centers for Disease Control and Prevention (CDC), developed and initiated a Cardiovascular Health Examination Survey (CHES) in the Mississippi Delta region. The Delta CHES will provide a baseline examination of CVD and related risk factors, which can be later replicated to assess progression and/or progress among adult residents of the Mississippi Delta region. The primary objectives of Delta CHES are (1) to determine the prevalence and distribution of CVD and CVD risk factors using self-reported and directly measured health metrics and (2) to assess environmental perceptions and existing policies that support or deter healthy choices. The secondary objectives are (1) to develop a replicable, regional-level data collection model for use in future studies and (2) to create a blood repository for use in future ancillary studies. Information gathered will help guide the state in the development, implementation, and evaluation of cardiovascular health promotion and risk factor control strategies. Here we describe the Delta CHES design and methods.

2. Materials and Methods

2.1. Development of the Model. The methods and model used in the Delta CHES were informed using comparable pilot surveys conducted in four US states (Washington [9], Arkansas [10], Kansas, and Oklahoma). Previous pilot surveys were undertaken to address a gap in available data at the local, regional, and state levels. The Delta CHES model was developed to provide regional estimates by using a detailed process and outcome evaluation conducted among the four pilot states and incorporating historical accounts of other local and regional data collection surveys (e.g., Survey of

TABLE 2: Age-adjusted death rates for major CVDs, heart disease, and stroke for non-Hispanic blacks and non-Hispanic whites, Mississippi Delta region, Mississippi, and the United States, 2008.

	All			Non-Hispanic black			Non-Hispanic white		
	Major CVDs death rate[ab] (95% CI)	Heart disease death rate[ac] (95% CI)	Stroke death rate[ad] (95% CI)	Major CVDs death rate[ab] (95% CI)	Heart disease death rate[ac] (95% CI)	Stroke death rate[ad] (95% CI)	Major CVDs death rate[ab] (95% CI)	Heart disease death rate[ac] (95% CI)	Stroke death rate[ad] (95% CI)
Delta Region[e]	369.0 (352.3–385.6)	279.6 (265.1–294.0)	56.2 (49.7–62.7)	443.8 (414.4–473.2)	311.0 (286.4–335.5)	79.1 (66.7–91.5)	314.7 (295.0–334.3)	256.8 (239.0–274.5)	40.6 (33.6–47.7)
Mississippi	338.9 (332.3–345.4)	264.3 (258.5–270.1)	52.7 (50.1–55.3)	419.1 (404.7–433.4)	308.6 (296.3–320.9)	74.8 (68.7–80.8)	310.7 (303.3–318.1)	249.5 (242.8–256.1)	44.2 (41.4–47.0)
United States	246.8 (246.2–247.3)	189.0 (188.6–189.5)	41.3 (41.1–41.5)	338.9 (336.7–341.1)	250.2 (248.3–252.1)	60.3 (59.4–61.2)	245.4 (244.8–246.0)	189.9 (189.3–190.4)	39.9 (39.6–40.1)

CVD: cardiovascular disease. Data source: Compressed Mortality File, CDC Wonder (http://wonder.cdc.gov/). [a]Rates are per 100,000 population, age-adjusted to the 2000 US standard population. [b]ICD-10 codes: I00–I78. [c]ICD-10 codes: I00–I09, I11, I13, and I20–I51. [d]ICD 10 codes: I60–I69. [e]Counties include Bolivar, Carroll, Coahoma, Desoto, Holmes, Humphreys, Issaquena, Leflore, Panola, Quitman, Sharkey, Sunflower, Tallahatchie, Tate, Tunica, Warren, Washington, and Yazoo.

the Health of Wisconsin [11]; New York City Health and Nutrition Examination Survey [12]).

Lessons learned from previous pilot surveys influenced the ordering of tasks during planning stages, the selection of a sampling method, and the choice for the Delta CHES model. Potential causes of delay identified by pilot surveys, such as institutional review board (IRB) approval, staffing, questionnaire development, and selection and use of contractors for data collection and management were prioritized during the initial phases of Delta CHES. Methods employed by prior examination surveys varied from in-home data collection for all aspects of the survey to telephone-based data collection of self-reported data and measured health data conducted at clinic sites. Variations in response rates and health outcome findings from prior surveys led to the selection of in-home data collection of self-reported and measured data for Delta CHES.

2.2. Study Design. Delta CHES is a population-based, cross-sectional study. Survey data, anthropometric measures, and blood samples are collected from individuals ≥18 years from the adult, noninstitutionalized population of the Mississippi Delta region. The MSDH IRB approved all Delta CHES procedures and documents. The planning phase began in 2011, and the implementation phase began in late 2012 with expectations of completion in early 2014.

2.3. Study Population. The Mississippi Delta region, an area the size of Connecticut in the Northwest part of Mississippi with a population of approximately 553,000, includes the following 18 counties: Bolivar, Carroll, Coahoma, Desoto, Holmes, Humphreys, Issaquena, Leflore, Panola, Quitman, Sharkey, Sunflower, Tallahatchie, Tate, Tunica, Warren, Washington, and Yazoo (Figure 1). Individuals are eligible to participate in Delta CHES if they are ≥18 years of age, nonpregnant, reside within the 18-county Mississippi Delta region, and are able to sign an informed consent form. Persons who cannot legally sign a consent form, persons with psychiatric, cognitive, or developmental disorders, persons with hemophilia, those undergoing treatment for cancer, non-English speakers, and those who are not expected to be in residence within 30 days of selection are excluded.

2.4. Sample Size and Power. One of our main interests is to compare prevalence estimates between non-Hispanic blacks and non-Hispanic whites, within the limits of sample size feasibility. Table 3 shows the sample sizes needed to have a power of 80% to detect a difference in leading CVD risk factor (i.e., dyslipidemia, hypertension, and, diabetes) prevalence between these two groups (Table 3). Based on a similar study conducted in Arkansas [10], we expect about one-third of contacted houses to have an eligible adult willing to participate and a 65% completion rate among surveys started. With 80% probability of detecting a true difference, at the 0.05 significance level, between equal-sized samples of non-Hispanic blacks and non-Hispanic whites, we estimate a total sample size of approximately 1,000 which will allow us to detect differences in selected CVD risk factors.

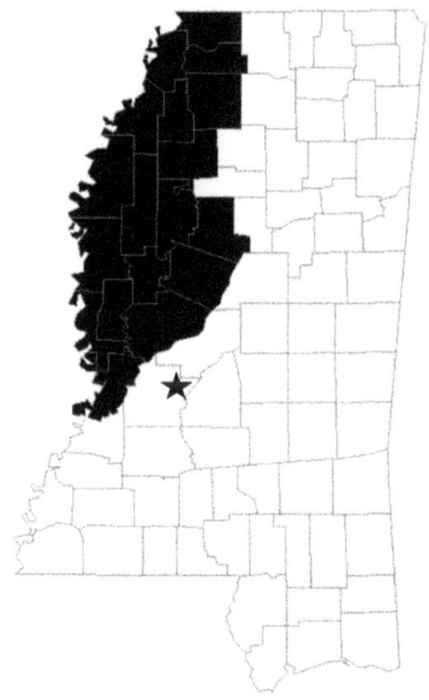

Figure 1: The 18-county Mississippi Delta region. The Mississippi Delta region (shaded in black) includes the following counties: Bolivar, Carroll, Coahoma, Desoto, Holmes, Humphreys, Issaquena, Leflore, Panola, Quitman, Sharkey, Sunflower, Tallahatchie, Tate, Tunica, Warren, Washington, and Yazoo.

2.5. Sampling and Recruitment. The Mississippi Delta region can be a difficult place to conduct health surveys due to many factors, including the rurality of the area, low landline telephone coverage, and low socioeconomic status of many residents. Therefore, innovative means are used to sample and recruit participants into Delta CHES. First, a two-stage address-based sampling method is used to sample households and participants. This approach reduces the potential coverage bias of traditional random-digit dialing. In the latter half of 2012, approximately 38% of US homes had only cellular phones [13]. In a recent comparison with other states, Mississippi had one of the highest proportions of adults in wireless-only households (42.3%) [14]. Further, adults living in cellular phone-only households tend to be younger, have lower incomes, and be members of minority populations [14], increasing the risk for coverage bias in Mississippi Delta communities with high percentages of non-Hispanic blacks and lower income households.

The frame for the first stage of sampling, which consisted of residential addresses in the Delta region, was purchased from a private vendor (Marketing Systems Group; http://www.m-s-g.com). The basis of this file is the US Postal Service Computerized Delivery Sequence File, which contains nearly all delivery-point addresses served by the US Postal Service [15]. Geographic information systems technology was used to construct an address frame that matched the geographies of the Delta CHES population and addresses were matched to telephone numbers (~47% matching rate). Approximately 6,000 households were randomly selected from the list of addresses.

Table 3: Power to detect statistically significant differences in rates of diabetes, dyslipidemia, and hypertension between non-Hispanic black and non-Hispanic white residents of the Mississippi Delta region.

Condition	Non-Hispanic blacks Prevalence (%)[a]	Non-Hispanic whites Prevalence (%)[a]	Power ($1-\beta$) for alpha = 0.05	Total sample size
Diabetes	16.0	10.2	0.80	1,006
Dyslipidemia	35.9	45.2	0.80	874
Hypertension	42.5	34.7	0.80	1,234

[a]From the 2007 and 2009 combined Mississippi Behavioral Risk Factor Surveillance System.

The second stage of sampling involves the selection of eligible adults for participation in Delta CHES. Each randomly selected household is mailed a letter which describes the study, identifies the household as being part of the survey sample, and informs residents that field staff would be calling the household. The letter also requests the household to contact study staff via a toll-free number to confirm the telephone number on file or to provide a telephone number so that they can be contacted regarding participation. This letter is particularly useful for those households where telephone matching is unsuccessful. Any returned or undeliverable letters are receipted into an electronic management system and the outcome of the mailing logged with an appropriate disposition code.

For addresses with an associated telephone number, trained telephone interviewers call the households to complete an enumeration survey. Interviewers make up to seven attempts to contact an adult household member at different times of the day and different days of the week including weekends. If contact is made, interviewers verify that they have reached the correct household, introduce and briefly explain Delta CHES, and administer the enumeration survey using a computer-assisted telephone interviewing (CATI) system. The name, age, sex, and phone number of each eligible household member is collected. Each contact attempt is tracked and households where telephone contact attempts are unsuccessful are reassigned for in-person enumeration.

An in-person household enumeration is used for any household for which there is not a valid telephone number or when telephone contact attempts are unsuccessful. Due to the high travel costs associated with in-person enumeration, only one visit is made to each home. The enumeration survey is programmed on handheld devices and allows for direct entry of information (i.e., name, age, sex, and phone number of each eligible household member) by interviewers. A door hanger is left at those houses where field staff are unable to reach a person during the visit. The door hanger describes Delta CHES and requests the household to call study staff via a toll-free telephone number to discuss participation in Delta CHES.

Once households are enumerated, one to two (depending on household size) eligible adults from each household are selected. Sampled residents are called to obtain verbal agreement to participate in Delta CHES. Up to seven attempts are made to reach each selected potential participant at different times of the day and different days of the week and a CATI recruitment script and data collection instrument is used to electronically capture all responses. If the randomly selected adult agrees to participate in Delta CHES, field-screening staff verify contact information and send this information to the data collection staff. At this time, each participant is assigned a unique identification number which is used throughout the study for tracking purposes.

To compensate for recruitment challenges of the random sampling strategy, recruitment of participants also includes a "self-selected" sample. Similar strategies have been used by other major CVD epidemiological studies, including the Framingham Heart Study [16] and the Jackson Heart Study [17]. Enrollment into Delta CHES is open to volunteers who meet census-derived age, sex, and race eligibility criteria for the 18-county region. An enrollment algorithm based on US Census data for each county determines anticipated recruitment for each age∗sex∗race subgroup. Individuals interested in participating in Delta CHES are asked to call the study's toll-free number to complete the screener questionnaire. The name and contact information of each recruited participant is subsequently sent to the data collection staff. The volunteer sample is targeted to not exceed the sample size of those randomly selected and at the end of the study, randomly and self-selected participants will be compared to assess differences in key characteristics.

2.6. Data Collection. Examination Management Services, Inc. (EMSI), a provider of specimen collection services for clinical trials and epidemiological studies, is responsible for scheduling and completing an interview and examination appointment at each participant's home. All field workers are required to complete training on the Delta CHES data collection protocol and adherence to National Institutes of Health data collection standards and protection of human subjects and obtain EMSI Human Participation and Protection certification prior to making any study visits. EMSI calls each participant 48 hours prior to the study visit to request a 9-hour fast. At the study home visit, written consent is obtained and questionnaire data, anthropometric measurements and blood samples are collected. The main Delta CHES questionnaire domains, physical measures, and blood tests are found in Table 4. A label containing the participant's unique identification number is placed on all study-related materials at each data collection visit.

2.6.1. Questionnaire. The Delta CHES questionnaire consists of up to 281 questions (depending on skip patterns) and is interviewer-administered with responses recorded directly on the paper form. The questionnaire includes questions

TABLE 4: Mississippi Delta Cardiovascular Health Examination Survey questionnaire domains, physical examination measures, and blood tests.

Category	
Questionnaire domains	Alcohol consumption; anxiety and depression; aspirin use; cholesterol; diabetes; diet and nutrition; general health and access to care; health insurance; hypertension; knowledge of signs and symptoms of heart attack and stroke; medical conditions and family medical history; community perception and environment; occupation; oral health; perceived stress; physical activity and physical fitness; reactions to race; social and emotional support; sociodemographic information and housing; tobacco use and exposure; vitamins and medications; weight history
Physical examination measures	Hip and waist circumference; blood pressure; height; pulse; weight
Blood tests	Complete blood count; comprehensive metabolic panel (alanine aminotransferase; albumin : globulin ratio; albumin, serum; alkaline phosphatase, serum; aspartate aminotransferase; bilirubin, total; bilirubin : creatinine ratio; calcium, serum; carbon dioxide, total; chloride, serum; creatinine, serum; globulin, total; glucose, serum; potassium, serum; protein, total, serum; sodium, serum); insulin; hemoglobin A1c; high sensitivity C-reactive protein; homocysteine; lipid profile (triglycerides, total cholesterol, low-density lipoprotein, high-density lipoprotein); nicotine and metabolite

related to medical history, CVD risk factors and behaviors (e.g., smoking, alcohol use, physical activity, and diet), and sociodemographics. Physical and built environments and community perceptions and existing health-related policies that support or deter healthy choices are also assessed. Participants are asked to present prescription and nonprescription medicines, including vitamins, supplements, and over-the-counter medications. The draft questionnaire was field-tested at a MSDH office in the Mississippi Delta region with community volunteers. Reactions, difficulties, and questions by respondents were noted systematically and discussed by Delta CHES staff and the questionnaire was revised accordingly. Many of the survey questions originated from established national (i.e., NHANES) or state-based surveys (e.g., BRFSS). The complete Delta CHES questionnaire is available on the study's website [18].

2.6.2. Physical Examination. The physical examination includes anthropometric and blood pressure measurements. Participants are measured for height, weight, and hip and waist circumference. Weight is measured on hard surface floor (if available) using a digital scale (Healthometer) and recorded in pounds to the nearest decimal. Height is measured on hard surface floor (if available) using a metal tape measure with the participant's heels and buttocks against a wall and recorded in feet and inches to the nearest half inch. Waist circumference is measured with a soft measuring tape at umbilicus level, keeping the tape parallel to the floor. The measurement is recorded in inches to the nearest half inch. Hip circumference is measured at the widest point of the participant's buttocks with the soft measuring tape parallel to the floor. It is recorded in inches to the nearest half inch. Resting blood pressure is measured in the right arm, if available, three times in the seated position with an American Diagnostic Corporation (Hauppauge, New York) sphygmomanometer. There is a five-minute waiting period before taking the first blood pressure and a 30-second period between measurements. Equipment is calibrated daily using standardized protocols and compared to the previous day's measurement.

2.6.3. Biological Specimen Collection. After administering the questionnaire and taking anthropometric measurements, interviewers collect approximately 36 mL of blood from each participant in a requested fasting state. All specimens are processed and shipped overnight to laboratories for analysis according to protocol (Table 5). The Mississippi Public Health Laboratory (Jackson, MS), a laboratory currently participating in the CDC Lipid Standardization Program [19], is responsible for the lipid assay. All remaining samples are analyzed by Laboratory Corporation of America (LabCorp) [20].

A portion of the blood collected during examination is stored for potential use in future health studies. Participants who provide consent for storage of blood have 5 mL of their serum stored at −70°C in a secure laboratory space at the Mississippi Public Health Laboratory. Future studies may be conducted using stored samples which will be identified using the participant's unique identification number. Researchers from public health agencies, universities, and other scientific centers can submit proposals to use the stored specimens, as well as other Delta CHES data. All research proposals will be reviewed for scientific merit and integrity by the MSDH IRB.

2.6.4. Food Frequency Questionnaire. At the end of the study visit, each participant is provided a food frequency questionnaire (FFQ), one-page instructions for completing the FFQ, a pencil, and a postage-paid preaddressed return envelope. The Delta CHES toll-free 800 number is included in the instructions and participants can call study staff with questions concerning the FFQ or to obtain assistance with completing it. The FFQ was developed by the Nutrition Assessment Shared Resource of Fred Hutchinson Cancer Research Center (Seattle, WA). This FFQ was chosen because it has an advantage of being comparable to the other CHES exam sites (i.e., Arkansas) and can provide an overall assessment of sodium intake, an important CVD risk factor.

TABLE 5: Mississippi Delta Cardiovascular Health Examination Survey specimen collection and processing.

Tube number	Tube type	Spin time (minutes)	Transfer	Ship	Ship temperature	Laboratory	Test
1	SST Gold top (5 mL)	15	None	Serum	Ambient	MPHL	Lipid profile
2	EDTA Lavender top (4 mL)	15	Plasma to 1 transfer tube	Plasma	Cold	LabCorp	Homocysteine
3 and 4	EDTA Lavender top (4 mL)	No spin	None	Whole blood	Cold	LabCorp	Hemoglobin Alc; complete blood count
5	Red top (10 mL)	15	Serum to 2 transfer tubes	Serum	Cold	LabCorp	Insulin; nicotine and metabolite
6	SST red/gray top (8.5 mL)	15	None	Serum	Cold	LabCorp	Metabolic panel; high sensitivity CRP

CRP: C-reactive protein; MPHL: Mississippi Public Health Laboratory; SST: Serum Separator Tube.

The self-administered FFQ booklet asks participants to report the frequency of consumption and portion size of approximately 120 line items over the past three months. Each line item is defined by a series of foods or beverages. Participants complete the FFQ and return it to MSDH. Approximately two weeks after the initial study visit, a call is made to nonresponding participants to remind them to complete the FFQ. Two weeks after the reminder call, a second call is made to nonresponding participants.

2.6.5. Pedometer and Daily Steps Diary. Following completion of the main Delta CHES data collection, participants are also given a pedometer kit to self-monitor physical activity for five consecutive days. Pedometers are a simple, inexpensive way to measure physical activity [21] and five consecutive days of data collection are enough to achieve a reliable and valid estimate of physical activity [22]. Kits include a pedometer, instructions on how to use the pedometer, a recording diary, and a postage-paid preaddressed return envelope. Interviewers provide assistance in opening and resetting the pedometers, if necessary. Study pedometers are the Yamax SW200 models, which demonstrate high concordance with accelerometers under laboratory conditions and in field settings [23]. The Yamax SW200 has been recommended in a number of validation studies as a preferred model for measuring daily steps in free-living populations [24, 25]. Participants are instructed to reset their pedometer to zero each morning, go about their typical activities, remove the pedometer only while bathing, showering, or swimming, and record their day-end steps taken on the provided diary. The completed diary is returned to MSDH; participants keep the pedometers. Approximately two weeks after the initial study visit, a call is made to nonresponding participants to remind them to complete the pedometer diary. Two weeks after the reminder call, a second call is made to nonresponding participants.

2.7. Data Integrity and Quality. Several steps are taken to ensure data integrity and quality. First, a 50% random subsample of respondents is telephoned after the study visit to assess the overall experience with the interviewers. Issues are reported to EMSI for resolution. Second, all data collection tools are hand-checked for readability, correct skip patterns and missing data as they are received by MSDH. Delta CHES staff call participants to verify information when needed. Lastly, laboratory analyses are conducted using industry recognized standards and are subjected to internal laboratory quality monitoring by the Mississippi Public Health Laboratory and LabCorp.

2.8. Data Management. MSDH acts as the data coordinating center for Delta CHES. At the end of the in-home data collection period, MSDH will collate all questionnaires. Data will be entered, processed, and weighed and results will be compiled into one dataset. MSDH logs and ships the FFQs, mailed back by participants, to the Fred Hutchinson Cancer Research Center for scanning and processing. The pedometer diary data are entered into a Delta CHES database as received, and laboratory results are transmitted electronically to MSDH. After data from all sources are received and entered, data will be merged into one master database, matched by the participant's unique identification number. The final analytic dataset will be in aggregate and void of personal identifiers. All subsequent data analyses will use this dataset to protect the confidentiality of participants.

2.9. Notification of Study Findings. A cover letter and a health report summarizing anthropometric measurements and clinically relevant laboratory results are mailed to each participant. Participants are encouraged to share results with their health care provider. A local telephone number is provided in the letter for medical provider referral information for individuals without a health care provider. Participants are called and advised to seek medical care when any laboratory results or blood pressure readings are above predetermined critical values. Participant feedback is based on the urgency for medical attention, using guidelines from the Seventh Report of the Joint National Committee on Prevention,

Detection, Evaluation, and Treatment of High Blood Pressure [26].

2.10. Incentives. In addition to the health report and pedometer, a $45 gift card is given to each participant as compensation for completing the study visit. Participants receive a $10 gift card for returning the FFQ and a $10 gift card for returning the pedometer diary. The incentives are mailed to the participant's home together with the cover letter, the health report, and CVD-related educational materials. If the FFQ and/or pedometer daily steps diary are received after the letter and report are mailed, then incentives are mailed immediately following receipt of the FFQ and/or pedometer daily steps diary.

2.11. Epidemiological Implications. While data from the national surveillance systems are used to provide reliable, directly measured health data for the nation, comparable state or regional-level data are not available to track leading health indicators and inform local-level policies and interventions. Since data collected by surveillance and monitoring systems allow for the appropriate allocation of limited resources and focused programmatic planning and intervention, localized systems are important.

Delta CHES is an integrated model designed to assess the burden of CVD and examine policy and environmental factors that influence CVD and its risk factors in the 18-county Mississippi Delta region. Delta CHES will fill a gap in applied population health by adding detailed information on chronic disease health outcomes and determinants at the regional level. Some of this information, such as levels of undiagnosed or uncontrolled disease and risk factors, is available for the first time at this level. Data can be used to develop localized CVD control strategies and to support policy and environmental interventions in the Mississippi Delta region that promote health. As the deleterious effects of CVD risk factors occur prior to a diagnosis or adverse health event, the identification and assessment of those unaware of major CVD risk factors, findings unavailable using a telephone-based survey, is a valuable example of one of the benefits of this data collection model. Finally, Delta CHES could serve as a demonstration project on how to successfully recruit, enroll, and collect data, including measured variables, from rural and other difficult to reach populations, and as a model for a future statewide CHES.

Conflict of Interests

There is no conflict of interests to declare. The findings and conclusions of this paper are those of the authors and do not necessarily represent the official position of the Centers for Disease Control and Prevention.

Authors' Contribution

Vanessa L. Short originated the paper and led the writing. Tameka Ivory-Walls, Larry Smith, and Fleetwood Loustalot assisted with paper preparation. All authors helped to conceptualize ideas, reviewed drafts of the paper, and read and approved the final paper.

Acknowledgments

This work was supported by the Centers for Disease Control and Prevention (Grant Award no. 1U50DP00308). The authors especially thank the Delta CHES participants as well as Etonne Bradford, Jane Campbell, Dr. Mary Currier, Cassandra Dove, Dr. Alfio Rausa, Dr. Victor Sutton, Dr. Evelyn Walker, Dr. Daphne Ware, and Dr. Lei Zhang (Mississippi State Department of Health) and Dr. Sharon Wyatt (University of Mississippi Medical Center). They thank the staff at the following institutions for their help in various aspects of the survey: EMSI, Fred Hutchinson Cancer Research Center, LabCorp, Mississippi State Department of Health, and Westat.

References

[1] M. Heron, D. L. Hoyert, S. L. Murphy, J. Xu, K. D. Kochanek, and B. Tejada-Vera, "Deaths: final data for 2006," *National Vital Statistics Reports*, vol. 57, no. 14, pp. 1–134, 2009.

[2] Institute of Medicine, *A Nationwide Framework For Surveillance of Cardiovascular and Chronic Lund Diseases*, The National Academies Press, Washington, DC, USA, 2011.

[3] United States Census Bureau: State and County QuickFacts, http://quickfacts.census.gov.

[4] D. D. Ingram and S. J. Franco, "National Center for Health Statistics urban-rural classification scheme for counties," *Vital and Health Statistics*, vol. 2, pp. 1–65, 2012.

[5] N. Schenker, T. E. Raghunathan, and I. Bondarenko, "Improving on analyses of self-reported data in a large-scale health survey by using information from an examination-based survey," *Statistics in Medicine*, vol. 29, no. 5, pp. 533–545, 2010.

[6] R. C. Gwynn, R. K. Garg, B. D. Kerker, T. R. Frieden, and L. E. Thorpe, "Contributions of a local health examination survey to the surveillance of chronic and infectious diseases in New York City," *American Journal of Public Health*, vol. 99, no. 1, pp. 152–159, 2009.

[7] M. Stommel and C. A. Schoenborn, "Accuracy and usefulness of BMI measures based on self-reported weight and height: findings from the NHANES & NHIS 2001–2006," *BMC Public Health*, vol. 9, article 421, 2009.

[8] A. Taylor, E. D. Grande, T. Gill et al., "Comparing self-reported and measured high blood pressure and high cholesterol status using data from a large representative cohort study," *Australian and New Zealand Journal of Public Health*, vol. 34, no. 4, pp. 394–400, 2010.

[9] J. Van Eenwyk, L. Bensley, E. M. Ossiander, and K. Krueger, "Comparison of examination-based and self-reported risk factors for cardiovascular disease, Washington state, 2006-2007," *Preventing Chronic Disease*, vol. 9, Article ID 110321, 2012.

[10] N. Zohoori, L. Pulley, C. Jones, J. Senner, H. Shoob, and R. K. Merritt, "Conducting a statewide health examination survey: the Arkansas Cardiovascular Health Examination Survey (ARCHES)," *Preventing Chronic Disease*, vol. 8, no. 3, p. A67, 2011.

[11] Survey of the Health of Wisconsin, http://www.med.wisc.edu/show/survey-of-the-health-of-wisconsin/35828.

[12] New York City Health and Nutrition Examination Survey, http://www.nyc.gov/html/doh/html/data/nyc-hanes.shtml.

[13] S. J. Blumberg and J. V. Luke, "Wireless substitution: early release of estimates from the National Health Interview Survey," 2012, http://www.cdc.gov/nchs/nhis.htm.

[14] S. J. Blumberg, J. V. Luke, N. Ganesh, M. E. Davern, M. H. Boudreaux, and K. Soderberg, "Wireless substitution: state-level estimates from the National Health Interview Survey, January 2007-June 2010," *National Health Statistics Reports*, no. 39, pp. 1–26, 2011.

[15] United States Postal Service, "Computerized delivery sequence file," http://www.usps.com/business/address-management -products.htm?.

[16] T. R. Dawber, G. F. Meadors, and F. E. Moore Jr., "Epidemiological approaches to heart disease: the Framingham Study," *American Journal of Public Health*, vol. 41, no. 3, pp. 279–281, 1951.

[17] S. R. Fuqua, S. B. Wyatt, M. E. Andrew et al., "Recruiting African-American research participation in the Jackson Heart Study: methods, response rates, and sample description," *Ethnicity and Disease*, vol. 15, no. 4, pp. S6–S6, 2005.

[18] The Mississippi Delta Cardiovascular Health Examination Survey, http://www.healthyms.com/deltaches.

[19] Centers for Disease Control and Prevention Lipid Standardization Program, http://www.cdc.gov/labstandards/lsp.html.

[20] Laboratory Corporation of America, http://www.labcorp.com.

[21] C. Tudor-Locke and D. R. Bassett Jr., "How many steps/day are enough? preliminary pedometer indices for public health," *Sports Medicine*, vol. 34, no. 1, pp. 1–8, 2004.

[22] C. Tudor-Locke, J. E. Williams, J. P. Reis, and D. Pluto, "Utility of pedometers for assessing physical activity: convergent validity," *Sports Medicine*, vol. 32, no. 12, pp. 795–808, 2002.

[23] P. L. Schneider, S. E. Crouter, and D. R. Bassett Jr., "Pedometer measures of free-living physical activity: comparison of 13 models," *Medicine and Science in Sports and Exercise*, vol. 36, no. 2, pp. 331–335, 2004.

[24] G. C. Le Masurier and C. Tudor-locke, "Comparison of pedometer and accelerometer accuracy under controlled conditions," *Medicine and Science in Sports and Exercise*, vol. 35, no. 5, pp. 867–871, 2003.

[25] C. Tudor-Locke, B. E. Ainsworth, R. W. Thompson, and C. E. Matthews, "Comparison of pedometer and accelerometer measures of free-living physical activity," *Medicine and Science in Sports and Exercise*, vol. 34, no. 12, pp. 2045–2051, 2002.

[26] A. V. Chobanian, G. L. Bakris, H. R. Black et al., "The seventh report of the joint national committee on prevention, detection, evaluation, and treatment of high blood pressure: the JNC 7 report," *The Journal of the American Medical Association*, vol. 289, no. 19, pp. 2560–2572, 2003.

18

Foodborne Infections and Intoxications in Hyderabad, India

R. V. Sudershan,[1] R. Naveen Kumar,[1] L. Kashinath,[1] V. Bhaskar,[2] and K. Polasa[1]

[1] *Food and Drug Toxicology Research Center, National Institute of Nutrition, Indian Council of Medical Research (ICMR), Jamai-Osmania, Tarnaka, Hyderabad 500007, India*
[2] *Statistical Division, National Institute of Nutrition, Indian Council of Medical Research (ICMR), Hyderabad 500007, India*

Correspondence should be addressed to R. V. Sudershan; vemulasr@yahoo.com

Academic Editor: Suminori Kono

Foodborne diseases are one of the health hazards and causes of morbidity and mortality in developing countries. In India there are no systematic studies to understand the types of foods involved and the etiological agent causing the disease. Therefore, a pilot study was proposed to investigate the food poisoning cases, undertaken by the Ronald Ross Institute of Tropical Diseases, which is a referral hospital for foodborne diseases in Hyderabad. Food and stool/rectal swabs of the patients affected were collected for microbiological examination. Odds ratio and 95% confidence interval were used to express the statistical significance of the differences. Epidemiological, environmental, and laboratory components indicated that *Staphylococcus aureus* was the etiological agent in most of the cases and in one case *Salmonella* spp. were the main cause of food poisoning. This study indicated the need to take up foodborne disease surveillance under the Indian context and to identify the common high-risk food commodities for microbial contamination and identification.

1. Introduction

Foodborne diseases cause morbidity and mortality in the general population and they have emerged as a growing public health and economic problem in many countries during the last 2 decades. Foodborne disease can be defined as any disease of an infectious or toxic nature caused by or thought to be caused by the consumption of food or water [1]. The global burden of foodborne disease is currently unknown but the World Health Organization (WHO) has responded to this data gap by launching a new initiative to provide better estimates. In 2005 it was reported that 1.8 million people died from diarrheal diseases largely due to contaminated food and water [2]. The scientific investigations/reports on outbreak of foodborne diseases in India for the past 29 (1980–2009) years indicated that a total of 37 outbreaks involving 3,485 persons have been affected due to food poisoning [3]. The estimated 47.8 million cases of foodborne diseases, resulting in 127,839 hospitalizations and 3037 deaths, transmitted through food each year in the United States of America (USA) alone [4].

In the United States, incidence of foodborne illness is documented through FoodNet, a reporting system used by public health agencies that capture foodborne illness in over 13% of the population. Of the 10 pathogens tracked by FoodNet, *Salmonella*, *Campylobacter*, and *Shigella* are responsible for most cases of foodborne illnesses. When both the estimated number of cases and mortality rate are considered for bacterial, viral, and parasitic cases of foodborne illness, *Salmonella* causes 31% of food related deaths, followed by *Listeria* (28%), *Campylobacter* (5%), and *Escherichia coli* O157:H7 (3%) [5].

Foodborne diseases are being investigated to prevent both ongoing transmissions of disease and similar outbreaks in the future. The importance of foodborne disease investigation includes control of ongoing outbreaks, detection and removal of implicated foods, identification of specific risk factors related to the host, the agent, and the environment, identification of factors that contribute to contamination, growth, survival, and dissemination of the suspected agent, prevention of future outbreaks and strengthening of food safety policies, acquisition of epidemiological data for risk assessment of foodborne pathogens, and stimulation of research that will help in the prevention of similar outbreaks [6].

In India foodborne diseases are not categorized separately in the Health Information of India. For example, in the official document of health information, Government of India for 2004, 9575112 cases of acute diarrhoel diseases including gastroenteritis with 2855 deaths have been recorded and cases of foodborne disease may have been categorized under gastroenteritis [7]. Foodborne disease surveillance is essential for estimating the burden of foodborne diseases and monitoring trends, identifying priorities, and setting policy in the control and prevention of foodborne diseases and their outbreaks, detection, and evaluation of control strategies [8].

At present as per Indian Food regulations, medical practitioners should report the occurrence of food poisoning to the food health authorities. State Food Laboratories are supposed to carry out food poisoning investigation. To carry out foodborne disease investigation epidemiological, environmental, and laboratory components should integrate closely at the beginning, during the course, and at the end of an investigation. This type of investigation system is lacking in India. In India there are no systematic studies to understand the types of foods involved and the etiological agent causing the disease. Therefore in order to create awareness among policy makers a pilot study was undertaken to investigate the food poisoning cases, with the support of Ronald Ross Institute of Tropical Diseases, a referral hospital for foodborne diseases in Hyderabad.

2. Materials and Methods

The investigation in Hyderabad was carried out after receiving information on food poisoning cases from the Institute of Tropical Diseases, which was a Government Fever Hospital earlier. Once a suspected outbreak of foodborne illness has been reported, a series of steps were taken as follows.

2.1. Receipt of Initial Data. The initial data on outbreak of suspected food poisoning during the period of 2003–05 was received by phone call from the Institute of Tropical Diseases.

2.2. Verification of the Diagnosis. The illness was confirmed by the doctor at the hospital and based on their symptoms and preliminary case history the investigation was done.

2.3. Determination of Whether an Outbreak Has Occurred. Initially the information on age, sex, symptoms, and type of food consumed was gathered from the patients at the hospital and also by visiting the affected area where ill persons are located and interviewing few persons and determining that food poisoning has occurred. Additional data was collected by using questionnaire which includes demographic information, occupation or disease setting, time of exposure, signs of symptoms and treatment, time of initial symptom, 74 hr food history, quantity of food taken, additional risk factor information, medical history and laboratory findings, and additional case reports.

2.4. Description of Cases in terms of Time, Place, and Person. The information on time of exposure and the time of onset of illness was collected and the incubation period was calculated directly. Assessment by place provided the information on the geographical extent of the outbreak and also provided important clues about its cause. Person characteristics were used to identify features that are common to cases as a clue to etiology or source of infection. Age, sex, ethnicity, and occupation were among the characteristic features that were used to describe the case studies.

2.5. Formulation of Hypothesis. In this stage the data was summarized and formulation of hypothesis was done to explain the outbreak. Based on the time of exposure and the time of onset of illness individual incubation period was calculated. These formed the bases for Hypothesis formulation. The mode and vehicle of transmission as well as the specific exposure that caused the disease were also considered. This hypothesis was strongly supported by epidemiological, laboratory, and food data.

2.6. Analytical, Epidemiological, Environmental, and Laboratory Studies. Analytical epidemiological studies determine a statistical association between certain food items and illness. Association of food items with the incident was analyzed. Odds ratio (OR) and their 95% confidence intervals were used to express the statistical significance of the differences. For environmental component studies a food preparation review was done to determine if foods involved could have been contaminated or otherwise abused in a manner that would have led to the illness being investigated. This review indicates what happened prior to the consumption of a suspect food that could have resulted in making someone ill.

2.7. Sample Handling and Processing. Stool samples/rectal swabs of the patients and the food samples at the site of outbreak were collected for microbiological examination. Consent was obtained from individual patient before the collection of biological sample. The samples were inoculated into Carry Blair transport medium and brought to the laboratory in an icebox. Aseptic condition was maintained during transportation of the biological samples. The samples were kept in refrigerator until further microbiological analysis. Direct microscopic examination of the samples and culture was carried out to see the kind and number of microorganisms present in them. Twenty-five grams of the food sample was taken in 225 mL of sterilized buffered peptone water. After thorough mixing of the sample 0.1 mL of the sample was inoculated on selective media like XLD (Xylose Lysine Deoxycholate Agar) for *Salmonella*, BPA (Baired Parker Agar) for *S. aureus*, BCA (Bacillus Cereus Agar) for *B. cereus*, TCBS (Thiosulfate Citrate Bile Sucrose Agar) for Vibrio spp., and MacConkey Agar for *Escherichia coli*. For isolation of *Salmonella* spp. approximately 1 g or 1 mL of each sample was transferred to selenite F broth (qualitative enrichment) and incubated at 37°C for 24 h. The enrichments were streaked on xylose lysine desoxycholate agar and incubated for 24 h at 37°C. Stool samples/rectal swabs were inoculated on these selective media to get pure culture. After incubation at 37°C for 24 hrs the colonies were observed and the identification of pure culture from food and stool samples was done by studying colony characteristics, microscopy, motility test,

Table 1: Age and sex distribution of recorded cases of food poisoning during 2003–2005.

Age group (years)	Male	Female	Total	Percentage
0–4	—	—	—	—
5–9	4	2	6	7.4
10–14	8	8	16	19.7
15–19	7	7	14	17.2
20–29	8	12	20	24.6
30–39	5	4	9	11.1
40–49	2	6	8	9.8
More than 50	5	3	8	9.8
Total	39	42	81	—

Table 2: Number of outbreaks (group size and sporadic cases) during 2003–2005.

Group size	2003	2004	2005	Total outbreaks	Percentage
2–5	1	—	3	4	40
6–10	—	1	1	2	20
11–15	—	—	—	—	—
16–20	—	3	—	3	30
More than 20	—	—	1	1	10
Sporadic	—	—	—	—	—
Total	1	4	4	10	—

and biochemical tests such as catalase, oxidase, coagulase, and carbohydrate fermentation tests. Ethical approval was obtained from the National Institute of Nutrition, Hyderabad, the Indian Council of Medical Research, and Ministry of Health and Family Welfare, Govternment of India.

2.8. Statistical Analysis. The statistical analysis was performed using SPSS 10.0 version. An association between intake of food and the presence of foodborne pathogen was found using chi-square analysis. Odds ratio values with 95% CI were computed to obtain the risk of presence of foodborne pathogen in a particular food. The odds ratio was calculated based on the presence of foodborne pathogen in food pertaining to ill and nonill patients.

3. Results and Discussions

The investigated cases of foodborne diseases in Hyderabad were 10 outbreaks involving 996 persons. A total of 81 patients were examined during the study. The patients aged between 5 and 9 are 7%, 10 and 14 were 19%, 15 and 19 were 17%, 20 and 29 were 24%, 30 and 39 were 11%, 40 and 49 were 9%, and more than 50 were 9% (Table 1). Most of the food poisoning affected persons had vomiting and diarrhoea symptoms. The type of food responsible for these outbreaks includes kaddu ka khee (sweet prepared from desiccated milk and bottle guard), milkshake, chicken biryani (dish prepared from rice and chicken), fruit salad, colostrum, mango juice, and jaggery rice and the etiological agent in most of the cases was *S. aureus* and in one case *Salmonella* species was isolated.

Food preparation review indicated that all the incriminated foods collected during food poisoning outbreaks were contaminated before consumption. During the investigation period the majority of the outbreaks (40%) involved group of 2–5 persons while 20% involved group of 6–10 persons (Table 2). Larger outbreak was involved in more than 15 persons (40%). Out of 10 cases investigated 9 were having incubation period ranging from 2 to 6 hrs which is typical of *S. aureus* food poisoning. The latent period of *S. aureus* is 30 mins–8 hrs; the latent period and symptoms of *S. aureus* were matching with most of the investigated food poisoning cases.

A total of 14 food samples and 12 rectal swab/stool samples were collected during the study period. Food and stool samples were subjected to microbiological analysis. Grams staining of the culture revealed the presence of Gram-positive cocci in most of the food and stool samples while in one case Gram-negative bacilli was observed. *S. aureus* was detected in most of the food and stool samples. The colonies of *S. aureus* in the food samples ranged from 4.0 to 9.5×10^8 cfu/g and in the stool/rectal swab samples it was 5–8.5×10^8 cfu/g. The *Salmonella* count was 3.0×10^4 cfu/g in the food sample and in the stool sample it was 2.5×10^6 cfu/g (Table 3)

Among all the cases investigated more outbreaks have been observed in marriage functions and at household level. Among the food poisoning cases investigated 7 cases were showing statistically significant association between illness and consumption of implicated food. No significant association was observed between illness and consumption of food in the other 3 cases. Analysis of the food items consumed showed that the odds ratio of food poisoning cases who had kaddu ka kheer was 5-6 times higher than those who did not consume, the 95% confidence interval being 2.1–11.2. The odds ratio of persons who had fruit salad was 4 times higher,

TABLE 3: Bacteriological analysis (cfu/g) of samples collected during food poisoning outbreaks in Hyderabad during 2003–2005.

Sample	*Staphylococcus aureus*	*Salmonella* spp.
Kaddu Ka Kheer	$4.5–5.5 \times 10^8$	ND
Fruit salad	6.5×10^8	ND
Milk shake	4.0×10^8	ND
Chicken biriyani	$8.5–9.5 \times 10^8$	ND
Colostrum	9.0×10^8	ND
Mango juice	ND	3.0×10^4
Jaggary rice	4.0×10^8	ND

ND: not detected.

TABLE 4: Risk estimate of different food samples using odds ratio and 95% confidence interval.

Sl. no	Food	Odds ratio	95% CI
1	Kaddu ka kheer	5.6	2.1–11.2
2	Fruit salad	4	1.8–8.5
3	Milk shake	4.5	1.9–10.2
4	Chicken biriyani	3.1	0.6–154.4
5	Colostrum	10	1.4–69.2
6	Mango juice	6	0.3–101.5
7	Jaggary rice	6	0.3–101.5

the 95% confidence interval being 1.8–8.5. The odds ratio of persons who had milk was 4.5 times higher, 95% confidence interval being 1.9–10.2. The odds ratio of the persons who had chicken biryani was 3 times higher, 95% confidence interval being 1.5–5.8. The odds ratio of the persons who had colostrum was 10 times higher, the 95% CI being 1.4–69.2 (Table 4).

It was noticed that kaddu ka kheer consistently appeared to have the highest risk of disease. There is a 95% chance that increased risk was associated with eating kaddu ka kheer between 2.1 and 11.2 times than for persons who did not eat kaddu ka kheer. Eating colostrum (OR = 10; 95% CI = 1.4–69.2) was identified as having a statistically significant association of being ill. These cases were 4 times riskier (95% CI = 1.8–8.5) than normal persons who have consumed fruit salad. In mango juice, jaggery rice, and chicken biryani measures of association (OR) were severalfold greater than one, although there was no statistical significance. Similar type of investigation of a large foodborne outbreak was reported in US; eating cucumber salad (OR = 12.1; 95% CI = 2.9–50.5) was identified as having statistically significant association with illness [9].

Various studies reported in India indicated the incidences of foodborne diseases, wherein the food implicated were sandwiches [10], soybean milk [11], stale rice [12], chicken [13], bread and vegetable curry, and butter milk [14], where as studies in other countries indicated the incidence of foodborne diseases wherein the foods implicated were Beef [15], Pork meat [16], frozen steaks [17], poultry, and other meat items [18]. Outbreak of food poisoning may be attributed to the type of food being consumed, which is based on the food habits of the people specific to the country problems associated during transport, climatic conditions, food storage, and awareness about food safety concerns.

The places of occurrence of most of the food poisoning cases were home (40%) and marriage functions (40%). Eating leftover food was one of the reasons for most of the food poisoning cases. Eating at commercial food establishments was one of the risk factors for sporadic cases of Salmonellosis [19] and Campylobacteriosis [20]. The present study indicated that in 9 out of 10 food poisoning outbreaks the bacteria were found to be *S. aureus*. Earlier individual investigation of foodborne disease in India reported variety of bacteria like *Vibrio parahaemolyticus, Vibrio vulnificus, Vibrio fluvialis, Escherichia coli,* and *Salmonella enteritidis* including *Staphylococcus aureus*. Some of the unusual bacteria like *Salmonella weltevreden* and *Salmonella bornum* also have been isolated where as other countries the incidence of foodborne diseases were due to *Salmonella typhimurium* [21], *Salmonella muenchen, Salmonella enteritidis, Escherichia coli* 0157:H7, and *Campylobacter*. *Salmonella* is one of the most important pathogens responsible for human food poisoning in the developing world and chicken products are widely acknowledged to be a significant reservoir of salmonella [22].

There is a 95% chance that foodborne disease outbreak in India is occasionally reported in newspapers, mostly from urban areas. The 10 outbreaks investigated during the study period probably represent a small proportion of those, which actually occurred in Hyderabad over this period. Outbreaks were recorded only when the patients are hospitalized. In most of the investigated cases *S. aureus* has been isolated. The high counts indicated the possible etiological role of *S. aureus* in the food poisoning outbreak as counts of more than 10^3 to 10^4/g in foods are considered to be contaminated and capable of causing food poisoning outbreak.

Out of the 10 food poisoning outbreaks investigated, only in 7 outbreaks consumption of particular food item and illness were associated significantly and it may be due to wrong perceptions of the affected people and the implicated foods such as mango juice and jaggery rice were not reported earlier. The investigated food poisoning cases could be less due to several reasons like discarding contaminated food, delay in reaching the outbreak site due to delay in communication, delay in analysis due to a failure to alert the lab in advance, and due to early discharge of the patients from the hospital. In addition to health consequences the economic consequences of foodborne disease such as loss of wages, cost of treatment, and loss of affected food articles are being overlooked. The economic cost of *Staphylococcus aureus* outbreak for 64 persons in Hyderabad was Rs 8.079 [23]. The economic impact of foodborne diseases on an annual basis in Canada, United States, and New Zealand ranges from 1.1 billion to 7 billion [24, 25].

4. Conclusions

The food poisoning cases investigated during 2003–05 in Hyderabad are an infective and intoxicating type of foodborne diseases caused by *Salmonella* spp. and *Staphylococcus aureus*. It is interesting that most of the food poisoning cases investigated are caused due to the organism *Staphylococcus aureus*. To prevent food poisoning outbreaks appropriate educative and preventive measures should be taken up. The health authorities should strengthen considerably the foodborne disease surveillance system and follow it with efficient education and extension activity or various aspects of food safety. The initiatives like epidemiological and laboratory components should be incorporated in our country to conduct appropriate surveillance programmes, so that the real burden of foodborne disease can be determined at various national levels.

Conflict of Interests

There is no conflict of interests regarding the publication of this paper.

Acknowledgments

The authors acknowledge the encouragement given during the course of study by the Director, National Institute of Nutrition (ICMR), Hyderabad, India, and also Superintendent, Ronald Ross Institute of Communicable Diseases, Hyderabad, for permitting them to collect the samples and data during the study. The authors also thank the subjects for their participation in the study.

References

[1] M. R. Adams and M. O. Moss, "Significance of food borne diseases," *Food Microbiology*, vol. 2, no. 163, pp. 160–164, 2003.

[2] D. G. Newell, M. Koopmans, L. Verhoef et al., "Food-borne diseases—the challenges of 20 years ago still persist while new ones continue to emerge," *International Journal of Food Microbiology*, vol. 139, supplement 1, pp. S3–S15, 2010.

[3] R. V. Sudershan, R. N. Kumar, and K. Polasa, "Foodborne diseases in India—a review," *British Food Journal*, vol. 114, no. 5, pp. 661–680, 2012.

[4] CDC, "Estimates of foodborne illness in the United States," 2011, http://www.cdc.gov/foodborneburden/2011-foodborne-estimates.html.

[5] P. S. Mead, L. Slutsker, V. Dietz et al., "Food-related illness and death in the United States," *Emerging Infectious Diseases*, vol. 5, no. 5, pp. 607–625, 1999.

[6] WHO, "Foodborne disease outbreaks. Guidelines for investigation and control," Tech. Rep., WHO, Geneva, Switzerland, 2007.

[7] Health Information of India. Central Bureau of Health Intelligence, Directorate General of Health Services, Ministry of Health and Family Welfare, Government of India, New Delhi, 2004.

[8] R. V. Bhat, "Safety and quality of processed foods," *Indian Food Industry*, vol. 23, no. 6, pp. 58–61, 2004.

[9] J. S. Yoder, S. Cesario, V. Plotkin, X. Ma, K. K. Shannon, and M. S. Dworkin, "Outbreak of enterotoxigenic *Escherichia coli* infection with an unusually long duration of illness," *Clinical Infectious Diseases*, vol. 42, no. 11, pp. 1513–1517, 2006.

[10] M. K. Lalitha, N. M. Walter, J. Mary, and V. I. Mathan, "An abstract of gastroenteritis due to *Vibrio parahaemolyticus* in Vellore," *The Indian Journal of Medical Research*, vol. 78, pp. 611–615, 1983.

[11] S. B. Kulshrestha, K. N. Kapoor, S. V. S. Malik, and P. N. Khanna, "Enterotoxigenic *Escherichia coli* from an outbreak with cholerigenic syndromes of gastroenteritis," *The Journal of Communicable Diseases*, vol. 21, no. 4, pp. 313–317, 1989.

[12] S. P. Choudhary, K. G. Narayan, S. N. Saxena, M. L. Mago, and P. C. John, "Isolation of *Salmonella bornum* (6, 7, 14: Z_{38}) for the first time in India," *Indian Journal of Medical Sciences*, vol. 39, no. 3, pp. 45–46, 1985.

[13] R. J. Thekdi, A. G. Lakhani, V. B. Rale, and M. V. Panse, "An outbreak of food poisoning suspected to be caused by *Vibrio fluvialis*," *Journal of Diarrhoeal Diseases Research*, vol. 8, no. 4, pp. 163–165, 1990.

[14] M. Abraham, M. Pai, G. Kang et al., "An outbreak of food poisoning in Tamil Nadu associated with *Yersinia enterocolitica*," *Indian Journal of Medical Research*, vol. 106, pp. 465–468, 1997.

[15] J. B. McLaughlin, L. J. Castrodale, M. J. Gardner, R. Ahmed, and B. D. Gessner, "Outbreak of multidrug-resistant *Salmonella typhimurium* associated with ground beef served at a school potluck," *Journal of Food Protection*, vol. 69, no. 3, pp. 666–670, 2006.

[16] U. Buchholz, B. Brodhun, S. O. Brockmann et al., "An outbreak of *Salmonella* München in Germany associated with raw pork meat," *Journal of Food Protection*, vol. 68, no. 2, pp. 273–276, 2005.

[17] E. S. Laine, J. M. Scheftel, D. J. Boxrud et al., "Outbreak of *Escherichi coli* O157:H7 infections associated with nonintact blade-tenderized frozen steaks sold by door-to-door vendors," *Journal of Food Protection*, vol. 68, no. 6, pp. 1198–1202, 2005.

[18] R. J. Meldrum, D. Tucker, R. M. M. Smith, and C. Edwards, "Survey of *Salmonella* and *Campylobacter* contamination of whole, raw poultry on retail sale in Wales," *Journal of Food Protection*, vol. 68, no. 7, pp. 1447–1449, 2005.

[19] J. M. Cowden, D. Lynch, C. A. Joseph et al., "Case-control study of infections with *Salmonella enteritidis* phage type 4 in England," *British Medical Journal*, vol. 299, no. 6702, pp. 771–773, 1989.

[20] P. Effler, M.-C. Ieong, A. Kimura et al., "Sporadic *Campylobacter jejuni* infections in Hawaii: associations with prior antibiotic use and commercially prepared chicken," *Journal of Infectious Diseases*, vol. 183, no. 7, pp. 1152–1155, 2001.

[21] M. Jacck, S. Ellen, P. Dennis et al., "A multistate outbreak of *Salmonella enterica* serotype Typhimurium infection linked to raw milk consumption," *Journal of Food Protection*, vol. 67, no. 10, pp. 2165–2170, 2004.

[22] G. Ozbey and H. B. Ertas, "*Salmonella spp.* isolation from chicken samples and identification by polymerase chain reaction," *Bulgarian Journal of Veternary Medicine*, vol. 9, no. 1, pp. 67–73, 2006.

[23] P. Sudhakar, R. Nageshwara, R. V. Bhat, and C. P. Gupta, "The economic impact of a foodborne disease outbreak due to *Staphylococcus aureus*," *Journal of Food Protection*, vol. 51, no. 11, pp. 898–900, 1988.

[24] E. C. Todd, "Costs of acute bacterial foodborne disease in Canada and the United States," *International Journal of Food Microbiology*, vol. 9, no. 4, pp. 313–326, 1989.

[25] W. G. Scott, H. M. Sutt, R. J. Lake, and M. G. Baker, "Economic cost to New Zealand of foodborne infectious disease," *The New Zealand Medical Journal*, vol. 14, pp. 281–284, 2000.

Sociodemographic Characteristics of Acne among University Students in Damascus, Syria

Waqar Al-Kubaisy,[1] Nik Nairan Abdullah,[1] Sabzali Musa Kahn,[2] and Maram Zia[3]

[1] *Population Health & Preventive Medicine, Faculty of Medicine, Universiti Teknologi MARA (UiTM), Sungai Buloh Campus, Jalan Hospital, 47000 Sungai Buloh, Selangor, Malaysia*
[2] *Cultural Centre, University of Malaya, Lembah Pantai, 50603 Kuala Lumpur, Malaysia*
[3] *Faculty of Medicine, Syrian International University for Science and Technology (SIUST), Dara'a, Damascus, Syria*

Correspondence should be addressed to Nik Nairan Abdullah; niknairan@yahoo.com

Academic Editor: Suminori Kono

To estimate the prevalence and identify risk factors that may be associated with acne among university students in Syria, a cross-sectional study was conducted in the Syrian International University for Science and Technology in December 2009. A sample of 500 students was chosen. Each participant was subjected to an interview and clinical examination of acne in addition to height and weight measurements. Acne prevalence was 34.7% (172/496). Male students had higher rate of acne compared to females (42.9% versus 23.6%, $P < 0.0001$) and their acne started significantly at a younger age (18.13 versus 19.04 years old, $P < 0.0001$). Face was the commonest site for acne in both males and females. Washing face frequently per day in both sexes has a significant relation with a decreased prevalence of acne. Moreover, psychological stress particularly when the students were away from family was associated with a significant higher rate of acne. We found that the prevalence of acne steadily increased with increasing body mass index. Acne is a health and psychological problem among university students particularly when affecting the face. Several factors such as gender, body mass index, and stress were found to be associated with acne formation.

1. Introduction

Vulgaris is a common skin disease which is a significant health problem among adolescents and young adults. It affects 85–100% of people at some point in their lives, and it usually begins at puberty. Acne can persist into the 30s and beyond. People of all ethnic backgrounds get acne [1]. More than half of those who experienced acne sought medical treatment. In USA, 61.9% of patients aged 18 years and older were seen in clinics for acne vulgaris [2]. Likewise in the university outpatient clinics, the most common complaint was acne vulgaris [3].

Acne formation is multifactorial. The four primary factors determining acne development are abnormal follicular epithelial desquamation, hyperactivity of the sebaceous glands, proliferation of Propionibacterium acnes, and follicular formation [4]. Furthermore, androgens play an important role in the pathogenesis of acne. Several studies in the Middle East reported that emotional stress, premenstrual factors (in females), and certain foods such as fatty food, sweets, and spices were believed to aggravate acne formation [5, 6]. On the other hand, in Syria, there is a lack of published studies on acne among university students. Studying acne is important because some forms of acne such as inflammatory acne may leave scarring and psychological consequences. Presence of acne has a negative impact on self-esteem and quality of life among adolescents. Therefore, increasing incidence of depression and other psychological disorders may be associated with acne [7]. Our objective of conducting this study was to estimate the prevalence of acne among the students in the Syrian International University for Science and Technology and also to identify some risk factors that may be associated with acne.

2. Methods

A cross-sectional study was conducted in Dara'a district of Damascus, Syria, from the 3rd to 28th of December 2009. The study was carried out on 2100 students of the Syrian International University for Science and Technology (SIUST). This new establishment (four years old) consists of six faculties: Medicine, Dentistry, Pharmacy, Petroleum Engineering, Business Administration, and Computer Science. A stratified cluster sampling method of three stages was implemented for the sample collection. In the first stage, students from each faculty were stratified according to their year level (first, second, third, and fourth) of study. Proportional to the number of students in each level, certain numbers of individuals were randomly chosen. In the second stage the individuals were stratified again and collected proportionally according to their sex. In the final stage, the chosen students from all faculties were grouped into clusters of manageable size.

A random sample of 500 students was chosen. The selected individuals were informed about the purpose of the study and assured about the confidentiality of the information gathered. Interviewing each participant was carried-out using a well-constructed questionnaire. The questionnaire included demographic (age, sex) and social information (living with or away from family) and life style such as washing body times per week (1-2, 3–5, and >5 times) and washing face times per day (1-2, 3–5 and >5 times) and information about stress frequency (absence, always, and occasional) was also included. In addition, female students were further asked whether acne formation was related to menstrual period. Moreover, clinical examination was carried out by trained two medical doctors who had experience in dermatology. They examined students for the presence and location of acne (such as on the face, shoulder, and others). The clinical examinations were performed at the same time and findings were confirmed between them. Beside that, height and body weight measurements were also taken. Body mass index was categorized into <20 kg/m^2, 20–24 kg/m^2, 25–29 kg/m^2, and ≥30 kg/m^2 [8].

This study received ethical approval from the Syrian International University for Science and Technology (SIUST). The data were analyzed using SPSS 16.0. The significant difference between proportions or means was tested using chi-square test (χ^2) and t-test, respectively, with P value ≤ 0.05 as the level of significance.

3. Results

Out of the 500 chosen students, only 496 (284 males and 212 females) participated, and hence the responding rate was 99.2%. The prevalence of acne among the students was 34.7% (172/496). As shown in Table 1, there was a significantly higher rate of acne among male students than that among females (42.9% versus 23.6%); χ^2 = 23.48, P < 0.0001. The mean age of students with acne was significantly younger in males (18.13 ± 0.59) than in females (19.04 ± 1.10); t = 6.8, P < 0.0001. The study also found a significant difference in acne location (χ^2 = 67.7, P < 0.001) in which both males (96.7%) and females (92%) demonstrated the highest rate of acne on the face followed by the shoulders.

Table 1: The Sociodemographic factors associated with acne formation.

Characteristics	Acne positive Male (%) N = 284	Acne positive Female (%) N = 212	χ^2	P value
Sex	122 (42.9)	50 (23.6)	23.48	<0.0001
Mean age ± S.D	18.13 ± 0.59	19.04 ± 1.106	t = 6.8	<0.0001
Location				
Face	118 (96.7)	46 (92)	67.7	<0.001
Shoulders	48 (39.3)	17 (34)		
Others	23 (18.9)	7 (14.0)		
Living with family				
Yes	50 (41)	33 (66)	54.9	<0.0001*
No	72 (59)	17 (34)	6.27	<0.05**
Stress				
Always	58 (47.5)	26 (52)	27.88	<0.0001*
Absence	23 (18.9)	10 (20)	19.64	<0.001**
Occasional	41 (33.6)	14 (28)		
Washing face/day				
1-2	47 (38.5)	19 (38)	8.1	<0.025*
3–5	47 (38.5)	20 (40)	11.21	<0.004**
>5	28 (23)	11 (22)		
Washing body/week				
1-2	42 (34.4)	8 (16)	14.0	<0.001*
3–5	51 (41.8)	11 (22)	4.44	>0.05**
>5	29 (23.8)	31 (62)		
BMI (Kg/m^2)				
<20	5 (18.5)	3 (8.1)	8.74	0.05*
20–24	55 (36.6)	29 (35.8)	22.6	<0.0001**
25–29	29 (47.5)	7 (10.5)		
≥30	6 (60)	3 (60)		
Menstrual cycles				
Yes		40		
No		10		

*Male, **female.

Students who wash their faces more than five time per day showed significantly lower prevalence of acne in males (23%, χ^2 = 8, P < 0.025) and females (22%, χ^2 = 11.21, P < 0.004).

On the other hand, significantly lower rate of acne was only demonstrated among those males washing their body more than five times per week (23.8%, χ^2 = 14.0, P < 0.001), while no significant association was found in females regarding body wash (62%, χ^2 = 4.44, P > 0.05).

Our study gave an evidence that acne prevalence significantly increased steadily (18.5%, 36.6%, 47.5%, 60%) and (8.1%, 35.8%, 10.5%, 60%) with the increased body mass index for BMI < 20, 20–24, 25–29 and >30 kg/m2; (χ^2 = 8.74, P = 0.05) and (χ^2 = 22.6, P < 0.0001) in both males and females respectively.

With respect to the relation between degree of stress and acne development, our study showed that the highest significant prevalence in both males (47.5%, $\chi^2 = 27.88$, $P < 0.0001$) and females (52%, $\chi^2 = 19.64$, $P < 0.001$) was among students who were always subjected to stress compared to those who were occasionally or not subjected to stress. Male students who were living away from their family demonstrated significantly higher rate of acne, $\chi^2 = 54.9$, $P < 0.0001$, but similar finding was not detected among females. Regarding female students, 80% reported acne formation appeared during their menstrual cycles.

4. Discussion

The good response rate (99.2%) reflected the interest of the students in this health problem. The prevalence of acne in this study was lower than reported among university students in Central Saudi Arabia (56.2%), Turkey (40.1%) and also among Singaporean adolescents (88%) [3, 6, 9]. This discrepancy could be attributed to variation in genetics, diet, or social factors (e.g., smoking).

The significant association between acne formation and sex of students that we detected was inconsistent with a study in Saudi [6]. However, similar finding was reported among school-aged adolescents in Malaysia, whereby acne was more common among males compared to females [10]. Males have higher prevalence of acne than females in our study and this conforms to studies in India, Dakar, Portugal, and Korea [11–14]. One of the reasons why men having more acne lesion may be due to increased sebum production [14].

Males with acne that of mean age was significantly younger than females. This finding is consistent with several studies [12, 15, 16]. The result most probably is attributed to the male sex hormones (androgen) which increase during adolescence period. Androgen stimulates sebaceous glands to produce sebum, so hyperandrogenism is closely associated with acne formation [17].

Our significant association between acne occurrence and washing face daily in both sexes is in disagreement with several studies in which they stated that poor hygiene does not cause acne [18, 19]. However, washing body frequently among males, but not in females, was found significantly associated with development of acne. There is a contradicting opinion about the association between acne formation and seasonal variation.

There is a conventional view that acne vulgaris exacerbates in winter, while South India study found acne prevalence is more in summer [12]. However, our study was conducted only during winter season in which, during cold weather, there is decrease in frequency of bathing among adolescents particularly male. That is why we observed significantly higher rate of acne among males with low frequency of bathing.

Degree of stress and its role with acne formation were stated by many authors [5, 14, 20]. They reported that emotional stress acts as an aggravating risk factor for development of acne. Moreover, Law et al., 2009, from his study in Hong Kong, found that higher perceived stress was positive predictor of acne among university students [21]. We confirmed the association between acne prevalence and degree of stress in which we found that students who always were subjected to continuous stress demonstrated higher rate of acne. Most probably, this relation could be attributed to the increased production of cortisol during emotional stress which in turn increased the sebum production [22, 23].

Male students living within their families have significantly lower prevalence of acne. This could be related to higher dependency of male students on their parents for providing better personal hygiene and nutrition compared to their female counterparts. In addition, less psychological stress could not be excluded. Menstruation and its association with the increase of acne were detected in 80% of our female students which is consistent with several studies that stated that hyperandrogenicity during the menstrual cycle may have contributed to the acne formation [16, 24]. With regard to acne location, face is the commonest site for acne and this conforms to several authors [11–13, 15]. The relation between acne formation and BMI has been studied by many authors [4, 17, 25, 26]. They found that acne was more prevalent among obese persons in women. We detected those obese students of both sexes to have higher acne rate.

Several explanations could explain the reasons and few of them are the excess androgens caused by obesity and psychological stress that could have resulted from being overweight which in turn cause surge of stress hormones that will worsen the acne [17, 25]. In addition, diet may play a role [5]. However, we did not explore the diet factors related to acne in our study.

Our study has several limitations. We did not assess the severity of acne or referred students with bad acne for further management. In addition, the questions on stress were a subjective assessment. A proper tool that measures the degree of stress should be taken into account. Furthermore, statistical analysis to identify the unconfounding factors was not applied.

5. Conclusion

Acne is a health and psychological problem among university students which is highly related to age of youth particularly among males. There were several significant factors associated with acne formation in the study which were gender, BMI, and stress. Locality of acne and frequency of washing were also significantly associated with acne formation.

Conflict of Interests

The authors declare that there is no conflict of interests regarding the publication of this paper.

Acknowledgments

The authors thank the president of the Syrian International University for Science and Technology (SIUST) and the Scientific Research Committee for granting them the approval and assistance in conducting the study.

References

[1] Y. Hussain, "Acne vulgaris in Nigerian adolescents—prevalence, severity, beliefs, perceptions, and practices," *International Journal of Dermatology*, vol. 48, no. 5, pp. 498–505, 2009.

[2] B. A. Yentzer, J. Hick, E. L. Reese, A. Uhas, S. R. Feldman, and R. Balkrishnan, "Acne vulgaris in the united states: a descriptive epidemiology," *Cutis*, vol. 86, no. 2, pp. 94–99, 2010.

[3] I. Ertam, Y. Babur, I. Unal, and S. Alper, "The frequency of skin diseases among students in a university clinic," *Skinmed*, vol. 8, no. 5, pp. 261–263, 2010.

[4] K. O. Abulnaja, "Changes in the hormone and lipid profile of obese adolescent Saudi females with acne vulgaris," *Brazilian Journal of Medical and Biological Research*, vol. 42, no. 6, pp. 501–505, 2009.

[5] Z. El-Akawi, N. A.-L. Nemr, K. Abdul-Razzak, and M. Al-Aboosi, "Factors believed by jordanian acne patients to affect their acne condition," *Eastern Mediterranean Health Journal*, vol. 12, no. 6, pp. 840–846, 2006.

[6] A. A. Al Robaee, "Prevalence, knowledge, beliefs and psychosocial impact of acne in university students in central Saudi Arabia," *Saudi Medical Journal*, vol. 26, no. 12, pp. 1958–1961, 2005.

[7] L. K. Dunn, J. L. O'Neill, and S. R. Feldman, "Acne in adolescents: quality of life, self-esteem, mood, and psychological disorders," *Dermatology Online Journal*, vol. 17, no. 1, 2011.

[8] *Global Database on Body Mass Index*, World Health Organization, Geneva, Switzerland, 2006, http://apps.who.int/bmi/index.jsp?introPage=intro_3.html.

[9] H.-H. Tan, A. W. Tan, T. Barkham, X.-Y. Yan, and M. Zhu, "Community-based study of acne vulgaris in adolescents in Singapore," *British Journal of Dermatology*, vol. 157, no. 3, pp. 547–551, 2007.

[10] A. Hanisah, K. Omar, and S. A. Shah, "Prevalence of acne and its impact on the quality of life in school-aged adolescents in Malaysia," *Journal of Primary Health Care*, vol. 1, no. 1, pp. 20–25, 2009.

[11] A. Kane, S. O. Niang, A. C. Diagne, F. Ly, and B. Ndiaye, "Epidemiologic, clinical, and therapeutic features of acnein Dakar, Senegal," *International Journal of Dermatology*, vol. 46, 1, pp. S36–S38, 2007.

[12] B. Adityan and D. M. Thappa, "Profile of acne vulgaris—a hospital-based study from South India," *Indian Journal of Dermatology, Venereology and Leprology*, vol. 75, no. 3, pp. 272–278, 2009.

[13] J. M. Amado, M. E. Matos, A. M. Abreu et al., "The prevalence of acne in the north of Portugal," *Journal of the European Academy of Dermatology and Venereology*, vol. 20, no. 10, pp. 1287–1295, 2006.

[14] D. H. Suh, J. W. J. Shin, S. U. Min et al., "Treatment-seeking behaviors and related epidemiological features in Korean acne patients," *Journal of Korean Medical Science*, vol. 23, no. 6, pp. 969–974, 2008.

[15] J. Hassan, S. Grogan, D. Clark-Carter, H. Richards, and V. M. Yates, "The individual health burden of acne: appearance-related distress in male and female adolescents and adults with back, chest and facial acne," *Journal of Health Psychology*, vol. 14, no. 8, pp. 1105–1118, 2009.

[16] S. Purdy, J. Langston, and L. Tait, "Presentation and management of acne in primary care: a retrospective cohort study," *British Journal of General Practice*, vol. 53, no. 492, pp. 525–529, 2003.

[17] M.-C. Tsai, W. Chen, Y.-W. Cheng, C.-Y. Wang, G.-Y. Chen, and T.-J. Hsu, "Higher body mass index is a significant risk factor for acne formation in schoolchildren," *European Journal of Dermatology*, vol. 16, no. 3, pp. 251–253, 2006.

[18] Mayo Clinic, Acne: causes, http://www.mayoclinic.com/health/acne/DS00169/DSECTION=causes.

[19] U.S. Food and Drug Administration, *Facing Facts about Acne*, Consumer Health Information. Department of Health and Human Services, http://www.fda.gov/Forconsumers/consumerUpdates/ucm174521.htm.

[20] N. Hunger and C. Kumar, "A clinico-epidemiological study of adult acne: is it different from adolescent acne?" *Indian Journal of Dermatology, Venereology and Leprology*, vol. 78, pp. 335–341, 2012.

[21] M. P. M. Law, A. A. T. Chuh, A. Lee, and N. Molinari, "Acne prevalence and beyond: acne disability and its predictive factors among chinese late adolescents in Hong Kong," *Clinical and Experimental Dermatology*, vol. 35, no. 1, pp. 16–21, 2009.

[22] C. W. Choi, J. W. Choi, K. C. Park, and S. W. Youn, "Facial sebum affects the development of acne, especially the distribution of inflammatory acne," *Journal of the European Academy of Dermatology and Venereology*, vol. 27, no. 3, pp. 301–306, 2013.

[23] G. Yosipovitch, M. Tang, A. G. Dawn et al., "Study of psychological stress, sebum production and acne vulgaris in adolescents," *Acta Dermato-Venereologica*, vol. 87, no. 2, pp. 135–139, 2007.

[24] C. N. Collier, J. C. Harper, W. C. Cantrell, W. Wang, K. W. Foster, and B. E. Elewski, "The prevalence of acne in adults 20 years and older," *Journal of the American Academy of Dermatology*, vol. 58, no. 1, pp. 56–59, 2008.

[25] A. O'Connor, Really? The claim: excess weight raises the risk of acne, http://well.blogs.nytimes.com/2012/01/23/really-the-claim-excess-weight-raises-the-risk-of-acne/?_r=1.

[26] J. A. Halvorsen, R. A. Vleugels, E. Bjertness, and L. Lien, "A population-based study of acne and body mass index in adolescents," *Archives of Dermatology*, vol. 148, no. 1, pp. 131–132, 2012.

Factors Associated with a Poor Treatment Outcome among Children Treated for Malaria in Ibadan, Southwest Nigeria

Adesola O. Sangowawa, Olukemi K. Amodu, Subulade A. Olaniyan, Folakemi A. Amodu, Peter E. Olumese, and Olayemi O. Omotade

Institute of Child Health, College of Medicine, University of Ibadan, Ibadan 200001, Nigeria

Correspondence should be addressed to Olukemi K. Amodu; amkemi@hotmail.com

Academic Editor: M. L. Wilson

We present data on factors associated with poor treatment outcome (death or recovery with a neurological complication) among children treated for malaria in Ibadan, Nigeria. A total of 2468 children (1532 with uncomplicated and 936 with severe malaria) were recruited from three government facilities. History was obtained from caregivers and malarial parasite test was carried out on each child. About 76.0% of caregivers had instituted home treatment. Following treatment, 2207 (89.5%) children recovered without complications, 9.1% recovered with neurological complications, and 1.4% died. The possibility of poor treatment outcome increased with decreasing child's age ($P < 0.0001$). A statistically significant proportion of children with pallor, jaundice, hepatomegaly, splenomegaly, respiratory distress, and severe anaemia had poor treatment outcome. Following logistic regression, child's age < 12 months compared to older age groups (O.R = 5.99, 95% C.I = 1.15–31.15, and $P = 0.033$) and loss of consciousness (O.R = 4.55, 95% CI = 1.72–12.08, and $P = 0.002$) was significantly associated with poor treatment outcome. We recommend interventions to improve caregivers' awareness on the importance of seeking medical care early. This will enhance early diagnosis and treatment and reduce the likelihood of complications that lead to poor treatment outcomes.

1. Introduction

Malaria remains an important cause of morbidity and mortality in Africa in spite of all efforts at prevention and control. In 2010, there were about 660, 000 malaria deaths around the world and, of these, approximately 86% were in children under five years of age [1]. The majority of cases (up to 80%) and deaths (up to 90%) due to malaria occur in Africa [1]. Malaria is still endemic in Nigeria with 97% of the population at risk of infection [2]. Findings from the 2010 Malaria Indicator Survey showed that about four out of ten children aged between six months and five years in Nigeria tested positive to malaria by blood smear test [3]. The Federal Ministry of Health estimates that every year malaria accounts for up to 110 million clinically diagnosed cases, 60% of outpatient visits, 30% of all hospitalizations, and more than 300,000 child deaths [2]. In addition to the high mortality, many children with the disease go on to develop short and long term complications such as anaemia, metabolic acidosis, hypoglycemia, hyperlacticacidemia, seizures, febrile convulsion and other complications affecting the central nervous system [4–6]. A number of factors have been suggested as predisposing to development of poor treatment outcomes among children with malaria. These include impaired consciousness, respiratory distress, hypoglycemia, and jaundice [7]. Knowledge of the factors that influence the outcome of malaria treatment is important in management of children with malaria in order to minimize morbidity and mortality from the disease. The paper discusses the factors associated with a poor outcome in children treated for malaria in Ibadan, Southwest Nigeria. Data for this paper was part of a larger study on genetic diversity and severe malaria.

2. Materials and Methods

The study was carried out in Ibadan, a city in southwest of Nigeria, a holoendemic area for malaria between 2007 and 2010. At the time of the study, the standard first-line treatment for uncomplicated malaria was artemether-lumefantrine or another artemisinin-based combination therapy. Drugs recommended for severe malaria included the following: quinine, artemether, or artesunate. These are to be commenced parenterally and changed to oral administration once the patient can take the drugs orally [8]. However, chloroquine injection and tablets were still available and could be purchased over-the-counter in drug stores within the country.

Children were recruited from the children's emergency ward of the University College Hospital, Ibadan, the Adeoyo Maternity Hospital, Ibadan, and the Oni Memorial Hospital, Ibadan. A total of 2468 children who were diagnosed with malaria (children presenting with fever and who had a positive malaria parasite test result or a clinical diagnosis of malaria) were recruited. Clinical categorization of all eligible children into "uncomplicated malaria (UM)," and "severe malaria" groups was done using World Health Organization criteria (WHO 2000). According to the WHO classification, cases of severe malaria included those with impaired consciousness, cerebral malaria, severe malaria anaemia, and jaundice [9]. Children were excluded from the study if informed consent was not obtained from a relative (primary caregiver) or if an alternative diagnosis was made clinically or by investigation (such as cerebrospinal fluid examination, chest radiography, or blood culture). All the children were managed in line with the National Malaria Treatment Policy [8]. All the 936 children with severe malaria were hospitalised and treated with quinine according to the National Malaria Treatment Policy, that is, parenteral quinine which was changed to oral as soon as the child was able to tolerate it orally [8]. Those with uncomplicated malaria were treated on an outpatient basis with an ACT. Their caregivers were asked to bring them back on days 2, 7, and 14 for follow-up which included a clinical assessment and repeat malaria parasite test. In line with routine care, caregivers were asked to return to hospital immediately if there was no improvement in symptoms or if their child's health got worse. Children with an initial diagnosis of uncomplicated malaria who subsequently presented with symptoms of severe malaria were admitted and treated appropriately as cases of severe malaria.

Ethical approval was obtained from the Joint University of Ibadan/University College Hospital, Ibadan Ethical Committee, and from the Oyo State Health board. Informed consent was obtained from the parents or guardian of the patients prior to recruitment.

Demographic information, clinical history information obtained from caregivers of children, and clinical examination done were recorded in a well-structured case record form. Patients body temperature was categorized as normal (36.6–37.2°C), febrile (>37.2°C), subnormal (36.6–35°C), and hypothermia (< 35°C) [10]. Thick blood smears stained with giemsa were prepared for each child and examined for trophozoites of *P. falciparum*. Parasite densities were calculated based on assumed total WBC of 8000/μL. Blood films were defined as negative if there were no asexual forms of *P. falciparum* in 100 high power fields examined. The parasite densities were log transformed and the geometric means of the parasite densities were calculated. Blood was also sampled for haematocrit or packed cell volume (PCV). Patients were classified as having severe (PCV ≤ 15%), moderate (PCV = 16–23%), mild (PCV = 24–33%), and no (PCV > 33%) anaemia. The Pediatric Glasgow Coma Scale was used to assess level of consciousness [11].

Statistical analysis was done with the SPSS 16.0 for Windows (SPSS Inc., Chicago, USA). The prevalence of malaria parasitaemia, spleen rate, liver rates, and anaemia (PCV < 33%) was calculated as a proportion of children with those indices. Poor treatment outcome was defined as recovery (resolution of fever, recovery of consciousness in children who were unconscious, and negative blood film) with a neurological complication at discharge or death. Chi-square was used for association between categorical variables. Logistic regression was used to determine the predictors of poor treatment outcome. Statistical significance was set at $P < 0.05$.

3. Results

Results of 2468 children aged 1–156 months, of mean age 42.9 ± 29.7 months, are presented. There were slightly more male (53.35) than female (46.7%) patients. The highest level of education of 49.0% of respondents' mothers and 51.1% of their fathers was secondary education and majority of the parents (71.8% of mothers and 63.7% of fathers) were semiskilled workers.

The medical histories of the children are shown in Table 1. The commonest symptoms that patients presented with were fever (97.9%), rigors (17.8%), loss of appetite (39.1%), cough (33.1%), and vomiting (30.1%). About 17.0% of caregivers reported that their children were pale and three percent were jaundiced (described by caregivers as yellowness of their child's eyes) prior to presentation in hospital. More than 200 (8.5%) presented with a history of loss of consciousness and 535 (21.7%) had at least an episode of convulsion prior to presentation in the health facility. More than three-quarters of caregivers (76.3%) had instituted some home treatments, of which the majority 1,457 (65.1%) gave paracetamol (PCM). Drugs also administered by mothers were chloroquine—CQ (16%), amodiaquine—AQ (4%), and others, including sulphadoxine-Pyrimethamine—SP (15%). Only 340 of the caregivers (15.4%) had not had a prior visit to a health provider such as a private hospital (19.2%), health centre (24.7%), patent medicine vendors (39.5%), and others (1.2%). The median number of days of onset of illness prior to a hospital visit was three. Two hundred and sixty-two children were reportedly semiconscious when they arrived to the hospital.

Clinical examination of the children at presentation revealed that 21.3% were pale and 3.7% were jaundiced. In all, 1532 (62.1%) of children were diagnosed with uncomplicated malaria and 936 (37.9%) were diagnosed with severe malaria. The mean parasite density was 1584.89 ± 15.49 [3235.94 ± 18.62 among those with severe malaria and 891.25 ± 11.48 among those with uncomplicated malaria $P < 0.0001$]. All the 2468 children were treated in line with malaria treatment guidelines. The 936 children diagnosed with severe malaria

TABLE 1: Child's medical history and history of illness.

Illness history	N	%
Symptoms prior to presentation (multiple responses) ($N = 2468$)		
Fever	2415	97.9
Loss of appetite	966	39.1
Cough	819	33.1
Vomiting	890	30.1
Convulsion	535	21.7
Catarrh	485	19.7
Rigors	438	17.8
Pallor	409	16.6
Lethargy	339	13.7
Loss of consciousness	211	8.5
Fast breathing	161	6.5
Diarrhoea	157	6.4
Body aches	154	6.2
Irritability	99	4.0
Jaundice	76	3.0
Any home treatment ($N = 2452$)		
Yes	1872	76.3
No	579	23.7
Level of consciousness (Paediatric Glasgow Coma Scale) ($N = 610$)		
15 (normal)	76	12.5
8–14 (altered sensorium)	462	75.7
7 and below (coma)	72	11.8

were admitted to hospital and treated with quinine (initially parenteral then changed to oral). The majority, 2207 (89.5%), of all 2468 children recovered fully without any neurological or other complications, 9.1% recovered but with neurological complications such as seizures and hearing deficit, and 1.4% died.

3.1. Sociodemographic Factors Associated with Treatment Outcome. Sociodemographic factors associated with a negative treatment outcome, recovery with a neurological complication (NC), or death are presented in Table 2. Child's age as well as the mother and fathers' level of education was significantly associated with an adverse treatment outcome. The possibility of adverse health income increased with decrease in child's age ($P < 0.0001$). The higher the level of education of a child's mother or father is, the less likely the occurrence of an adverse outcome will be ($P < 0.0001$).

3.2. Association between Illness History and Treatment Outcome. Illness history and prior treatment associated with a negative treatment outcome, recovery with a NC, or death are presented in Table 3. Use of PCM prior to presentation was significantly associated with a better treatment outcome ($P < 0.001$). More children with a history of jaundice, loss

TABLE 2: Sociodemographic factors associated with treatment outcome.

	Full recovery	Recovery + NC or death	Chi-square	P value
Sex ($N = 2466$)				
Male	1168 (88.8)	147 (11.2)	1.369	0.263
Female	1039 (90.3)	112 (9.7)		
Age group (months)				
<12	193 (74.8)	65 (25.2)	81.014	<0.0001*
12–23	425 (88.2)	57 (11.8)		
24–35	402 (89.5)	47 (10.5)		
36–47	333 (92.0)	29 (8.0)		
48–59	278 (95.2)	14 (4.8)		
≥60	576 (92.9)	44 (7.1)		
Mother's level of education ($N = 2450$)				
No formal	83 (50.9)	80 (49.1)	301.3	<0.0001*
Primary	528 (83.3)	106 (16.7)		
Secondary	1137 (95.1)	58 (4.9)		
Tertiary	455 (99.3)	3 (0.7)		
Father's level of education ($N = 2435$)				
No formal	51 (49.5)	52 (50.5)	303.251	<0.0001*
Primary	349 (76.4)	108 (23.6)		
Secondary	1168 (93.9)	76 (6.1)		
Tertiary	627 (99.4)	4 (0.6)		

NC: neurological complications.
*Statistically significant.

of consciousness, and convulsion had a negative treatment outcome ($P < 0.0001$). However, more of those who did not have a history of rigors (11.2%, $P < 0.01$), loss of appetite (13.6%, $P < 0.0001$), vomiting (11.5%, $P < 0.040$), or pallor (11.1%, $P < 0.022$) had negative treatment outcomes.

3.3. Association between Clinical Examination and Laboratory Findings and Treatment Outcome. Negative treatment outcome was observed more in patients with pallor (19%, $P < 0.0001$), jaundice (33.3%, $P < 0.0001$), subnormal temperature (20.0%, $P < 0.0001$), hepatomegaly (26.7%, $P < 0.0001$), splenomegaly (26.9%, $P < 0.0001$), and severe anaemia defined as PCV ≤ 15% (20.1%, $P < 0.0001$) at presentation than among their counterparts who did not have these findings on examination at the hospital (see Table 4).

Following bivariate analysis, factors significantly associated with poor treatment outcome ($P < 0.05$) were entered into the regression model and logistic regression analysis carried out. Child's age less than 12 months (O.R = 5.99, 95% C.I = 1.15–31.15, and $P = 0.033$), history of loss of consciousness (O.R = 4.55, 95% CI = 1.72–12.08, and $P = 0.002$), and subnormal temperature (O.R = 11.52, 95% CI =

TABLE 3: Illness history associated with outcome.

	Full recovery	Recovery + NC or death	Chi-square	P value
Any home treatment				
Yes	1683 (89.9)	189 (10.1)		
No	524 (90.5)	55 (9.5)	0.936	0.776
Any drug used prior to presentation (N = 2240)				
Yes	1553 (98.9)	17 (1.1)		
No	649 (96.9)	21 (3.1)	11.852	0.001
Drug used prior to presentation				
PCM				
Yes	1442 (99.0)	15 (1.0)		
No	757 (97.1)	23 (2.9)	11.206	0.001
CQ				
Yes	346 (98.3)	6 (1.7)		
No	1853 (98.3)	32 (1.7)	0.000	1.000
AQ (2237)				
Yes	93 (97.9)	2 (2.1)		
No	2106 (98.3)	36 (1.7)	0.098	1.000
SP				
Yes	21 (95.5)	1 (4.5)		
No	2178 (98.3)	37 (1.7)	1.078	0.315
Symptoms prior to presentation				
Fever (n = 2468)				
Yes	2165 (89.6)	250 (10.4)	2.426	0.116
No	44 (83.0)	9 (17.0)		
Rigors (n = 2468)				
Yes	407 (92.9)	31 (7.1)	6.618	0.010*
No	1802	228 (11.2)		
Loss of appetite (n = 2468)				
Yes	912 (94.4)	54 (5.6)	40.644	<0.0001*
No	1297 (86.4)	205 (13.6)		
Vomiting (n = 2468)				
Yes	812 (91.2)	78 (8.8)	4.437	0.040*
No	1397 (88.5)	181 (11.5)		
Diarrhoea (n = 2468)				
Yes	142 (90.4)	15 (9.6)	0.158	0.788
No	2067 (89.4)	244 (10.6)		
Jaundice (n = 2468)				
Yes	56 (73.7)	20 (26.3)		
No	2153 (90.0)	239 (10.0)	20.897	0.0001*
Pallor (n = 2467)				
Yes	379 (92.7)	30 (7.3)	5.222	0.022*
No	1829 (88.9)	229 (11.1)		
Fast breathing (N = 2468)				
Yes	140 (87.0)	21 (13.0)	1.192	0.286
No	2069 (89.7)	238 (10.3)		
Lethargy (n = 2468)				
Yes	298 (87.9)	41 (12.1)	1.071	0.295
No	1911 (89.8)	218 (10.2)		
Loss of consciousness (n = 2240)				
Yes	197 (93.4)	14 (6.6)	34.069	<0.0001*
No	2005 (98.8)	24 (1.2)		
Convulsion (n = 2466)				
Yes	449 (83.9)	86 (16.1)	22.566	<0.0001*
No	1758 (91.0)	173 (9.0)		

*Statistically significant.

1.07–123.64, and P = 0.044) were significant predictors of a poorer treatment outcome (Table 5).

4. Discussion

Despite intensified programs in disease control, malaria still remains a public health burden in Sub-Saharan Africa [1]. Although several factors were associated with a poor outcome, after conducting multiple logistic regression analysis, history of loss of consciousness and a child's age less than 12 months were significant predictors of a poorer treatment outcome. These conditions are recognized as pointers to severe malaria [9] and thus emphasize the need for prompt diagnosis and institution of appropriate treatment in the management of malaria. Children who were less than a year old were the most susceptible to neurological complications or even death after treatment and this susceptibility decreased with increasing age, with the lowest susceptibility recorded among children who aged 48–59 months. Riley et al. noted that, while research suggests that neonates and infants are relatively protected against malaria infection and death from severe malaria, this protection was not infallible and could be undermined in the presence of high transmission [12]. Thus infants could still be infected and could suffer from adverse outcomes and this was in keeping with our study findings. Our study also found that children with subnormal temperature at presentation had poorer outcomes than those with normal temperatures and febrile patients. However, the small number of patients in this subcategory could have accounted for this finding.

TABLE 4: Examination findings at presentation associated with outcome.

	Full recovery	Recovery with NC or death	Chi-square	*P* value
Pallor (*n* = 2445)				
Yes	423 (81.0)	99 (19.0)	51.096	<0.0001*
No	1766 (91.8)	157 (8.2)		
Jaundice (*n* = 2441)				
Yes	60 (66.7)	30 (33.3)	53.820	<0.0001*
No	2130 (90.6)	221 (9.4)		
Temperature (°C)				
Febrile (>37.2)	1133 (88.1)	153 (11.9)		
Normal (36.6–37.2)	1032 (94.7)	58 (5.3)		
Subnormal (36.6–35)	8 (80.0)	2 (20.0)		
Hypothermia (<35)	5 (100.0)	0	34.581	<0.0001*
Paediatric GCS				
≤7	68 (94.4)	4 (5.6)		
8–14	439 (95.0)	23 (5.0)		
15	73 (96.1)	3 (3.9)	0.219	0.896
Hepatomegaly (*n* = 2312)				
Yes	381 (73.3)	139 (26.7)	255.3	<0.0001*
No	1722 (96.3)	70 (3.9)		
Splenomegaly (*n* = 2253)				
Yes	209 (73.1)	77 (26.9)	216.4	<0.0001*
No	1894 (96.3)	73 (3.7)		
Anaemia packed cell volume (*n* = 2468)				
Severe (≤15%)	290 (79.9)	73 (20.1)		
Moderate (16–23%)	291 (82.2)	63 (17.8)		
Mild (24–33%)	863 (91.7)	78 (8.3)		
Normal (>33%)	765 (94.4)	45 (5.6)	81.736	<0.0001*

*Statistically significant.

The level of education of both the father and mother of the children surveyed was significantly related to the adverse outcome recorded. Gakidou et al. (2010) in their paper on the effect of increased educational attainment on child mortality in 175 countries between 1970 and 2009 noted that the education of women of reproductive age may account for as much as half of the reduction in under-5 mortality observed in their review [13]. Other studies have also found a relationship between higher levels of maternal education and better child heath outcome [14, 15].

Our study suggests a beneficial effect of prior administration of paracetamol as a lower proportion of children who

TABLE 5: Multivariate analysis of factors associated with poor treatment outcome.

	Odds ratio	95% C.I	*P* value
Sociodemographic characteristics			
Age group			
<12	5.99	1.15–31.15	0.033*
12–23	3.05	0.62–14.88	0.169
24–35	2.54	0.51–12.65	0.254
36–47	3.02	0.62–14.80	0.174
48–59	1		
≥60	1.08	0.16–6.85	0.939
Mother's highest level of education			
No formal	0.000	0.000	0.997
Primary	1.11	0.19–6.57	0.905
Secondary	1.19	0.23–6.11	0.835
Tertiary	1		
Father's highest level of education			
No formal	0.000	0.000	0.998
Primary	1.62	0.31–8.39	0.565
Secondary	2.0	0.48–8.35	0.342
Tertiary	1		
Illness history given by caregiver			
Any drug used prior to presentation			
Yes	1		
No	1.43	0.29–6.93	0.657
Use of PCM prior to presentation			
Yes	1		
No	1.31	0.27–6.44	0.738
Symptoms prior to presentation			
Rigors			
Yes	1		
No	1.51	0.57–4.03	0.409
Loss of appetite			
Yes	1		
No	1.70	0.78–3.70	0.180
Vomiting			
Yes	1		
No	0.64	0.31–1.32	0.226
Jaundice			
Yes	1.26	0.27–5.87	0.767
No	1		
Pallor			
Yes	1		
No	1.58	0.60–4.13	0.353
Loss of consciousness			
Yes	4.55	1.72–12.08	0.002*
No	1		

Table 5: Continued.

	Odds ratio	95% C.I	*P* value
Convulsion			
Yes	1.61	0.66–3.94	0.296
No	1		
Clinical examination findings			
Pallor			
Yes	2.54	0.90–7.16	0.078
No	1		
Jaundice			
Yes	2.05	0.55–7.64	0.284
No	1		
Patients' temperature			
Febrile	1.89	0.77–4.63	0.163
Normal	1		
Sub-normal	11.52	1.07–123.64	0.044*
Hypothermia	—		
Hepatomegaly			
Yes	1.17	0.51–2.68	0.709
No	1		
Splenomegaly			
Yes	1.95	0.82–4.62	0.129
No	1		
Respiratory distress			
Yes			
No			
Anaemia			
Severe	2.62	0.67–10.18	0.165
Mild	0.87	0.21–3.72	0.854
Moderate	1.50	0.45–5.01	0.507
No anaemia	1		

*Statistically significant.

had been given paracetamol developed negative outcomes after treatment compared to their counterparts who were not given paracetamol. Russel et al. (2003) in their review of the use of paracetamol in febrile children submitted that there was no clear evidence in support of its use in treating febrile children [16]. However, early diagnosis of malaria and institution of prompt treatment remain the gold standard for reducing morbidity and mortality from the disease.

Caregivers listed rigors, loss of appetite, vomiting, jaundice, pallor, loss of consciousness, and convulsion as symptoms they observed in their wards. These indicate that many caregivers recognized these symptoms. However more children were noted to be jaundiced, pale, and anaemic on clinical examination and following laboratory investigations conducted at the hospital compared with the caregivers self-report of these symptoms. This implies that many of these symptoms were missed by the caregivers and would therefore explain why a higher percentage of children who were not pale or jaundiced based on their caregivers report had a negative health outcome. This might also explain why a higher percentage of those who had jaundice, pallor, and severe anaemia on clinical examination and/or following laboratory investigations died or developed neurological disorders compared with those who did not have these symptoms or signs.

The study findings also revealed that more children who had not experienced rigors, lost appetite, or vomited had adverse health outcomes. It is thus possible that the caregivers had associated the lack of these symptoms with mild illness leading to delayed presentation at hospital and ultimately delay in commencement of appropriate treatment.

5. Conclusion

A history of loss of consciousness and child's age less than 12 months were significant predictors of poorer treatment outcome in our study sample. Although the caregivers mentioned a number of symptoms that their children had prior to presentation which were associated with poor outcome, the numbers of children who actually had these symptoms was higher on clinical examination and following laboratory investigation. Many of these symptoms such as pallor, jaundice, and severe anemia were positively associated with adverse treatment outcomes. This has implications for programmes that advocate for home management of malaria because commencement of home management relies on the caregivers ability to recognize mild symptoms of malaria. This approach might be counterproductive as complications may then set in especially when caregivers do not recognize symptoms of severe disease. In view of the study findings, we recommend that caregivers be properly educated so that they can seek medical care promptly in order to prevent progression to severe disease which is associated with poor treatment outcomes.

Conflict of Interests

The authors declare that there is no conflict of interests regarding the publication of this paper.

Acknowledgments

The authors are grateful to all study participants and their parents/guardians. They appreciate all the field and laboratory staff of the malaria pathogenesis unit, Institute Child Health, University of Ibadan. The research leading to these results has received funding from the European Community under Grant agreement LSHP-CT-2004-503578.

References

[1] World Health Organization, "World Malaria Report, 2012 Summary," 2013, http://www.who.int/malaria/publications/world_malaria_report_2012/wmr2012_summary_en.pdf.

[2] Federal Ministry of Health, "National Malaria Control Program Strategic Plan 2009–2013," Federal Ministry of Health, Abuja, Nigeria, 2009.

[3] National Population Commission (NPC), "National Malaria Control Programme (NMCP), Measure DHS," Nigeria Malaria Indicator Survey 2010, 2012.

[4] P. W. Njuguna and C. R. J. C. Newton, "Management of severe falciparum malaria," *Journal of Postgraduate Medicine*, vol. 50, no. 1, pp. 45–50, 2004.

[5] S. Ahmed, F. Adil, T. Shahzad, and Y. Yahiya, "Severe malaria in children: factors predictive of outcome and response to Quinine," *Journal of the Pakistan Medical Association*, vol. 61, no. 1, pp. 54–58, 2011.

[6] S. K. Mishra and C. R. J. C. Newton, "Diagnosis and management of the neurological complications of falciparum malaria," *Nature Reviews Neurology*, vol. 5, no. 4, pp. 189–198, 2009.

[7] K. Marsh, D. Forster, C. Waruiru et al., "Indicators of life-threatening malaria in African children," *The New England Journal of Medicine*, vol. 332, no. 21, pp. 1399–1404, 1995.

[8] Federal Ministry of Health, "National Antimalarial Treatment Policy," Federal Ministry of Health, National Malaria and Vector Control Division, Abuja ,Nigeria, May 2005.

[9] WHO, "Severe falciparum malaria," *Transactions of the Royal Society of Tropical Medicine and Hygiene*, vol. 94, supplement 1, pp. S1–S90, 2000.

[10] M. Swash, *Hutchison's Clinical Methods*, ELBS with Bailliere Tindall, London, UK, 19th edition, 1989.

[11] F. J. Kirkham, C. R. J. C. Newton, and W. Whitehouse, "Paediatric coma scales," *Developmental Medicine and Child Neurology*, vol. 50, no. 4, pp. 267–274, 2008.

[12] E. M. Riley, G. E. Wagner, B. D. Akanmori, and K. A. Koram, "Do maternally acquired antibodies protect infants from malaria infection?" *Parasite Immunology*, vol. 23, no. 2, pp. 51–59, 2001.

[13] E. Gakidou, K. Cowling, R. Lozano, and C. J. Murray, "Increased educational attainment and its effect on child mortality in 175 countries between 1970 and 2009: a systematic analysis," *The Lancet*, vol. 376, no. 9745, pp. 959–974, 2010.

[14] A. R. Joshi, "Maternal schooling and child health: preliminary analysis of the intervening mechanisms in rural Nepal," *Health Transition Review*, vol. 4, no. 1, pp. 1–28, 1994.

[15] D. Buor, "Mothers' education and childhood mortality in Ghana," *Health Policy*, vol. 64, no. 3, pp. 297–309, 2003.

[16] F. M. Russell, F. Shann, N. Curtis, and K. Mulholland, "Evidence on the use of paracetamol in febrile children," *Bulletin of the World Health Organization*, vol. 81, no. 5, pp. 367–372, 2003.

Identifying At-Risk Subpopulations of Canadians with Limited Health Literacy

Takashi Yamashita,[1] A. John Bailer,[2,3] and Douglas A. Noe[2]

[1] *Department of Sociology, University of Nevada, Las Vegas, Las Vegas, NV 89154, USA*
[2] *Department of Statistics, Miami University, Oxford, OH 45056, USA*
[3] *Scripps Gerontology Center, Miami University, Oxford, OH 45056, USA*

Correspondence should be addressed to Takashi Yamashita; takashi.yamashita@unlv.edu

Academic Editor: Wolfgang Ahrens

Background. Health literacy, the set of skills for locating, understanding, and using health-related information, is associated with various health outcomes through health behaviors and health care service use. While health literacy has great potential for addressing health disparities stemming from the differing educational attainment in diverse populations, knowledge about subpopulations that share the same risk factors is useful. *Objective.* This study employed a logistic regression tree algorithm to identify subpopulations at risk of limited health literacy in Canadian adults. *Design.* The nationally representative data were derived from the International Adult Literacy and Skills Survey (n = 20,059). The logistic regression tree algorithm splits the samples into subgroups and fits logistic regressions. *Results.* Results showed that the subpopulation comprised of individuals 56 years and older, with household income less than $50,000, no participation in adult education programs, and lack of reading activities (i.e., newspaper, books) was at the greatest risk (82%) of limited health literacy. Other identified subgroups were displayed in an easily interpreted tree diagram. *Conclusions.* Identified subpopulations organized in tree diagrams according to the risk of limited health literacy inform not only intervention programs targeting unique subpopulations but also future health literacy research.

1. Identifying At-Risk Subpopulations of Canadians with Limited Health Literacy

Health literacy (HL) describes the set of abilities to locate, understand, and use health-related information to make better health decisions throughout one's life [1]. Along with rapidly advancing medical/health sciences and changing health care systems, being able to obtain timely health-related information is critical for health maintenance/promotion [2]. Limited HL is prevalent in many adult populations and is directly and indirectly associated with lack of knowledge about health/diseases, miscommunication in healthcare settings, and adverse health behaviors (e.g., infrequent preventive healthcare service use and sedentary lifestyle) and, in turn, poorer health outcome [2–4]. Nearly half of the adult populations in developed nations like the US and Canada have insufficient HL skills [5, 6]. Improving HL is one strategy suggested for addressing health disparities [7].

The Rootman and Ronson HL conceptual model [8] depicts predictors of HL and theoretical pathways between HL and health. In this model, community-/societal-level (e.g., community development and public policy) and individual-level (e.g., aging and primary language) HL determinants are called "Actions" and "Determinants," respectively. HL may directly influence one's health, for instance, due to misunderstanding/misuse of medications [9]. At the same time, HL may influence health through various well-known health determinants including healthcare service use, health and disease management behaviors (e.g., smoking), economic resource access, and living environments [10–14]. Additionally, previous studies found that social factors such as access to quality education early in life and continuous opportunities for continuous literacy improvement (e.g., work-related literacy tasks) and health literacy proficiency are interrelated [15, 16]. In short, the Rootman and Ronson HL conceptual model suggests the complex associations of demographic, socioeconomic and geographic factors on health and, in turn, emphasizes the diversity of limited HL risk factors as well as theoretical pathways to health.

The health disparities research model suggests that identification of populations at risk of adverse health should be the first step in public health research [17]. Generally, public health intervention programs can be categorized as either a homogeneous intervention program for a large target population (i.e., population approach) or as a tailored program for each individual at risk (i.e., individual-at-high-risk approach) [18, 19]. However, a review of recent public health interventions suggests that both approaches have not yet made significant impacts on health disparities [20, 21]. Arguably, lack of attention to the intrinsic variability in populations in the population approach and resource-/labor-intensiveness in the individual-at-high-risk approach partially explain some unsuccessful interventions. A reasonable compromise between the population and individual intervention targeting options would be to target at-risk subpopulations identified by a series of risk factors.

Guided by the Rootman and Ronson HL conceptual model (2005) and the health disparities research framework [17], this study identifies subpopulations at risk of limited HL in Canadian adults using the International Adult Literacy and Life Skills Survey data (described later). Specifically, the following research question is addressed: what characteristics define subpopulations at high risk of limited HL in the Canadian adult population? While a combination of bivariate analyses may identify some reasonable subpopulations, more insight is likely to be provided by simultaneously considering a large collection of potentially relevant predictors of limited HL.

2. Methods

2.1. Data. The data come from the International Adult Literacy and Skills Survey (IALSS). IALSS data include a nationally representative sample of Canadian adults (n = 20,059) and provide measures in literacy skills; the data also include information regarding demographic, socioeconomic, lifestyle, and health conditions [22]. The definition of each literacy domain is described elsewhere [23]. HL measure is derived from a subset of health-related prose literacy, document literacy, and numeracy test items. The score ranges from zero to 500. The respondents were categorized according to their HL scores into 5 levels (level 1 (very poor skills) = 0–225; level 2 (poor skills) = 226–275; level 3 (adequate skills) = 276–325; level 4 (Strong skills) = 326–375; level 5 (strongest skills) = 376–500) [6, 24]. The literacy measurement tool was jointly developed by the Educational Testing Service (ETS) in the US and Statistics Canada and is comparable to other major national-level adult literacy assessments such as the National Assessment of Adult Literacy (NAAL) and the International Adult Literacy Survey (IALS), assessment tools also developed by the same organization (ETS) [25].

2.2. Outcome Variable. The outcome variable is a dichotomous variable coded as [1] if individuals have the lowest category of HL, limited HL (*level 1*) defined in the IALSS, and (0) if individuals have the basic, intermediate or proficient HL skills (*levels 2–5*). Assuming that limited HL translates into higher risk of adverse health outcomes we believe is an appropriate emphasis. In our preliminary analyses (results now shown) which are to compare the respondents with limited HL *level 1* to those with all other levels (each level separately), those with limited HL *level 1* had significantly lower scores in all widely used physical health indicators and most of mental health indicators except two emotional problems indicators (i.e., feeling depressed or anxious; did not do work or other activity as carefully as usual) than those with upper level HL skills (i.e., SF-12; 26). In this regard, focusing on *level 1* as the highest risk group is empirically supported by a variety of health indicators.

2.3. Predictor Variables. The model includes predictor variables that reflect "determinants" factors from the Rootman and Ronson model (2005). We focus on the "determinants" factors due to unavailability of "actions" or community/society-level factors in the IALSS. In this model, the determinants include "Education," "Early child development," "Aging," "Personal capacity," "Living/working condition," "Gender," and "Culture." Although the variables from the IALSS may not always reflect each component, this study preserves the terminologies in the Rootman and Ronson model.

Education. College education is an indicator variable recording whether the respondents completed a college degree. *Adult education* records whether the respondents attended any postsecondary education or training including any educational/training program, course, private lessons, workshops, and so forth in last 12 months. The following three variables are used to reflect the respondents' everyday literacy-related activities. *Reading Newspapers* records whether a respondent reads newspapers at least once a week. *Watching TV* records the hours per day a respondent watches TV, video, or DVD: categories (1) 1 hour or less, (2) over 1 hour to 2 hours, (3) more than 2 but less than 5 hours, and (4) 5 or more hours. *Reading Books* records whether a respondent reads books at least once a week.

Early Child Development. English as first language learned records whether the first language a respondent learned was English. *English as a primary language* records whether the primary language spoken at home was English when a respondent grew up.

Aging. Age group records the six age groups (age 16–25; 26–35; 36–45; 46–55; 56–65; 66 and older) according to the respondents' age at the time of the survey in 2003. Age in years was not available for all IALSS respondents.

Personal Capacity. Self-rated health records whether a respondent reported his/her health is (5) excellent, (4) very good, (3) good, (2) fair, or (1) poor. While health status is not a common indicator of personal capacity including literacy skills, several studies found that health status indicators can serve as a surrogate measure of chronic conditions (e.g., diabetes and disease-caused visual impairment) that are negatively associated with one's HL [26, 27]. *Emotional problem* records whether the respondent reported any emotional problems (e.g., depressed feeling and feeling anxious) during the past 4 weeks. *Life satisfaction* records whether a respondent reported his/her life satisfaction as (5) extremely satisfied, (4) satisfied, (3) neither satisfied nor unsatisfied, (2) unsatisfied, or (1) extremely unsatisfied.

Living/Working Condition. Household Income records the respondent's annual household income (converted to the US dollar unit) as (1) $25,000 or less, (2) $25,001 to $50,000, (3) $50,001 to 90,000, and (4) more than $90,000. *Employment* records whether a respondent was working at least part-time at the time of the study. *Urban area* indicates whether a respondent lived in an urban area. *Region* records one of the five regions where the respondents reside and includes Atlantic, Quebec, Ontario, West, and North. Health insurance was not taken into account due to the universal health care coverage in Canada. Also, marital status information was not available in IALSS. *Student* records whether a respondent was a student (including work programs).

Gender. Female records if a respondent is female or not.

Culture. Immigrants records whether a respondent was an immigrant. *Born in Canada* records whether a respondent reported that they were born in Canada. *Immigrants* indicates whether a respondent was born outside of Canada and moved to Canada at some point of their lives. A value = 1 for *Immigrants* also identifies individuals who become Canadian citizens by naturalization.

2.4. Statistical Methods. This study employs a logistic regression tree approach, which has several advantages over commonly used traditional methods such as bivariate testing and logistic regression in epidemiologic research [28]. Compared to standard logistic regression, the logistic regression tree approach allows a more flexible model structure, including the incorporation of complex interactions, for describing how predictor variables impact the odds of limited HL. This approach implements a method that identifies subpopulations with similar HL and then allows for the fitting of a logistic regression model with potentially different predictor variable for each subpopulation. In addition, this method does not require imputation or case-wise deletion to deal with missing values.

2.5. Logistic Tree with Unbiased Selection—LOTUS. This study employs the logistic regression tree algorithm named Logistic Tree with Unbiased Selection (LOTUS) [29]. LOTUS is designed specifically to deal with binary responses (limited HL versus not limited HL in this study) and has advantages (e.g., unbiased split variable selection) over other classification and regression tree algorithms such as CART [30] and CHAID [31]. LOTUS can be considered a combination of classification trees and logistic regression. LOTUS merges the desirable capabilities of these two methods in such a way that logistic regressions are fit in recursively split subdata (i.e., subpopulations).

To determine the final size (i.e., number of subpopulations) of the logistic regression tree, LOTUS employs an overfit-and-prune approach. The recursive process of splitting nodes continues until no further splits are possible due to either homogeneity (e.g., a subgroup has 100% limited HL) or a lack of sufficient numbers of cases. Obviously, such a complete, unpruned tree provides an excellent fit to the provided data but may not generalize well to new observations. To prune back the overgrown tree in this study, 10-fold cross-validation using the 1-SE rule is used as described by Breiman et al. [30]. More technically, detailed descriptions of LOTUS are provided in Chan and Loh [29] and Loh [32]. The LOTUS algorithm version 2.3 was applied for the IALSS respondents to identify subgroups at high risk of limited HL.

3. Results

Table 1 includes descriptive summaries of candidate predictor variables for the individuals with and without limited HL. Approximately 29% of the respondents had limited HL, the lowest, Level 1 category of HL. As expected, a series of bivariate comparisons showed that higher education, learning/reading activities (e.g., adult education, reading newspapers), English as the first language, younger age, higher income, employment, and nonimmigrants and being born in Canada are more common in individuals with greater HL skills than in individuals with limited HL.

The results of the LOTUS analysis are summarized in a tabular form listing all identified subpopulations (Table 2) ordered from highest percentage to lowest percentage of limited HL. In addition, a graphical display of these subpopulations is presented in tree diagrams (Figure 1(a) (left half of the diagram) and Figure 1(b) (right half of the diagram)). The pathway to the highest risk groups is in bold in Figures 1(a) and 1(b). The respondents aged 56 and older with household income less than $50,000 who read books less than once a week, read newspapers less than once a week, and report no adult education program participation last 12 months were at the highest risk (81.8%) of limited HL (see Figure 1(b)).

Among each subpopulation (i.e., terminal nodes or rectangular boxes in the tree diagram) identified according to the risk of limited HL, further within-subpopulation differences were detected by simple logistic regression models; 5 out of 15 subpopulations had household income as the predictor variable in the simple logistic regression models. Also, a noteworthy interaction effect between reading newspapers and having a college education on the odds of limited HL was detected in the subgroup of people aged 56 and older with household income less than $50,000 who read books less than once a week and report no participation in adult education programs in the last 12 months. In this particular subpopulation, the respondents who read a newspaper more than once a week had 0.18 times odds of having limited HL when they had college education compared to those who did not. On the other hand, respondents who read a newspaper less than once a week had 0.29 times the odds of having limited HL when they had college education compared to those who did not. In other words, college education was

TABLE 1: Descriptive summary statistics, 95% confidence interval, and bivariate tests by the IALSS respondents with and without limited health literacy.

Variables	All respondents (n = 23,038)			Difference (95% CL: LL, UL,)	X^2 (DF, P value)
	Total	Limited HL	Not limited HL		
Limited HL[d]	29.3%	—	—		
College education[c]	40.0%	18.6%	48.5%	30.0 (28.6, 31.2)	1780.2 (1, $P < .0001$)
Adult education[c]	45.1%	20.7%	55.1%	34.3 (33.0, 35.7)	2182.8 (1, $P < .0001$)
Read newspapers[c]	75.2%	65.9%	79.0%	13.1 (11.9, 14.3)	421.6 (1, $P < .0001$)
Read books[d]	41.7%	25.2%	48.4%	23.3 (21.9, 24.7)	1020.5 (1, $P < .0001$)
Watch TV				NA	908.9 (3, $P < .0001$)
1 hour or less per day	25.0%	*18.8%*	*27.6%*	—	—
Over 1 hour to 2 hours per day	33.0%	*27.9%*	*35.1%*	—	—
More than 2 hours but less than 5	33.5%	*37.1%*	*32.1%*	—	—
5 or more hours per day	8.5%	*16.3%*	*5.3%*	—	—
English was the first language learned[c]	50.2%	40.5%	54.1%	13.6 (12.2, 15.1)	341.6 (1, $P < .0001$)
English is the primary language[c]	62.0%	55.2%	64.7%	9.6 (8.1, 11.0)	163.9 (1, $P < .0001$)
Age group				NA	2256.8 (5, $P < .001$)
16–25	16.8%	*10.9%*	*19.2%*	—	—
26–35	15.5%	*10.3%*	*17.7%*	—	—
36–45	21.3%	*16.5%*	*23.3%*	—	—
46–55	20.2%	*17.4%*	*21.3%*	—	—
56–65	13.3%	*17.1%*	*11.7%*	—	—
66 and older	12.9%	*27.9%*	*6.7%*	—	—
Self-rated health				NA	1322.6 (4, $P < .0001$)
Poor	3.9%	*7.8%*	*2.3%*	—	—
Fair	11.5%	*19.2%*	*8.4%*	—	—
Good	29.0%	*33.7%*	*27.1%*	—	—
Very good	33.3%	*25.0%*	*36.7%*	—	—
Excellent	22.2%	*14.3%*	*25.4%*	—	—
Emotional problem[c]	8.9%	12.8%	7.3%	−5.6 (−6.4, −4.7)	175.1 (1, $P < .0001$)
Life satisfaction				NA	396.9 (4, $P < .0001$)
Extremely unsatisfied	1.8%	*2.7%*	*1.4%*	—	—
Unsatisfied	6.5%	*9.9%*	*5.1%*	—	—
Neither	9.6%	*9.8%*	*9.5%*	—	—
Satisfied	61.3%	*62.7%*	*60.7%*	—	—
Extremely satisfied	21.0%	*15.0%*	*23.4%*	—	—
Household income				NA	1739.6 (3, $P < .0001$)
$25,000 or less (bottom quintile)	25.3%	*43.4%*	*18.2%*	—	—
$25,000.01 to $50,000	30.7%	*33.7%*	*29.5%*	—	—
$50,000.01 to $90,000	28.5%	*16.6%*	*33.1%*	—	—

TABLE 1: Continued.

Variables	All respondents (n = 23,038)			Difference (95% CL: LL, UL,)	X^2 (DF, P value)
	Total	Limited HL	Not limited HL		
More than $90,000.01 (top quintile)	15.6%	*6.3%*	*19.2%*	—	—
Employed[c]	61.9%	41.5%	70.4%	29.0 (27.6, 30.3)	1696.4 (1, P < .0001)
Student[c]	5.7%	3.2%	6.7%	3.6 (2.9, 4.2)	113.3 (1, P < .0001)
Urban areas[c]	74.4%	72.3%	75.3%	3.0 (1.7, 4.4)	18.5 (1, P < .0001)
Regions				NA	
Atlantic	20.3%	23.0%	19.2%	−3.8 (−5.0, −2.7)	43.0 (1, P < .0001)
Quebec	18.1%	14.5%	20.0%	5.1 (4.0, 6.1)	82.3 (1, P < .0001)
Ontario	21.5%	23.8%	20.5%	3.0 (1.7, 4.4)	31.0 (1, P < .0001)
West	28.9%	26.4%	30.0%	3.6 (2.3, 4.9)	30.2 (1, P < .0001)
North	11.2%	12.3%	10.8%	−1.5 (−2.4, −0.6)	11.2 (1, P < .0008)
Gender (female)[c]	54.5%	53.4%	55.0%	1.7 (0.3, 3.1)	5.2 (1, P < .022)
Immigrants[c]	18.2%	25.7%	15.1%	−10.6 (−11.7, −9.4)	315.5 (1, P < .0001)
Born in Canada[c]	71.8%	64.4%	74.9%	10.6 (9.3, 11.8)	263.1 (1, P < .0001)

[a]Data source: International Adult Literacy and Skills Survey (IALSS) 2003.
[b]All descriptive summary statistics are unweighted
[c]Dummy variables (1 versus 0).
[d]Limited health literacy: health literacy level 1; nonlimited health literacy: health literacy level 2,3, and 4.
NA: not applicable; HL: health literacy; CL: confidence interval; UL: upper limit; LL: lower limit; DF: degrees of freedom; IALSS = International Adult Literacy and Life Skills Survey.

associated with lower chance of limited health literacy in both of these subpopulations although the effect of college education varied between individuals who read a newspaper more than once a week and those who did not.

4. Discussion

Building on the HL conceptual model [8] and the public health disparities research model [17], this study employs a logistic regression tree analysis and identifies the subpopulations at risk of having limited HL in the Canadian adult population aged 16 years and older. The proportions of limited HL in the identified subpopulations range from 12% to 82% (see Figures 1(a) and 1(b)). Approximately 82% of the subpopulation of Canadian adults aged 56 years and older with household income less than $50,000 who read books and newspapers less than once a week and report no participation in adult education last 12 months exhibited limited HL, the highest percentage among all 15 subpopulations identified.

Combinations of demographic and other relevant factors clearly identified subpopulations at risk of limited HL. The identified risk factors can be roughly classified into two groups: (1) the demographic/socioeconomic factors of age and household income; (2) everyday learning activities: reading books, participation in adult education programs, and reading newspapers. These risk factors are also reflected in the "Determinants" domain of Rootman and Ronson's model. Although the observational data in this study do not allow causal inference, a lack of regular learning activities may further increase the risk of limited HL in particular subgroups (e.g., older age and low income) with individuals who are already at greater risk [12]. At the same time, it is also possible that some aging-related physical or cognitive declines and/or a lack of resources (e.g., time for reading and money to buy new books) might influence opportunities for learning activities and, in turn, resulted in limited HL [33, 34].

In addition, earlier educational attainment (lack of college education was the best predictor of limited HL in the highest risk subpopulation) is likely to determine one's socioeconomic status (e.g., income and occupation) and put those with lower educational attainment are put at risk of limited HL [35–38]. Arguably, from a long-term perspective, lack of

Table 2: Identified subpopulations and predictor variables by the risks of limited health literacy.

Subpopulations	% Limited HL (n)	Age	Household income	Read books	Adult education	Read newspaper	College education	Employed	Immigrants	Born in Canada
1	81.8% (817)	≥56	≤$50,000	No	No	No	—	—	—	—
2	64.9% (1,775)	≥56	≤$50,000	No	No	Yes	—	—	—	—
3	63.5% (365)	≤55	—	No	No	—	No	Yes	Yes	—
4	58.7% (1,160)	≤55	—	No	No	—	No	No	—	—
5	52.3% (779)	≥66	≤$50,000	Yes	No	—	—	—	—	—
6	37.7% (245)	≥56	≥$50,000	—	—	—	No	—	—	—
7	36.5% (679)	≤55	—	No	No	—	No	Yes	No	—
8	35.1% (262)	≥56	≤$50,000	No	Yes	—	—	—	—	—
9	34.0% (586)	56–65	≤$50,000	Yes	No	—	—	—	—	—
10	33.5% (477)	≥56	≤$50,000	Yes	Yes	—	—	—	—	—
11	26.3% (864)	≤55	—	—	No	—	Yes	—	—	No
12	25.4% (1,501)	≤55	—	—	No	—	Yes	—	—	—
13	16.6% (692)	≥56	≥$50,000	—	—	—	Yes	—	—	—
14	13.9% (9,622)	≤55	—	—	Yes	—	—	—	—	—
15	12.0% (197)	≤55	—	—	No	—	Yes	—	—	Yes

Note: see Figures 1(a) and 1(b) for simple logistic regression results for terminal nodes (i.e., identified sub-populations).
HL: health literacy.

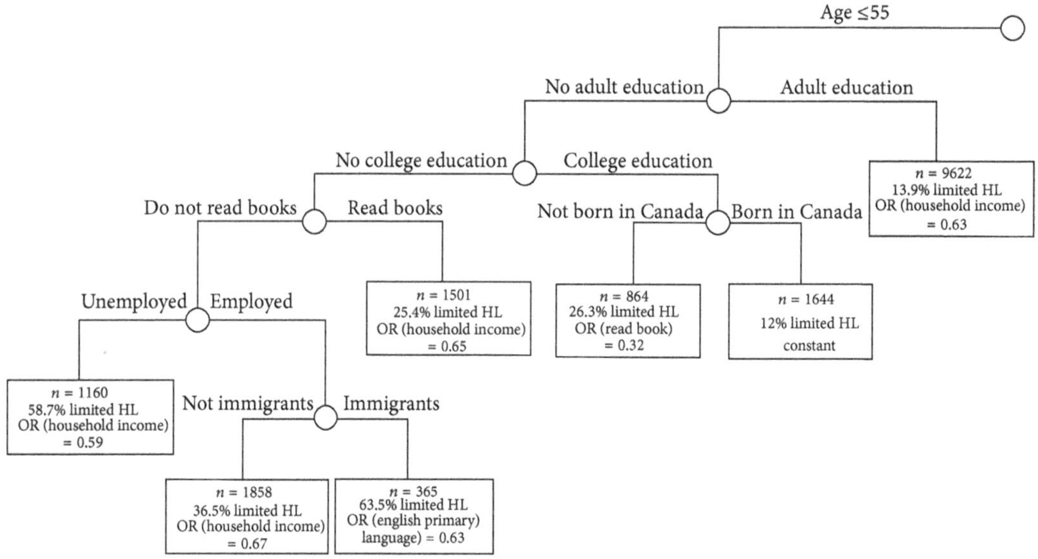

Notes:
Data source: international adult literacy and life skill survey (IALSS)
OR: estimated odds ratio for a predictor variable of simple logistic regression in each terminal node.

(a)

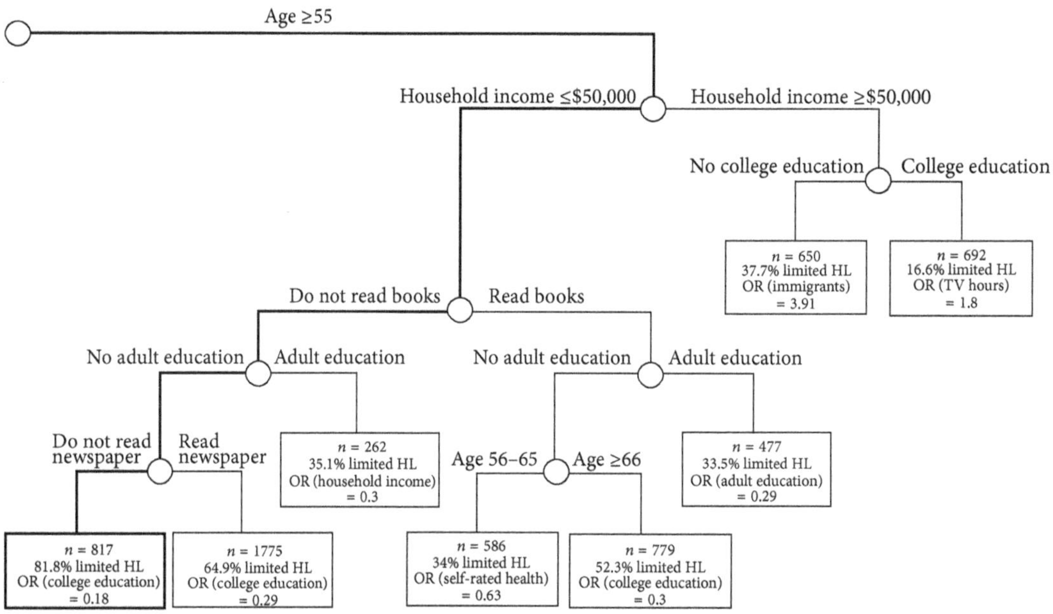

Notes:
Data source: international adult literacy and life skill survey (IALSS)
OR: estimated odds ratio for a predictor variable of simple logistic regression in each terminal node.
Bold lines lead to the sub-population at the highest risk of limited health literacy

(b)

FIGURE 1: (a) Logistic regression tree diagrams of limited health literacy: the entire International Adult Literacy and Life Skills Survey (ILASS) respondents (left half). (b) Logistic regression tree diagrams of limited health literacy: the entire International Adult Literacy and Life Skills Survey (ILASS) respondents (right half).

literacy skills (e.g., health literacy) could impact social status determinants like educational attainment and employment, and vice versa. Therefore, individuals with poor initial literacy skills may experience cumulative disadvantages over the life course [15, 39]. As suggested in Rootman and Ronson's model, formal education contributes to one's general literacy as well as other types of literacy skills (e.g., scientific literacy) and, in turn, HL skills. In this regard, life-long (i.e., mostly occupation-related formal programs) and life-wide (i.e., informal education programs) learning activities such as participation in adult education programs and reading newspapers/books might have acted as mediators of the association between limited HL and possible risk factors, particularly after participation in formal schooling ends [15]. Indeed, those who reported frequent reading/learning activities were less likely to have limited HL.

It should be noted that the national level efforts to address limited HL have been made by the governments and national organizations last few decades [40, 41]. In most cases, the health systems (e.g., healthcare providers and health organizations) provide customized materials and additional services to individuals with limited HL. Such "downstream" approach (i.e., assisting existing health illiterates) is a critical part of national health goals because even individuals with mid-level HL skills often face difficulties in healthcare settings [42]. Especially, unfamiliar health-related literacy tasks may be challenging. At the same time, efforts to prevent limited health literacy (i.e., "upstream" approach) are necessary for sustainable long-term HL interventions as more than half of Canadian adults may have difficulties with health-related literacy tasks [6]. Results of this study could inform not only interventions for existing limited HL prevalence but also for preventing future health illiterates. HL and/or literacy education interventions in earlier lives are key for successful prevention strategies considering the identified risk factors like older age and lack of learning activities. As one's health needs and necessary health knowledge change over the life course, identified risk factors in this study may help target potential health illiterates. Finally, a more health literate population may require less case management and direct HL education which could translate into health care cost savings.

4.1. Implications. The findings from this study have several implications for future research and practice to improve HL. First, this analysis identifies subpopulations with higher risk of limited HL; these findings can guide resource allocations for interventions from public health practitioners and heath policy makers. Targeting the highest risk subgroups for interventions is an efficient and, hopefully, effective alternative. Second, the information about multiple risk factors and their relationships with each other in the tree diagrams provide useful insights for designing intervention programs. For instance, for individuals who are older and in lower income households, HL intervention programs need to be sensitive to their needs including familiar communication styles and logistics (e.g., transportation) [43–45]. For example, given the identified reading-related risk factors, multiple interventions such as offering a series of educational opportunities and/or making reading activities more accessible to the high risk groups may improve one's literacy and ultimately health literacy [46]. Additionally, the risk factor of older age suggests that intervention programs/materials should be accessible (e.g., larger font and familiar examples) to mid-aged to older adults with limited health literacy. On a related note, careful examination of tree diagrams generates possible hypotheses for future inquiries. Arguably, each subpopulation has different processes that lead individuals to limited HL. Therefore, more detailed subpopulation analyses could improve understanding about etiological pathways to limited HL.

Third, logistic regression tree algorithms like LOTUS can be applied for various other populations such as community members, hospital patients, and individuals with diseases (e.g., diabetes and arthritis) and data routinely collected by political boundaries [28]. Finally, the identified subpopulations in order of the risk of limited HL (see Table 2) need to be systematically compared in future research. Such a comparative study may further advance practically relevant HL research. Also, the subpopulation strategy may be further tailored to reflect local demographic characteristics (e.g., race and ethnicity), culture, politics, and education systems. In short, while the findings in this study are not conclusive, they will guide current practice and research related to limited HL prevalence that is a serious public health concern by proposing a novel approach for identifying subpopulations.

4.2. Limitations. Possible omitted variable bias might exist due to the information availability in the IALSS data. Other types of education measurement, cognitive skills, more detailed community-level information (i.e., "Actions" domain in Rootman and Ronson's model) besides *regions*, health care utilization, and other health conditions are important to be included in future data collection. Also, although the IALSS is arguably one of only few nationally representative datasets that provides methodologically sound estimate of health literacy skill levels, the evaluation of specific level has not been established, and therefore, the results may need to be verified in future research. Moreover, the statistical method (LOTUS) employed in this study has some advantages over traditional methods, but LOTUS could still benefit from several features for further improvement. Such options might include more flexible options for split point selection of a continuous variable (instead of specific percentile points), the capability to incorporate survey sampling weights, the provision of additional model fit indices (e.g., c-statistic), and features to analyze longitudinal data. Finally, the logistic regression tree approach does not replace traditional methods but adds new analytic capabilities.

5. Conclusion

This study identified specific subpopulations that share the same characteristics and are at risk of limited HL. Specifically, older Canadian adults (56 years and older) earning less than $50,000 household income who read infrequently and who do not participate in adult education programs are at the highest risk of having limited HL. As demonstrated in this study, the logistic regression tree algorithm (LOTUS) generates an easily interpreted tree diagram and provides insights such as splitting points and/or potential interaction effects of key risk factors. In addition, possible hypotheses about distinct associations and etiological relationships between limited HL and risk factors across age groups should be on the future research agenda. The findings in this study, particularly the idea of a subpopulation approach, provide promising leads for targeting future intervention programs to address the issue of highly prevalent limited HL in adult populations.

References

[1] M. Kutner, E. Greenberg, Y. Jin, and C. Paulsen, *The Health Literacy of America's Adults: Results from the 2003 National Assessment of Adult Literacy*, U.S. Department of Education, Washington, DC, USA, 2006.

[2] L. Nielsen-Bohlman, A. M. Panzer, and D. A. Kindig, *Health Literacy: A Prescription to End Confusion*, National Academy Press, Washington, DC, USA, 2004.

[3] D. Schillinger, A. Bindman, F. Wang, A. Stewart, and J. Piette, "Functional health literacy and the quality of physician-patient communication among diabetes patients," *Patient Education and Counseling*, vol. 52, no. 3, pp. 315–323, 2004.

[4] S. C. Ratzan, "Health literacy: communication for the public good," *Health Promotion International*, vol. 16, no. 2, pp. 207–214, 2001.

[5] M. Kutner, E. Greenberg, and J. Baer, *A First Look at the Literacy of America's Adult in the 21st Century*, U.S. Department of Education, Washington, DC, USA, 2005.

[6] T. S. Murray, J. Hagey, J. D. Willms, and R. Shillington, *Health Literacy in Canada: A Healthy Understanding 2008*, Canadian Council on Learning, Ottawa, Canada, 2008.

[7] C. L. Bennett, M. R. Ferreira, T. C. Davis et al., "Relation between literacy, race, and stage of presentation among low-income patients with prostate cancer," *Journal of Clinical Oncology*, vol. 16, no. 9, pp. 3101–3104, 1998.

[8] I. Rootman and B. Ronson, "Literacy and health research in Canada: where have we been and where should we go?" *Canadian Journal of Public Health*, vol. 96, no. 2, pp. S62–S77, 2005.

[9] T. C. Davis, M. S. Wolf, P. F. Bass et al., "Literacy and misunderstanding prescription drug labels," *Annals of Internal Medicine*, vol. 145, no. 12, pp. 887–894, 2006.

[10] D. W. Baker, "Reading between the lines: deciphering the connections between literacy and health," *Journal of General Internal Medicine*, vol. 14, no. 5, pp. 315–317, 1999.

[11] M. S. Wolf, J. A. Gazmararian, and D. W. Baker, "Health literacy and health risk behaviors among older adults," *American Journal of Preventive Medicine*, vol. 32, no. 1, pp. 19–24, 2007.

[12] Statistics Canada and Organisation for Economic Co-operation Development, *Literacy, Economy and Society: Results of the First International Adult Literacy Survey*, OECD Publications and Information Center, 1995.

[13] D. Schillinger and T. Davis, "A conceptual framework for the relationship between health literacy and health care outcomes: the chronic disease exemplar," in *Understanding Health Literacy: Implications for Medicine and Public Health*, J. G. Schwartzberg, J. VanGeest, and C. Wang, Eds., American Medical Association Press, Chicago, Ill, USA, 2005.

[14] S. C. Kalichman, B. Ramachandran, and S. Catz, "Adherence to combination antiretroviral therapies in HIV patients of low health literacy," *Journal of General Internal Medicine*, vol. 14, no. 5, pp. 267–273, 1999.

[15] R. Desjardins, "Determinants of literacy proficiency: a lifelong-lifewide learning perspective," *International Journal of Educational Research*, vol. 39, no. 3, pp. 205–245, 2003.

[16] S. R. Schecter and J. Lynch, "Health learning and adult education: in search of a theory of practice," *Adult Education Quarterly*, vol. 61, no. 3, pp. 207–224, 2011.

[17] A. M. Kilbourne, G. Switzer, K. Hyman, M. Crowley-Matoka, and M. J. Fine, "Advancing health disparities research within the health care system: a conceptual framework," *American Journal of Public Health*, vol. 96, no. 12, pp. 2113–2121, 2006.

[18] G. Rose, K. T. Khaw, and M. Marmot, *Rose's Strategy of Preventive Medicine: The Complete Original Text*, Oxford University Press, Oxford, UK, 2008.

[19] P. A. Braveman, C. Cubbin, S. Egerter et al., "Socioeconomic status in health research: one size does not fit all," *Journal of the American Medical Association*, vol. 294, no. 22, pp. 2879–2888, 2005.

[20] B. D. Smedley and S. L. Syme, "Promoting health: intervention strategies from social and behaviroral research," in *Commiittee on Capitalizing on Social Science and Behaviroral Research to Improve the Public's Health*, Division of Health Promotion and Disease Prevention, Ed., National Academy Press, Washington, DC, USA, 2000.

[21] P. Braveman and E. Tarimo, "Social inequalities in health within countries: not only an issue for affluent nations," *Social Science and Medicine*, vol. 54, no. 11, pp. 1621–1635, 2002.

[22] T. S. Murray, Y. Clermont, and M. Binkley, *Measuring Adult Literacy and Life Skills: New Frameworks for Assessment*, Statistics Canada, Ottawa, Canada, 2005.

[23] "The international adult literacy and skills survey, 2003," Public Use Microdata File User's Manual, Statistics Canada, Ottawa, Canada, 2002.

[24] Statistics Canada, *Literacy in the Information Age: Final Report of the International Adult Literacy Survey*, OECD, Ottawa, Canada, 2000.

[25] I. Kirsch and M. Lennon, "The ICT literacy framework," in *Measuring Adult Literacy and Life Skills: New Framework for Assessment*, T. S. Murray, Y. Clermont, and M. Binkley, Eds., Statistics Canada, Ottawa, Canada, 2005.

[26] D. Schillinger, K. Grumbach, J. Piette et al., "Association of health literacy with diabetes outcomes," *Journal of the American Medical Association*, vol. 288, no. 4, pp. 475–482, 2002.

[27] T. L. Scott, J. A. Gazmararian, M. V. Williams, and D. W. Baker, "Health literacy and preventive health care use among medicare enrollees in a managed care organization," *Medical Care*, vol. 40, no. 5, pp. 395–404, 2002.

[28] S. C. Lemon, J. Roy, M. A. Clark, P. D. Friedmann, and W. Rakowski, "Classification and regression tree analysis in public health: methodological review and comparison with logistic regression," *Annals of Behavioral Medicine*, vol. 26, no. 3, pp. 172–181, 2003.

[29] K. Y. Chan and W. Y. Loh, "Lotus: an algorithm for building accurate and comprehensible logistic regression trees," *Journal of Computational and Graphical Statistics*, vol. 13, no. 4, pp. 826–852, 2004.

[30] L. Breiman, J. H. Friedman, R. A. Olshen, and C. J. Stone, *Classification and Regression Trees*, Chapman & Hall/CRC, New York, NY, USA, 1984.

[31] G. V. Kass, "An exploratory technique for investigating large quantities of categorical data," *Applied Statistics*, vol. 29, no. 2, pp. 119–127, 1980.

[32] W.-Y. Loh, "Logistic regression tree analysis," in *The Handbook of Engineering Statistics*, H. Pham, Ed., Springer, London, UK, 2006.

[33] K. F. Ferraro and T. P. Shippee, "Aging and cumulative inequality: how does inequality get under the skin?" *Gerontologist*, vol. 49, no. 3, pp. 333–343, 2009.

[34] I. Rootman and J. Wharf-Higgins, "Literacy and health: implications for active living," *Well Spring*, vol. 18, no. 4, pp. 1–3, 2007.

[35] V. A. Freedman, L. G. Martin, and R. F. Schoeni, "Recent trends in disability and functioning among older adults in the United States: a systematic review," *Journal of the American Medical Association*, vol. 288, no. 24, pp. 3137–3146, 2002.

[36] I. S. Kickbusch, "Health literacy: addressing the health and education divide," *Health Promotion International*, vol. 16, no. 3, pp. 289–297, 2001.

[37] M. Marmot, "Social determinants of health inequalities," *Lancet*, vol. 365, no. 9464, pp. 1099–1104, 2005.

[38] D. Nutbeam, "The evolving concept of health literacy," *Social Science and Medicine*, vol. 67, no. 12, pp. 2072–2078, 2008.

[39] D. Dannefer, "Cumulative advantage/disadvantage and the life course: cross-fertilizing age and social science theory," *Journals of Gerontology B*, vol. 58, no. 6, pp. S327–S337, 2003.

[40] I. Rootman and D. Gordon-El-Bihbety, *A Vision for a Health Literate Canada*, Canadian Public Health Association, Ottawa, Canada, 2008.

[41] *Healthy People 2010 with Understanding and Improving Health and Objectives for Improving Health*, U.S. Department of Health and Human Services, Washington, DC, USA, 2nd edition, 2000.

[42] P. Franks and K. Fiscella, "Reducing disparities downstream: prospects and challenges," *Journal of General Internal Medicine*, vol. 23, no. 5, pp. 672–677, 2008.

[43] D. Haber, *Health Promotion and Aging: Practical Applications for Health Professionals*, Springer, New York, NY, USA, 2007.

[44] G. A. Mensah and M. J. Glover, "Epidemiology of racial and ethnic disparities in health and healthcare," in *Eliminating Healthcare Disparities in America*, R. A. Williams, Ed., pp. 21–40, Humana Press, Totowa, NJ, USA, 2007.

[45] S. J. Shaw, C. Huebner, J. Armin, K. Orzech, and J. Vivian, "The role of culture in health literacy and chronic disease screening and management," *Journal of Immigrant and Minority Health*, vol. 11, no. 6, pp. 460–467, 2009.

[46] N. D. Berkman, S. Sheridan, K. E. Donahue et al. et al., *Health Literacy Interventions and Outcomes: An Updated Systematic Review*, Agency for Healthcare Research and Quality, Rockville, Md, USA, 2007, contract no. 199.

22

Robust Medical Test Evaluation Using Flexible Bayesian Semiparametric Regression Models

Adam J. Branscum,[1] Wesley O. Johnson,[2] and Andre T. Baron[3]

[1] *Biostatistics Program, College of Public Health and Human Sciences, Oregon State University, Corvallis, OR 97331, USA*
[2] *Department of Statistics, University of California, Irvine, CA 92697, USA*
[3] *Tumor Biology Investment Group, Inc., Richmond, KY 40475, USA*

Correspondence should be addressed to Adam J. Branscum; adam.branscum@oregonstate.edu

Academic Editor: Leo J. Schouten

The application of Bayesian methods is increasing in modern epidemiology. Although parametric Bayesian analysis has penetrated the population health sciences, flexible nonparametric Bayesian methods have received less attention. A goal in nonparametric Bayesian analysis is to estimate unknown functions (e.g., density or distribution functions) rather than scalar parameters (e.g., means or proportions). For instance, ROC curves are obtained from the distribution functions corresponding to continuous biomarker data taken from healthy and diseased populations. Standard parametric approaches to Bayesian analysis involve distributions with a small number of parameters, where the prior specification is relatively straight forward. In the nonparametric Bayesian case, the prior is placed on an infinite dimensional space of all distributions, which requires special methods. A popular approach to nonparametric Bayesian analysis that involves Polya tree prior distributions is described. We provide example code to illustrate how models that contain Polya tree priors can be fit using SAS software. The methods are used to evaluate the covariate-specific accuracy of the biomarker, soluble epidermal growth factor receptor, for discerning lung cancer cases from controls using a flexible ROC regression modeling framework. The application highlights the usefulness of flexible models over a standard parametric method for estimating ROC curves.

1. Introduction

Bayesian analysis is often used in the support of epidemiologic research [1–7]. A contemporary area of research in the population health sciences involves the development and application of statistical methods for evaluating the accuracy of medical tests. With binary outcome data, statistical methods focus on estimating sensitivity and specificity, while with quantitative data, standard objects of interest are the receiver operating characteristic (ROC) curve and area under the curve (AUC).

The ROC curve can be regarded as a graphical portrayal of the degree of separation between the distributions of test outcomes for "diseased" and nondiseased populations. The formula for an ROC curve depends on Se(k) and Sp(k), the sensitivity and specificity of the test at classification threshold k. We proceed under the innocuous assumption that test outcomes tend to be higher for individuals in the diseased population. Let y denote a continuous test outcome for a disease D, where disease status is labeled as $D = 0$ for disease absent and $D = 1$ for disease present. In general, y can be any continuously measured classifier that varies according to a cumulative distribution function G_0 for nondiseased individuals and varies according to G_1 for diseased individuals. The ROC curve is a plot of true positive probability versus false positive probability across all classification thresholds, that is, a plot of pairs $(1 - \text{Sp}(k), \text{Se}(k))$ for all k. Since $\text{Se}(k) = \Pr(y > k \mid D = 1) = 1 - G_1(k)$ and $1 - \text{Sp}(k) = \Pr(y > k \mid D = 0) = 1 - G_0(k)$, accurate direct estimation of the ROC curve depends crucially on accurate estimation of the distribution functions G_0 and G_1.

This motivates the use of flexible data-driven methods for estimating functions, which is a central goal of nonparametric Bayesian analysis. The standard parametric approach imposes the strong condition that G_0 and G_1 be members of the normal family (i.e., the normal-normal model), while a flexible nonparametric approach treats them as arbitrary continuous distribution functions. A flexible method is desirable because G_0 and/or G_1 could exhibit unanticipated right or left skewness, multimodality, or they could be symmetric but not bell-shaped. As a result, the methodology we present has the flexibility to handle data from many different settings, and notably it will be designed to include the normal-normal model as a special case.

The development of modern nonparametric and semiparametric Bayesian procedures for ROC analysis is an active area of research [8–17]. The main goals of this paper are (i) to use flexible Bayesian models and ROC curves to evaluate the accuracy of a biomarker that may depend on patient characteristics and (ii) to provide a nontechnical description of Polya tree priors and show how they can be implemented in epidemiological research using standard statistical software.

2. Materials and Methods

Robust inference for ROC curves stems from allowing G_0 and G_1 to be members of broad classes of distributions. Our approach is to model them using Mixtures of Finite Polya Trees (MFPT) priors, which have been carefully discussed in the statistics literature [18, 19]. We avoid a full technical description because it requires considerable mathematical detail. Instead, a conceptual introduction appears in Appendix A.

Briefly, a major advantage beyond flexibility is that MFPT priors for G_0 and G_1 can be "centered" on separate parametric families. In part, this means that the flexible model generalizes the standard parametric model since the normal-normal model is allowed as a special case. Additionally, it means that the expected value of G_ℓ under the prior will be the distribution function that corresponds to the centering family. In our illustrations, the centering families will be $F_\ell \equiv \{N(\mu_\ell, \sigma_\ell^2) : \mu_\ell \in \mathbb{R}, \sigma_\ell^2 \in \mathbb{R}^+\}, \ell = 0, 1$. The MFPT priors will also have positive weight parameters, c_0 and c_1, and positive integers J_0 and J_1 that define the (finite) length of the trees. Large values for the weights indicate higher prior confidence in the centering distributions, while values near zero allow for considerable flexibility around the centering family. To aid the selection of a weight parameter, consider that the parametric model F_ℓ is the special case obtained when $c_\ell \to \infty$. Hence, using a large weight value is similar to fitting the parametric centering model to the data (possible oversmoothing). The opposite extreme of setting $c_\ell \doteq 0$ produces empirical estimates (possible undersmoothing). In our experience, a weight parameter between 0.5 and 1 is often a positive compromise between these extremes. Tree lengths generally range between 4 and 10, depending on the sample size. Small values for J_ℓ tend to oversmooth the data. A fully nonparametric prior is obtained as $J_\ell \to \infty$, but large values of J_ℓ can substantially increase computing time. Finally, there will be priors on (μ_ℓ, σ_ℓ); write them as $p_\ell(\mu_\ell, \sigma_\ell)$, for $\ell = 0, 1$. We assume G_0 and G_1 are independent, with priors denoted by $G_\ell \sim$ MFPT (F_ℓ, p_ℓ, c_ℓ), for $\ell = 0, 1$.

2.1. Models. In the absence of covariates, consider two independent samples of continuous biomarker measurements, where $y_1, y_2, \ldots, y_{n_0}$ constitute a random sample from an unknown distribution G_0, and $z_1, z_2, \ldots, z_{n_1}$ are realizations from G_1. We regard the y_i's as biomarker outcomes from n_0 nondiseased individuals and the z_j's as outcomes from n_1 diseased individuals. Our model is represented as $y_i \mid G_0 \overset{\text{indep}}{\sim} G_0$ with $G_0 \sim \text{MFPT}(F_0, p_0, c_0)$ and similarly for the z_j's. The prior $p_\ell(\mu_\ell, \sigma_\ell)$ in our illustrations involves a normal distribution on μ_ℓ and an independent uniform distribution on σ_ℓ.

There are many possible extensions of this two-group model depending on the complexity of the data. We describe a semiparametric regression model that can be easily adapted to handle a variety of scenarios. The model specifies separate linear regressions with arbitrary residual distributions for the data from the nondiseased and diseased populations:

$$\begin{aligned} y_i &= \beta_1 x_{i1} + \beta_2 x_{i2} + \cdots + \beta_g x_{ig} + \epsilon_i \equiv x_i\beta + \epsilon_i, \\ \epsilon_i \mid G_0 &\sim G_0, \quad G_0 \sim \text{MFPT}\left(N\left(\mu_0, \sigma_0^2\right), p_0, c_0\right); \\ z_j &= \alpha_1 \tilde{x}_{j1} + \alpha_2 \tilde{x}_{j2} + \cdots + \alpha_h \tilde{x}_{jh} + \tilde{\epsilon}_j \equiv \tilde{x}_j\alpha + \tilde{\epsilon}_j, \\ \tilde{\epsilon}_j \mid G_1 &\sim G_1, \quad G_1 \sim \text{MFPT}\left(N\left(\mu_1, \sigma_1^2\right), p_1, c_1\right). \end{aligned} \tag{1}$$

There are no intercepts in the regression part of the models since each residual distribution has an arbitrary unknown mean. The covariate vectors x_i and $\tilde{x}_j$ can be distinct or have some overlap (e.g., both might include age) or complete overlap ($x_i = \tilde{x}_j$). In the absence of available prior information, independent normal prior distributions with mean 0 and large variance can be used for the regression coefficients. Alternatively, when prior information is available, we recommend conditional means priors [20]. Special cases include a model with no covariates for the nondiseased population (no x_{ir} variables), a model with no covariates for the diseased population (no $\tilde{x}_{js}$ variables) and a model without covariates (the two-group model).

Our model can be used to estimate covariate-specific ROC curves and AUC. Let $x^* = (x, \tilde{x})$ define two particular subpopulations of nondiseased and diseased people. Then, ROC(x^*) and its corresponding AUC(x^*) are measures of the tests' accuracy when applied to nondiseased people with covariate vector x and diseased people with covariate vector $\tilde{x}$ (often, the researcher will set x equal to $\tilde{x}$). Approximate posterior inference for ROC curves can be made by calculating posterior summaries of $(1 - G_0(k - x\beta), 1 - G_1(k - \tilde{x}\alpha))$ across a fine grid of values for k that spans the sample space.

3. Results

3.1. Fitting MFPT Models in SAS. The SAS 9.3 (SAS Institute, Inc., Cary, North Carolina) code that was used to fit a one-sample MFPT model to the simulated data described in Appendix A is in Appendix B.

3.2. ROC Analysis of sEGFR Data. We investigated a soluble isoform of the epidermal growth factor receptor (sEGFR) as a biomarker for lung cancer in premenopausal and postmenopausal women. sEGFR also has been associated with ovarian cancer [21, 22]. The data were collected from a case-control study conducted at the Mayo Clinic in Rochester, Minnesota between 1998 and 2003. There were 140 controls and 101 lung cancer cases, and 92 premenopausal and 149 postmenopausal women enrolled in the study.

In a preliminary analysis, we found no clear evidence of a difference in the distributions of $y = \sqrt{\text{sEGFR}}$ for premenopausal versus postmenopausal lung cancer cases (Wilcoxon $P = 0.15$). However, there was evidence for a statistical difference in the distribution of y for controls based on menopausal status (Wilcoxon $P < 0.01$). We thus included menopausal status as a covariate in models for the control data. A flexible approach is supported over the standard parametric approach because normal quantile plots (not shown) indicated a right skew in the distributions of y for cases and postmenopausal controls.

We compared two analyses. The first analysis had menopausal status as a covariate for the control group in an ROC regression model. The second analysis modeled outcomes among pre- and postmenopausal controls with completely separate (flexible) distributions, without regression structure. We compared these models using the log pseudomarginal likelihood (LPML) [23], [24, Section 4.9].

For all models that used Polya trees, we set weight parameters (the c_ℓ's) equal to 0.5 and tree lengths (the J_ℓ's) equal to 5. In this setting, values of y tended to be higher among controls instead of cases, so we reversed the roles for cases and controls. Let $\tilde{x} = 1$ for premenopausal women and $\tilde{x} = 0$ for postmenopausal women. For both models under consideration, the data from cases were modeled as independently distributed according to an unknown distribution G_0. The prior was $G_0 \sim \text{MFPT}(N(\mu_0, \sigma_0^2), p_0, c)$, with $p_0(\mu_0, \sigma_0)$ selected to be $\mu_0 \sim N(50, 400)$ independent of $\sigma_0 \sim \text{Uniform}(0, 100)$. The prior mean of 50 for μ_0 was chosen because that was approximately the mean of y for male lung cancer cases in a similar study, but we allowed for a high degree of uncertainty about the value of μ_0 through a large prior variance.

For controls, model 1 for the data was the regression

$$\begin{gathered} z_j = \alpha_1 \tilde{x}_j + \tilde{\epsilon}_j, \\ \tilde{\epsilon}_j \mid G_1 \sim G_1, \\ G_1 \sim \text{MFPT}\left(N\left(\mu_1, \sigma_1^2\right), p_1, c\right), \end{gathered} \tag{2}$$

where, independently, $\alpha_1 \sim N(0, 400)$, $\mu_1 \sim N(50, 400)$, and $\sigma_1 \sim \text{Uniform}(0, 100)$.

Model 2 specified separate distributions for data from premenopausal and postmenopausal controls. Denote the distributions by G_2 and G_3, respectively, where G_w was assigned an MFPT prior that was centered at $N(\mu_w, \sigma_w^2)$, with $\mu_w \sim N(50, 400)$ and $\sigma_w \sim$ Uniform $(0, 100)$, for $w = 2, 3$. Using the same priors, we also considered the standard parametric analysis (model 3) in which G_0, G_2, and G_3 were normal distributions with distinct means and variances.

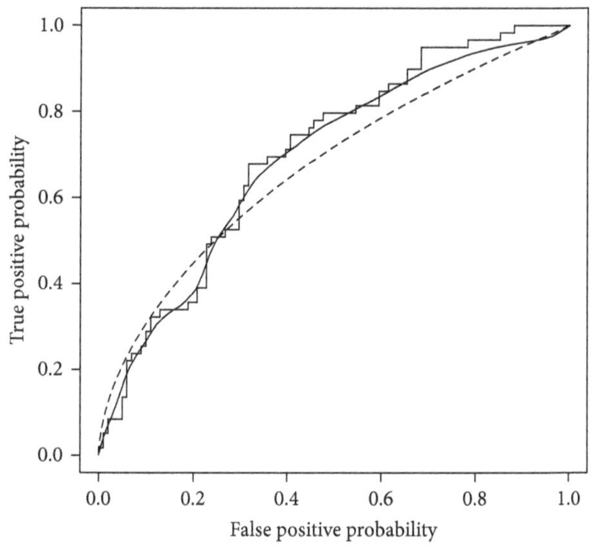

Figure 1: Empirical ROC curve for postmenopausal women and estimates of the ROC curve from a parametric normal model (dashed line) and a mixture of finite Polya trees analysis (smooth solid line).

The LPML statistics were similar for models 1 and 2 (LPML $\doteq -1187$). We therefore selected the more flexible model 2 that had separate distributions across $\tilde{x}$. For the standard parametric model 3, LPML $= -1201$, indicating a strong preference for the more flexible models (pseudo-Bayes factor $= e^{14}$).

Estimated ROC curves were obtained from model 2, together with estimates from the parametric normal model 3 and from nonparametric empirical distribution functions. The estimated ROC curve from the parametric analysis differs drastically from estimates obtained from the MFPT and empirical distribution functions for postmenopausal women (Figure 1). Not surprisingly, the parametric model fails to track either of the data-driven estimates. Note that although the parametric model is its prior expectation, the MFPT model has the flexibility to allow the data to reallocate probability mass away from a bell-curve to produce an appropriately smooth and flexible estimate of the ROC curve. For premenopausal women, the parametric and Polya tree models also give different inferences, including at clinically important cutoffs corresponding to false positive probabilities up to 10% (Figure 2). The empirical partial AUC over that region was 0.026, while the estimate from the parametric analysis was increased by 37% to 0.041. A 90% posterior interval for the partial AUC from the parametric model was (0.027, 0.055), which does not contain the empirical estimate. The Polya tree analysis is a middle ground between these extremes, with an estimated ROC curve that is essentially a smoothed version of the empirical curve and an estimated partial AUC of 0.019 (0.009, 0.036). Similar results were obtained from a sensitivity analysis that placed diffuse Gamma priors with mean 1 and variance 10000 on the μ_ℓ's and σ_ℓ's.

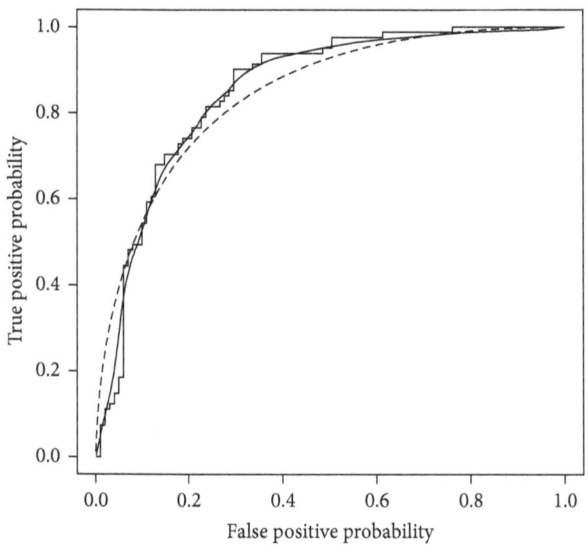

FIGURE 2: Empirical ROC curve for premenopausal women and estimates of the ROC curve from a parametric normal model (dashed line) and a mixture of finite Polya trees analysis (smooth solid line).

<table>
<tr><td colspan="8">Sample space</td></tr>
<tr><td colspan="4">$B_{1,1}$</td><td colspan="4">$B_{1,2}$</td></tr>
<tr><td colspan="2">$B_{2,1}$</td><td colspan="2">$B_{2,2}$</td><td colspan="2">$B_{2,3}$</td><td colspan="2">$B_{2,4}$</td></tr>
<tr><td>$B_{3,1}$</td><td>$B_{3,2}$</td><td>$B_{3,3}$</td><td>$B_{3,4}$</td><td>$B_{3,5}$</td><td>$B_{3,6}$</td><td>$B_{3,7}$</td><td>$B_{3,8}$</td></tr>
</table>

FIGURE 3: Partition structure of a Polya tree with three levels.

4. Conclusions

We have described the use of MFPT priors in Bayesian analysis. Even when a parametric model is thought to hold, a Polya tree analysis offers a way to assess parametric assumptions and to perform a sensitivity analysis to address deviations from them. For example, a simple approach to sensitivity analysis involves comparing estimated ROC curves and AUC from the normal-normal and semiparametric models.

A finite Polya tree prior is not technically nonparametric. Bayesian nonparametric models are characterized by having an infinite number of parameters. Such models often use finite approximations, as in our case. It is thus more accurate to view models that contain finite Polya tree priors as parametric, with a large number of parameters. In fact, Bayesian statistical analysis with finite Polya tree priors has been called "parametric nonparametric statistics," because it uses parametric models (with many parameters) that maintain flexibility [25]. In our experience, finite approximations of Polya trees are sufficiently flexible and scalable to perform well for a wide variety of complex settings.

Appendices

A. Polya Tree Priors

A.1. Finite Polya Tree Priors. A random sample $y_1, \ldots, y_n$ is obtained from an unknown distribution G. We describe informally what it means to place a finite Polya tree prior on G. Polya tree priors place a distribution on a collection of cumulative distribution functions. The first step in constructing a finite Polya tree prior is to create nested partitions of the sample space. The first partition splits the sample space into two nonoverlapping intervals. In the second partition, those two intervals are each split, yielding a finer partition that contains four intervals. Then, these four intervals are each split to give an 8 interval third-level partition of the sample space. This sequential process of splitting the sample space into finer and finer partitions continues up to a certain (finite) level J.

An analogy is to a convention center with J floors. The rooftop encompasses the entire sample space. Down one level is a floor with two large meeting rooms. Two levels down is a floor with four meeting rooms, then a floor with 8 rooms, and so on until we get to the ground floor J levels down, which contains 2^J meeting rooms (Figure 3 contains an example with $J = 3$). Suppose the unknown distribution G assigns multiple people (the y_i's in this analogy) to rooms on the ground floor, and our task is to use the observed distribution of people to rooms to estimate G. Although all levels (floors) of the tree (convention center) are important for the purpose of estimating G, of primary importance is level J (the ground floor).

The goal is to produce a data-driven estimate of G that assigns high probability to intervals (rooms) that contain lots of data (people), assigns low probability to empty intervals, and assigns midrange probability to intervals that contain some (but not a lot) of the data. Consider first the simplest case where the convention center has only one floor ($J = 1$). Then, people are assigned to one of two meeting rooms on floor 1. Call them rooms $B_{1,1}$ and $B_{1,2}$. The probability of being assigned to the first room on floor 1 is $G(B_{1,1}) = \Pr(y_i \in B_{1,1})$, which, since G is a cumulative distribution function and $B_{1,1}$ is an interval of the form (L, U), is to be interpreted as $G(B_{1,1}) = G(U) - G(L)$. Denote this unknown probability by the parameter $\pi_{1,1}$. Then, by the complement rule, $\pi_{1,2} = 1 - \pi_{1,1}$ is the probability of being assigned to room 2 on floor 1. In notation, $\Pr(y_i \in B_{1,1}) = G(B_{1,1}) = \pi_{1,1}$ and $\Pr(y_i \in B_{1,2}) = G(B_{1,2}) = \pi_{1,2}$. Since G is unknown, $\pi_{1,1}$ and $\pi_{1,2}$ are unknown. To help interpret these parameters, suppose the data arise from a right-skewed distribution (lots more people in room 1 than room 2), then $\pi_{1,1}$ would be large and hence $\pi_{1,2}$ would be small, and vice-versa for left-skewed data. In practice, $J = 1$ is never used because it would lead to a crude estimate of the density function g, much like estimating a density using a relative frequency histogram that contains only two bins. In our experience, setting J equal to 4, 5, or 6 often works well in practice. Another option is to select J so that roughly $2^J \doteq n$ [18].

Now suppose we return a year later to find that the convention center has expanded and contains a second floor ($J = 2$). Suppose the new ground floor has four rooms,

$B_{2,1}$, $B_{2,2}$, $B_{2,3}$, and $B_{2,4}$ (third row of Figure 3). Moreover, suppose that room assignments are made based on whether the individual was in room $B_{1,1}$ or $B_{1,2}$ during the previous visit. If the previous assignment was to room $B_{1,1}$, then the individual is assigned again to the left side of the convention center, namely, to either room $B_{2,1}$ with unknown probability $\pi_{2,1}$ or to room $B_{2,2}$ with probability $\pi_{2,2} = 1 - \pi_{2,1}$. Similarly, define $\pi_{2,3}$ and $\pi_{2,4}$ $(= 1 - \pi_{2,3})$ to be the probability of being assigned to room $B_{2,3}$ or $B_{2,4}$, respectively, given that the previous assignment was to room $B_{1,2}$.

The $\pi_{j,k}$'s are *conditional* probability parameters, since $\pi_{2,1} = \Pr(y_i \in B_{2,1} \mid y_i \in B_{1,1})$ and $\pi_{2,3} = \Pr(y_i \in B_{2,3} \mid y_i \in B_{1,2})$. To relate the $\pi_{j,k}$'s to G, we must determine the *marginal* probability of assignment to the various ground-floor rooms. Observe that interval $B_{2,1}$ is a subset of interval $B_{1,1}$ (see Figure 3), so the marginal probability of interval $B_{2,1}$ is

$$\begin{aligned} G(B_{2,1}) &= \Pr(y_i \in B_{2,1}) \\ &= \Pr(y_i \in B_{2,1}, y_i \in B_{1,1}) \\ &= \Pr(y_i \in B_{2,1} \mid y_i \in B_{1,1}) \Pr(y_i \in B_{1,1}) \\ &= \pi_{2,1}\pi_{1,1}. \end{aligned} \quad (A.1)$$

Similar steps lead to $G(B_{2,2}) = (1 - \pi_{2,1})\pi_{1,1}$, $G(B_{2,3}) = \pi_{2,3}\pi_{1,2}$, and $G(B_{2,4}) = (1 - \pi_{2,3})\pi_{1,2}$. Suppose again that G is right skewed. Then the data will estimate $\pi_{1,1}$ to be large, and it will estimate $\pi_{2,1}$ to be large since most of the n people will be assigned to room $B_{2,1}$. Therefore, the estimate of $G(B_{2,1})$ will be (relatively) large.

Notice that level 1 has only one unique parameter ($\pi_{1,1}$) associated with it because $\pi_{1,2}$ is completely determined by $\pi_{1,1}$; similarly, level 2 has two unique parameters ($\pi_{2,1}$ and $\pi_{2,3}$) associated with it. We can continue the convention center storyline to any level J. For $J = 3$ (Figure 3), we add conditional probability parameters $\pi_{3,1}$, $\pi_{3,2}$, $\pi_{3,3}$, $\pi_{3,4}$, $\pi_{3,5}$, $\pi_{3,6}$, $\pi_{3,7}$, and $\pi_{3,8}$, but only 4 of these are unique. For instance, $\pi_{3,1}$ is the probability that y_i is in interval $B_{3,1}$ given that it is in interval $B_{2,1}$, and $G(B_{3,1}) = \Pr(y_i \in B_{3,1}) = \Pr(y_i \in B_{3,1}, y_i \in B_{2,1}) = \Pr(y_i \in B_{3,1} \mid y_i \in B_{2,1}) \Pr(y_i \in B_{2,1}) = \pi_{3,1}\pi_{2,1}\pi_{1,1}$.

The key point is that if we can estimate all of the $\pi_{j,k}$'s, then we can estimate the probability that is allocated by G to each interval at level J. Estimating continuous G requires continuing ad infinitum as J grows. However, in practice we truncate to a fixed J, hence the term, finite Polya tree. But this is incomplete for the purpose of estimating a continuous G, because we have not modeled how probability mass is distributed *within* each interval at level J. In terms of the convention center analogy, we have modeled the probability of assignment to each of the ground-floor rooms, but we have not modeled how people are distributed within those rooms. For instance, they could all be clustered in the middle of the room (all the y_i's clumped together in the center of the interval). Alternatively, the data could be uniformly distributed, clumped to the right or left side of the interval, or have any other dispersion pattern within each interval. To address this issue, we model the data according to how a user-specified distribution G^* allocates probability mass within the intervals at level J.

The distribution G^* is important in two other ways. First, it is used to determine the lower and upper endpoints of all intervals in the tree. The median of G^* is used to split the sample space into two intervals at level 1 of the tree. The quartiles of G^* define cutpoints for intervals at level 2. Writing the 25th percentile as $G^{*-1}(1/4)$, the median as $G^{*-1}(2/4)$, and the 75th percentile as $G^{*-1}(3/4)$, we have for a sample space that covers the real line

$$\begin{aligned} B_{2,1} &= \left(-\infty, G^{*-1}\left(\frac{1}{4}\right)\right), \\ B_{2,2} &= \left(G^{*-1}\left(\frac{1}{4}\right), G^{*-1}\left(\frac{2}{4}\right)\right), \\ B_{2,3} &= \left(G^{*-1}\left(\frac{2}{4}\right), G^{*-1}\left(\frac{3}{4}\right)\right), \\ B_{2,4} &= \left(G^{*-1}\left(\frac{3}{4}\right), +\infty\right). \end{aligned} \quad (A.2)$$

In general, the (j,k)th interval is $B_{j,k} = (G^{*-1}((k-1)/2^j), G^{*-1}(k/2^j))$, for $j = 1, \ldots, J$ and $k = 1, \ldots, 2^j$.

Second, G^* is the prior expectation of the unknown distribution function G. This provides guidance for selecting G^*; we select it based on our best prior assessment of the data-generating distribution G. If our prior assessment is that the data will be governed by a certain normal distribution, we use that normal for G^*. If our prior assessment is accurate, the posterior estimate of G from the finite Polya tree model will take the shape of that normal distribution. But the real advantage of Polya tree priors is their flexibility to allow for data-driven prior-to-posterior reallocation of probability mass away from the shape of G^* to any shape supported by the data. This happens by estimating the $\pi_{j,k}$'s that were equated to G.

The collection $\{\pi_{j,k} : j = 1, \ldots, J;\ k = 1, \ldots, 2^j\}$ constitutes the unknown parameters corresponding to G. We need to specify a prior distribution over this collection. Recall that when k is an even number between 2 and 2^j, $\pi_{j,k} = 1 - \pi_{j,k-1}$. Therefore, priors are needed only on $\pi_{j,k}$ when k is odd. It is standard to use independent beta priors, specifically $\pi_{j,k} \sim \text{Beta}(cj^2, cj^2)$ for k odd and all j. The prior mean of 0.5 gives equal weight to the left and right intervals formed by splitting a parent interval. The positive constant c is often set equal to 0.5 or 1. The value of c reflects our confidence in the prior estimate G^* for the unknown G. Large values of c (e.g., $c \geq 10$) translate into higher prior confidence in the particular G^*, so a relatively larger amount of data are needed in order for the posterior estimate to stray from G^* if the data conflict with it. A low value (e.g., $c = 0.1$) will often lead to an estimate of G that is similar to the empirical distribution function. We have found that $c = 0.5$ or 1 performs well in practice because it often is a middle ground between a purely data-based and model-based estimate.

```
proc mcmc data=MFPT nbi=5000 nmc=50000 thin=10 monitor=(G littleg mu sigma);
begincnst; J=4; c=1; endcnst;
parms pi11 pi21 pi23;
parms pi31 pi33 pi35 pi37;
parms pi41 pi43 pi45 pi47 pi49 pi411 pi413 pi415;
parms mu sigma / t(3);
array p[16];
p1 = pi11*pi21*pi31*pi41; p2 = pi11*pi21*pi31*(1-pi41);
p3 = pi11*pi21*(1-pi31)*pi43; p4 = pi11*pi21*(1-pi31)*(1-pi43);
p5 = pi11*(1-pi21)*pi33*pi45; p6 = pi11*(1-pi21)*pi33*(1-pi45);
p7 = pi11*(1-pi21)*(1-pi33)*pi47; p8 = pi11*(1-pi21)*(1-pi33)*(1-pi47);
p9 = (1-pi11)*pi23*pi35*pi49; p10 = (1-pi11)*pi23*pi35*(1-pi49);
p11 = (1-pi11)*pi23*(1-pi35)*pi411; p12 = (1-pi11)*pi23*(1-pi35)*(1-pi411);
p13 = (1-pi11)*(1-pi23)*pi37*pi413; p14 = (1-pi11)*(1-pi23)*pi37*(1-pi413);
p15 = (1-pi11)*(1-pi23)*(1-pi37)*pi415; p16 = (1-pi11)*(1-pi23)*(1-pi37)*(1-pi415);
prior pi11 ~ beta(c,c); prior pi21 pi23 ~ beta(c*2**2,c*2**2);
prior pi31 pi33 pi35 pi37 ~ beta(c*3**2,c*3**2);
prior pi41 pi43 pi45 pi47 pi49 pi411 pi413 pi415 ~ beta(c*4**2,c*4**2);
prior mu ~ normal(50,sd=10); prior sigma ~ uniform(0,20);
k = int(2**J * cdf("normal", y, mu, sigma) + 1);
llike=J*log(2) + log(p[k]) + lpdfnorm(y, mu, sigma);
model general(llike);
array setID[52]; array G[52]; array littleg[52];
do i = 1 to dim(G) by 1;
setID[i] = int(2**J * cdf("normal", 39 + i/2, mu, sigma) + 1);
G[i] = p1*(setID[i] ge 2) + p2*(setID[i] ge 3) + p3*(setID[i] ge 4)
      + p4*(setID[i] ge 5) + p5*(setID[i] ge 6) + p6*(setID[i] ge 7)
      + p7*(setID[i] ge 8) + p8*(setID[i] ge 9) + p9*(setID[i] ge 10)
      + p10*(setID[i] ge 11) + p11*(setID[i] ge 12) + p12*(setID[i] ge 13)
      + p13*(setID[i] ge 14) + p14*(setID[i] ge 15) + p15*(setID[i] ge 16)
      + p[setIDi] *(2**J * cdf("normal", 39 + i/2, mu, sigma)- setID[i] + 1);
littleg[i] = 2**J * p[setIDi] * pdf("normal", 39 + i/2, mu, sigma);
end; run;
```

Algorithm 1

Once we have selected J, G^*, and c, we have all the elements needed to specify a finite Polya tree prior for G. Formulas for G and its corresponding density function g are

$$G(y) = \sum_{i=1}^{k(y)-1} p(B_{J,i}) + p(B_{J,k(y)}) \times \left[2^J G^*(y) - k(y) + 1\right], \qquad g(y) = 2^J p(B_{J,k(y)})\, g^*(y), \tag{A.3}$$

where $k(y)$ is an integer between 1 and 2^J that identifies the interval at level J containing y, and $p(B_{J,k(y)})$ is the probability of that interval (it is the product of J of the $\pi_{j,k}$'s) [19]. The interval that contains y at level J can be determined using the formula $k(y) = \mathrm{Int}(2^J G^*(y)+1)$, where the function $\mathrm{Int}(\cdot)$ returns the integer portion of a decimal number (e.g., $\mathrm{Int}(3.14) = 3$).

To motivate an extension to *mixtures* of finite Polya tree priors, consider Figure 4(a), where g is estimated using a finite Polya tree analysis of 200 simulated data values from a mixture of two normal distributions (70% of observations from $N(70,4)$ and 30% from $N(57,2.25)$). The prior mean, G^*, was the $N(50,25)$, and we set $J = 4$. The estimate from the finite Polya tree analysis is choppy, which turns out to be the result of using a fixed G^*. These bumps get smoothed over if instead we replace G^* with a parametric distribution G^*_θ, where θ denotes a collection of unknown parameters that is assigned a prior distribution. The posterior estimate of g in Figure 4(b) was obtained using a $N(\mu,\sigma^2)$ for G^*_θ, with $\mu \sim N(50,100)$ and $\sigma \sim U(0,20)$. This is an example of our preferred prior in nonparametric Bayesian statistics, namely, the mixture of finite Polya trees prior. The model is $y_i \mid G \sim G$, $G \sim \mathrm{MFPT}(G^*_\theta, p, c)$, where p is a prior distribution on θ. With large c, the model for y_i is simply $N(\mu,\sigma^2)$ and the analysis becomes completely parametric. For a more elaborate but still elementary description, see [25].

B. SAS Code

SAS 9.3 code to fit the one-sample MFPT model to simulated data from the mixture of two normal distributions described in Appendix A is presented in Algorithm 1. The SAS data step is not shown in the code; in it, the variable y is read into a data set that was named MFPT, where y contains 200 evenly spaced percentiles from the true mixture distribution. The

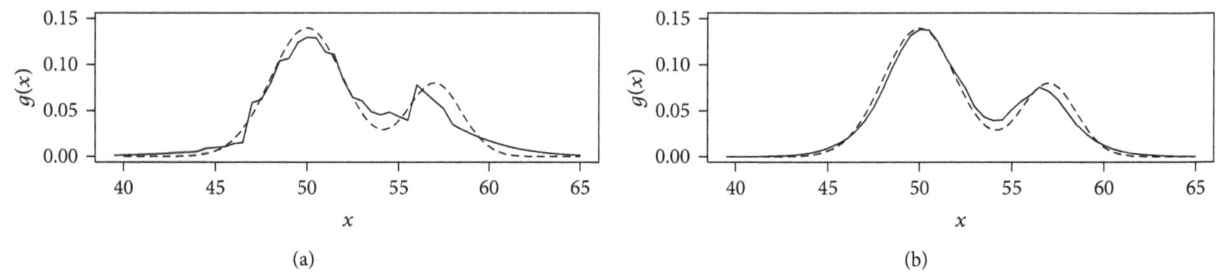

FIGURE 4: Posterior estimates of g from simulated bimodal data using a finite Polya tree prior ((a), solid line) and a mixture of finite Polya trees prior ((b), solid line). The dashed lines represent the true data density g.

first line instructs the mcmc procedure to use the data in `MFPT` and specifies options for the number of burn-in iterates (`nbi`), the number of iterates to simulate post burn-in (`nmc`), to retain every 10th iterate (`thin=10`), and the parameters to monitor for posterior inference. Constants that are used in the program appear in line 2; in this example we set $J = 4$ and $c = 1$. Each parameter $\pi_{j,k}$ is coded as `pijk`, with the appropriate numbers substituted for `j` and `k`. The marginal probabilities at level $J = 4$ are named `pk`, where `k` ranges from 1 to 16; these variables represent $p(B_{J,k(y)})$ as defined in Appendix A. Priors on the $\pi_{j,k}$'s, μ, and σ follow. SAS code to fit the finite Polya tree model described in Appendix A can be obtained by omitting the `prior` and `parms` lines associated with μ and σ and setting `mu` and `sigma` equal to constants in line 2 of the code. The variable `k` identifies the set each y_i belongs to at level 4. The log likelihood (`llike`) is obtained by taking the natural log of the formula for g that appears in (A.3). The remaining code is used to estimate the distribution function (`G`) and the density function g (coded as `littleg` since SAS is not case sensitive).

The model is fit using Gibbs sampling with block updating occurring for the groups of parameters that are defined in the `parms` statements. The posterior distributions of $g(y)$ and $G(y)$ are evaluated at $y = 39.5, 40, 40.5, \ldots, 65$. Figure 4(b) plots the posterior means of $g(39.5), g(40), g(40.5), \ldots, g(65)$, and a continuous density is obtained by interpolation.

Disclosure

Andre Baron is a coinventor of patents related to sEGFR and cofounder of Tumor Biology Investment Group, Inc., a biotechnology company that holds the rights to several sEGFR patents. Of note, Dr. Baron was not involved in the statistical analyses or interpretation of the statistical results of these analyses.

Acknowledgments

This work was supported by National Institutes of Health (Grants K07 CA76170, R21 CA82520, and RO3 CA82091 to A.T.B). The authors thank both referees for their helpful and encouraging comments.

References

[1] D. B. Dunson, "Commentary: practical advantages of Bayesian analysis of epidemiologic data," *American Journal of Epidemiology*, vol. 153, no. 12, pp. 1222–1226, 2001.

[2] S. Greenland, "Bayesian perspectives for epidemiological research: I. Foundations and basic methods," *International Journal of Epidemiology*, vol. 35, no. 3, pp. 765–775, 2006.

[3] S. Greenland, "Bayesian perspectives for epidemiological research. II. Regression analysis," *International Journal of Epidemiology*, vol. 36, no. 1, pp. 195–202, 2007.

[4] S. Greenland, "Bayesian perspectives for epidemiologic research: III. Bias analysis via missing-data methods," *International Journal of Epidemiology*, vol. 38, no. 6, pp. 1662–1673, 2009.

[5] A. Lawson, *Bayesian Disease Mapping: Hierarchical Modeling in Spatial Epidemiology*, CRC Press, Boca Raton, Fla, USA, 2009.

[6] R. F. MacLehose, J. M. Oakes, and B. P. Carlin, "Turning the Bayesian crank," *Epidemiology*, vol. 22, no. 3, pp. 365–367, 2011.

[7] S. R. Cole, H. Chu, S. Greenland, G. Hamra, and D. B. Richardson, "Bayesian posterior distributions without Markov chains," *American Journal of Epidemiology*, vol. 175, no. 5, pp. 368–375, 2012.

[8] A. Erkanli, M. Sung, E. J. Costello, and A. Angold, "Bayesian semi-parametric ROC analysis," *Statistics in Medicine*, vol. 25, no. 22, pp. 3905–3928, 2006.

[9] T. E. Hanson, A. Kottas, and A. J. Branscum, "Modelling stochastic order in the analysis of receiver operating characteristic data: Bayesian non-parametric approaches," *Journal of the Royal Statistical Society C*, vol. 57, no. 2, pp. 207–225, 2008.

[10] A. J. Branscum, W. O. Johnson, T. E. Hanson, and I. A. Gardner, "Bayesian semiparametric ROC curve estimation and disease diagnosis," *Statistics in Medicine*, vol. 27, no. 13, pp. 2474–2496, 2008.

[11] T. E. Hanson, A. J. Branscum, and I. A. Gardner, "Multivariate mixtures of Polya trees for modeling ROC data," *Statistical Modelling*, vol. 8, no. 1, pp. 81–96, 2008.

[12] J. Gu, S. Ghosal, and A. Roy, "Bayesian bootstrap estimation of ROC curve," *Statistics in Medicine*, vol. 27, no. 26, pp. 5407–5420, 2008.

[13] C. Wang, B. W. Turnbull, Y. T. Gröhn, and S. S. Nielsen, "Nonparametric estimation of ROC curves based on Bayesian models when the true disease state is unknown," *Journal of Agricultural, Biological, and Environmental Statistics*, vol. 12, no. 1, pp. 128–146, 2007.

[14] G. T. Fosgate, H. M. Scott, and E. R. Jordan, "Development of a method for Bayesian nonparametric ROC analysis with

application to an ELISA for Johne's disease in dairy cattle," *Preventive Veterinary Medicine*, vol. 81, no. 1–3, pp. 178–193, 2007.

[15] V. Inácio, A. A. Turkman, C. T. Nakas, and T. A. Alonzo, "Nonparametric Bayesian estimation of the three-way receiver operating characteristic surface," *Biometrical Journal*, vol. 53, no. 6, pp. 1011–1024, 2011.

[16] I. V. de Carvalho, A. Jara, T. E. Hanson, and M. de Carvalho, "Bayesian nonparametric ROC regression modeling," *Bayesian Analysis*, vol. 8, no. 3, pp. 623–646, 2013.

[17] M. Ladouceur, E. Rahme, P. Bélisle, A. N. Scott, K. Schwartzman, and L. Joseph, "Modeling continuous diagnostic test data using approximate Dirichlet process distributions," *Statistics in Medicine*, vol. 30, no. 21, pp. 2648–2662, 2011.

[18] T. Hanson and W. O. Johnson, "Modeling regression error with a mixture of Polya trees," *Journal of the American Statistical Association*, vol. 97, no. 460, pp. 1020–1033, 2002.

[19] T. E. Hanson, "Inference for mixtures of finite Polya tree models," *Journal of the American Statistical Association*, vol. 101, no. 476, pp. 1548–1565, 2006.

[20] E. J. Bedrick, R. Christensen, and W. Johnson, "A new perspective on priors for generalized linear models," *Journal of the American Statistical Association*, vol. 91, no. 436, pp. 1450–1460, 1996.

[21] A. T. Baron, J. M. Lafky, C. H. Boardman et al., "Serum sErbB1 and epidermal growth factor levels as tumor biomarkers in women with stage III or IV epithelial ovarian cancer," *Cancer Epidemiology Biomarkers and Prevention*, vol. 8, no. 2, pp. 129–137, 1999.

[22] A. T. Baron, C. H. Boardman, J. M. Lafky et al., "Soluble epidermal growth factor receptor (SEG-FR) and cancer antigen 125 (CA125) as screening and diagnostic tests for epithelial ovarian cancer," *Cancer Epidemiology Biomarkers and Prevention*, vol. 14, no. 2, pp. 306–318, 2005.

[23] S. Geisser and W. F. Eddy, "A predictive approach to model selection," *Journal of the American Statistical Association*, vol. 74, pp. 153–160, 1979.

[24] R. Christensen, W. Johnson, A. Branscum, and T. Hanson, *Bayesian Ideas and Data Analysis: An Introduction for Scientists and Statisticians*, CRC Press, Boca Raton, Fla, USA, 2010.

[25] R. Christensen, T. Hanson, and A. Jara, "Parametric nonparametric statistics: an introduction to mixtures of finite Polya trees," *The American Statistician*, vol. 62, no. 4, pp. 296–306, 2008.

Behavioural Risk Factors of Noncommunicable Diseases among Nepalese Urban Poor: A Descriptive Study from a Slum Area of Kathmandu

Natalia Oli,[1] Abhinav Vaidya,[1] and Gobardhan Thapa[2]

[1] *Department of Community Medicine, Kathmandu Medical College, Sinamangal, Kathmandu, Nepal*
[2] *Kathmandu Medical College, Sinamangal, Kathmandu, Nepal*

Correspondence should be addressed to Natalia Oli; olinatalia@hotmail.com

Academic Editor: Ana Marice Ladeia

There has been a rapid rise in the burden of noncommunicable diseases in low-income countries like Nepal. Political and economical instability leading to internal migration give rise to haphazard urbanization in Nepal. This, coupled with negative effects of globalization, is largely responsible for changing lifestyle and developing risky behaviour among the urban poor that put them at high risk of developing noncommunicable diseases. A descriptive cross-sectional quantitative study was conducted from September to December 2012 in an urban slum of Kathmandu to explore the prevalence of four major behaviour risk factors namely physical inactivity, low fruit and vegetable consumption, and tobacco and alcohol use and to measure the burden of obesity and hypertension in the population. We used WHO NCDs Risk Factor steps 1 and 2 questionnaires in all the 689 households of the slum. The major behavioral risk factors for noncommunicable diseases were very common with at least a quarter of the population having the major risk factors. The results may serve to form a framework to future planning, policy-making, implementation, and evaluation of any measures undertaken to reduce these risk factors, especially as the government is planning to unveil the National Urban Health Policy soon.

1. Introduction

It is well established that noncommunicable diseases (NCDs) are the leading cause of adult mortality and morbidity worldwide including the Southeast Asia region (SEAR) [1]. Four main NCDs, namely cardiovascular diseases (CVDs), diabetes, cancers, and chronic respiratory diseases, are mainly responsible for this high mortality and morbidity. Of the estimated 14.5 million total deaths in 2008 in SEAR, more than half (55%) of them were due to NCDs, mainly cardiovascular disease (25%) [1].

From the beginning, NCDs and particularly CVDs were termed diseases of the rich in the developed countries [2]. However, over the past two decades, CVD deaths have been declining in the high-income countries but increasing significantly in the low- and middle-income countries (LMICs) [3]. One of the reasons for this increase is the rising life expectancy like the one being seen in South Asia region which leads to shifting disease burden towards NCDs [4]. Moreover, at the same time, the trend of urbanization is drastically increasing in this region causing changes in lifestyle of the people. For example, shifting lifestyle towards low physical activity and unhealthy diet leads to a rise in prevalence of obesity and NCDs among urban population [5]. For this reason, NCDs have also been called "diseases of urbanization". Risk factors of NCDs such as high blood pressure are found more commonly among urban communities compared to rural in the developing countries [6].

In 2008, half of the world's population lived in urban areas and if this trend continues, 70 percent of the global population will be living in urban areas by 2050 [7]. No doubt that one of the negative impacts of this demographic transition is formation of slum and squatter settlements in the urban area. UN-HABITAT has estimated some 38 percent of the LMIC population lives in slums with 433 million of them living in Asia [8]. Slum communities are defined as a wide range of low-income settlements with inadequate living conditions and substandard facilities. The residents of slums areas generally own their land and house and have formal title papers. On the other hand, squatter settlements are those communities where people have settled on land without any legal right to be there. But as the patterns of living in both these settlements are similar, the term slum is often used to describe both. The urban poor have the most disadvantageous position among all the urban population. This is because they adopt urban lifestyle that put them at a higher risk of developing NCDs and at the same time, lack of knowledge and information regarding health, poor access to healthcare, and poor economic status worsen the situation among them [6].

Nepal is not an exception in regard to urbanization. According to the national census 2011, about 17 percent of the total Nepalese population live in urban areas [9]. Most of the urban population is concentrated in the capital Kathmandu and its rapid growth has led to increasing pressure in Kathmandu. At present, there are 63 slum and squatter settlements in Kathmandu, and their population is estimated to be growing by 25 percent per year [10]. Most of the slums settlements are located in the centre of the city along the river banks of Bagamati, Bishnumati, and Manohara Rivers. People in slum areas have high levels of health risks and problems due to inadequate water supply, basic sanitation, and proper nutrition, amongst others.

Facing the epidemiological transition like many LMICs, Nepal is also experiencing double burden of communicable and noncommunicable diseases [11]. CVDs are the most common cause of NCD admissions in Nepal (38%) according to a 2010 hospital-based study [12]. It is well known that up to 80% of heart disease, stroke, and type 2 diabetes and over a third of cancers could be prevented by eliminating common risk factors, mainly tobacco use, unhealthy diet, physical inactivity, and the harmful use of alcohol [13]. These unhealthy behaviours lead to metabolic changes such as raised blood pressure, obesity, raised blood sugar, and lipids. Moreover, coexistence of modifiable behavioural and metabolic risk factors in the same person increases the individual's total risk of developing acute vascular events such as heart attacks and strokes [3].

Studies and interventions in the Nepalese slums deal mainly with communicable diseases, environmental, and sanitation problems, while NCDs have remained largely neglected [10, 14–16]. Thus, very little is known about the spectrum and burden of NCD morbidity in the Nepalese slum population. Because people from slum do come to hospitals with late complications of NCDs, it is obvious that NCDs exist among urban poor as well [17, 18]. Reasons for this late presentation could be their low health seeking behaviour due to lack of health knowledge and information and poor purchasing ability [17].

A number of studies have been conducted in Nepal using WHO steps risk factors questionnaire in different urban and rural areas [19]. These studies have however eluded slum and squatters areas. Hence, we undertook the present study to measure the prevalence of four major behaviour risk factors, namely physical inactivity, low fruit and vegetable consumption, and tobacco and alcohol use, in a slum population of Kathmandu. Additionally, we also aimed to find out the level of two major physical risk factors, obesity, and hypertension, in this study.

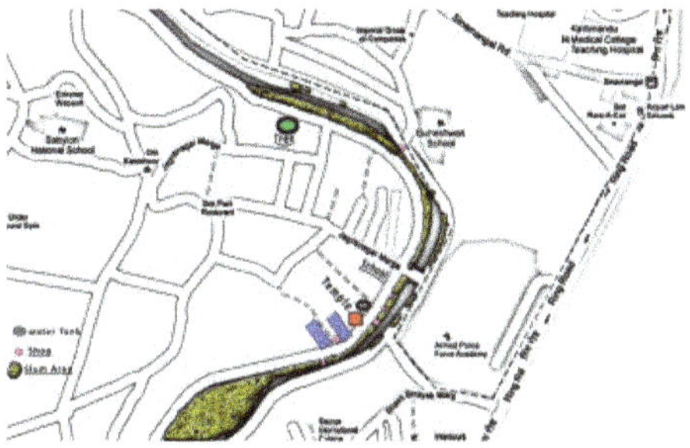

Figure 1: Map of the Sinamangal slum area, Kathmandu. The study area is shown as the shaded area (yellow) along the banks of the river (grey) across the middle of the map.

2. Methods

2.1. Study Site and Population. The study was of descriptive cross-sectional quantitative design. It was conducted in the Sinamangal squatter area in Kathmandu Metropolitan City along the banks of Bagmati River, from September to December 2012 (Figure 1). The study area was purposively selected because it is a predefined study area for Family Health Advisory Programme for medical students under the Department of Community Medicine, Kathmandu Medical College. The study area is about one kilometre away from the medical college. As the squatter area has settlements scattered both upstream and downstream, the area of the squatter settlement falling in the Sinamangal area was first demarcated. It was then arbitrarily divided into four clusters.

The study population included household members aged 15–64 years living for at least 6 months in the defined squatter area and who consented to participate in the study. Because there was no official information about the number of households in the squatter area to construct a sampling frame, nonprobability convenient sampling technique was used.

2.2. Data Collection. Data was collected by third-year medical students of Kathmandu Medical College. The eighty medical students were divided in to four groups of 20 for each of the four clusters. The students were trained by the researchers in taking informed consent, administering questionnaire, interview techniques, and physical measurements. Each household was visited and the person available at that time was interviewed. If nobody was present in the household during the first visit, the student revisited it again at the time when the resident of the house would be available.

If there was more than one eligible respondent in a household, a lottery method was used to select one respondent. The students were continuously supervised by the researchers during the data collection process.

2.3. Study Tools

2.3.1. Questionnaire. Data was collected through face-to-face interviews using questions based on WHO NCD risk factor steps 1 and 2 questionnaires [20]. Biochemical measurements of step 3 were not performed because of logistic limitations. The questionnaire included questions regarding demographic characteristic of the respondents, tobacco and alcohol consumption, physical activity, and fruit and vegetable consumption.

2.3.2. Physical Measurements. Height, weight, waist, and hip circumferences were measured. The instructions given in the step 2 were followed while taking the measurements. Weight was measured with Microlife BR-9201 weighing machine (Microlife AG Swiss Corporation, Widnau, Switzerland). Height, waist, and hip circumferences were measured with nonstretchable measuring tapes (Jonson Tapes Ltd., New Delhi, India). Aneroid sphygmomanometers (Doctor Aneroid Sphygmomanometer, Japan) were used for blood pressure recording. Blood pressure was recorded three times with a gap of 5 minutes between the recordings. Average of the three readings was taken as the final blood pressure measurement.

2.3.3. Operational Definitions. The definitions used for the study were based on the WHO steps survey manual and are briefly described below [20]. Occupation and educational categories are also based on the WHO steps survey manual. Classification of ethnic group is based on the National Central Bureau of Statistics of Nepal [9]:

(a) current drinkers: respondents who consumed alcohol in the previous 30 days;

(b) one serving of vegetable: one cup of raw, leafy green vegetables (spinach, salad, etc.), one half cup of other vegetables, cooked or raw (tomatoes, pumpkin, beans etc.), or half cup of vegetable juice;

(c) one serving of fruit: one medium-sized piece of fruit (banana, apple, etc.) or half cup of raw, cooked or canned fruit, or a half cup of juice from a fruit (not artificially flavoured);

(d) physical activity: it included questions on number of days and time spent on vigorous and/or moderate activities at work, travel to and from places, and recreational activities. The responses were then converted to MET minutes/week. The respondents were labelled as having vigorous activity or moderate activity if they achieved certain MET minutes as given in the WHO steps manual. Someone was termed as having low physical activity (LBA) if s/he did not fulfil the criteria of having vigorous or moderate activity;

(e) hypertension: it included those who self-reported as having hypertension or those who had high blood pressure according to JNC-VII classification [21] during the time of survey;

(f) combined risk factors: the following risk factors were considered while counting the number of risk factors present:

  (i) current daily smoker,

  (ii) less than 5 servings of fruits and vegetables per day,

  (iii) low physical activity (<600 MET minutes),

  (iv) overweight or obese (BMI $\geq 25\,kg/m^2$),

  (v) raised BP (SBP $\geq$ 140 and/or DBP $\geq$ 90 mmHg or currently on medication for raised BP).

2.4. Data Management and Analysis. The filled questionnaires were thoroughly checked by the researchers for any inconsistencies. Data coding and cleaning were done. Data was entered and analysed with SPSS version 20.0 (IBM, Armonk, New York, USA). Descriptive analysis was done; mean with standard deviations was calculated for continuous variables, and percentages were calculated for categorical variables.

2.5. Ethical Consideration. The study obtained approval from Ethical Review Committee of Kathmandu Medical College. All principles of Helsinki Declaration were ensured during the study. Informed consent was obtained from each participant after the objectives of study had been explained. Privacy and confidentiality were thoroughly maintained during the interview. Filled questionnaires were securely placed in the Department of Community Medicine. There were no physical risks as there was no intervention such as blood sampling done during the study. However, there was possible psychological risk due to questions related to income and personal behaviours, and the students were trained to sensitively handle them. Those who were found to have the risk factors under the study were counselled and/or referred to Kathmandu Medical College for the needful.

3. Results and Discussion

Altogether 689 households were identified in the defined study area and we included one person from each household; thus, we had a sample size of 689. There were no non-responders. Based on the response given by the respondents about the number of adults aged 15–64 years in his/her house, we calculated that there were 2356 adults of age 15–64 residing in the area. Thus, our study covered 29.24% of the adults aged 15–64 years living in the area.

3.1. Demographic Characteristics. The demographic characteristics of the study population are described in Table 1. Half of the respondents were aged less than 35 years. About 60% were women. About 40% had no formal education. About one third of the respondents were self-employed, while a quarter of the women were housewives. Thirteen percent of the respondents were unemployed though they were able to work. Majority (72.3%) of them had been staying there for more than five years. More than one third of the respondents had a monthly income of less than NRs. 5000 (1 US Dollar = approximately 85 Nepalese Rupees). Most of them had come to live in the squatter because of economic reasons, in search of a job, because of natural calamities like flood in their native places, or due to marriage. They had migrated mainly from other parts of Kathmandu district (22%), or from

TABLE 1: Demographic characteristics of the study population ($N = 689$). Classification of ethnic group is based on the National Central Bureau of Statistics [9]. Primary and secondary schooling indicate education up to grades 4 and 10, respectively. Other ethnic group includes Terai Dalit, disadvantaged Janajatis (Terai), disadvantaged non-Dalit Terai caste groups, and religious minorities. Other occupations include nonpaid, retired, and unemployed ones (unable to work).

	Male		Female		Total	
	N	%	*N*	%	*N*	%
Age (years)						
15–24	75	26.5	117	28.8	192	27.9
25–34	56	19.8	109	26.8	165	23.9
35–44	61	21.6	87	21.4	148	21.5
45–54	48	17.0	53	13.1	101	14.7
55–64	29	10.2	23	5.7	52	7.5
≥65	14	4.9	17	4.2	31	4.5
Ethnicity						
Hill Dalit	33	11.7	66	16.3	99	14.4
Disadvantaged Janajatis (Hill)	113	39.9	185	45.6	298	43.3
Relatively advantaged Janajatis	34	12.0	30	7.4	64	9.3
Upper caste groups	89	31.4	112	27.6	201	29.2
Others	14	49	13	3.2	27	3.9
Highest education						
No formal education	71	25.1	209	51.5	280	40.6
Less than primary	27	9.5	19	4.7	46	6.7
Primary completed	109	38.5	106	26.1	215	31.2
Secondary completed	58	20.5	55	13.5	113	16.4
High school or more	18	6.4	17	4.2	35	5.1
Occupation						
Employed (government/nongovernment)	59	20.8	32	7.9	90	13.1
Self-employed	137	48.4	109	26.8	246	35.7
Student	21	7.4	38	9.4	59	8.6
Housewife	0	0.0	159	39.2	163	23.7
Unemployed (able to work)	46	16.3	45	11.1	89	12.9
Others	20	7.1	23	5.7	42	6.1
Migration (years)						
<1	28	9.9	38	9.4	66	9.6
1–5	43	15.2	82	20.2	125	18.1
5–10	98	34.6	139	34.2	237	34.4
>10	114	40.3	147	36.2	261	37.9
Income status (NRs) ($n = 391$)						
1st quartile (≤5000)	55	27.9	91	46.9	146	37.3
2nd quartile (5001–7000)	32	16.2	35	18.0	67	17.1
3rd quartile (7001–10000)	51	25.9	42	21.6	93	23.8
4th quartile (≥10000)	59	29.9	26	13.4	85	21.7

NRs: Nepalese rupees.

other nearby districts such as Kavrepalanchok (6%) and Sindhupalchowk (3%), or from Eastern Nepal districts such as Sindhuli (10%), Jhapa (7%), and Morang (5%).

3.2. Behavioural Risk Factors. The urban poor remain neglected part of urban population in terms of exploring their burden of behaviour risk factors and prevalence of NCDs among them. During the present study, it was found that the four important behavioural risk factors of NCDs—tobacco consumption, harmful use of alcohol, low fruit and vegetable consumption, and physical inactivity—are rampant in the slum population. Moreover, hypertension and obesity are also prevalent in the study population.

3.2.1. Tobacco Consumption. Age-sex distribution of smoking is presented in Figure 2. Prevalence of smoking in men, women, and both sexes is 51.9%, 24.1%, and 35.6%. The overall (both sexes) prevalence of smoking in the present study is higher than the national data (23.8%) [19]. The smoking rate in the population is higher than that in the urban population

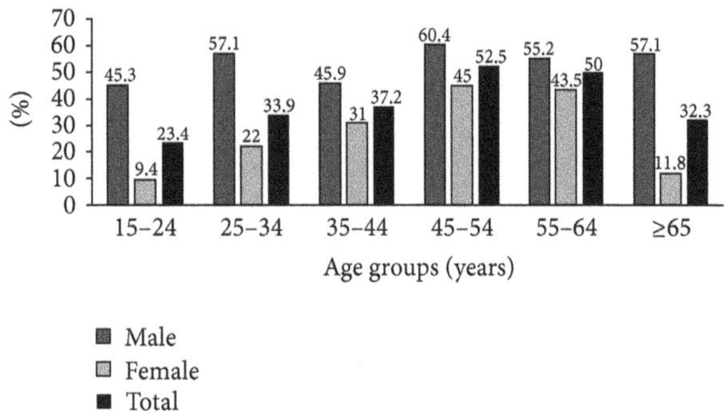

Figure 2: Prevalence (%) of current smokers in the study population according to the age group (n = 689). The categories are based on the WHO NCD risk factor steps survey manual [20]. Current smokers included those who responded "yes" to "Do you smoke?". Dark and light grey bars are for men and women, respectively, while the black bars represent both sexes.

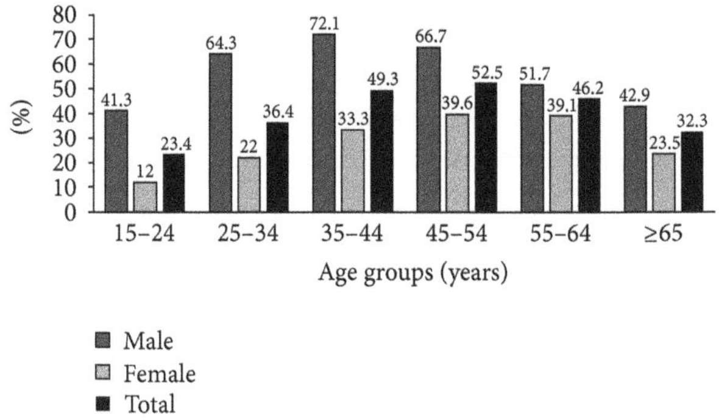

Figure 4: Prevalence (%) of current drinkers in the study population according to the age group (n = 689). The categories are based on the WHO NCD risk factor steps survey manual [20]. Current drinkers refer to the ones that consumed alcohol within the previous month. Dark and light grey bars are for men and women, respectively, while the black bars represent both sexes.

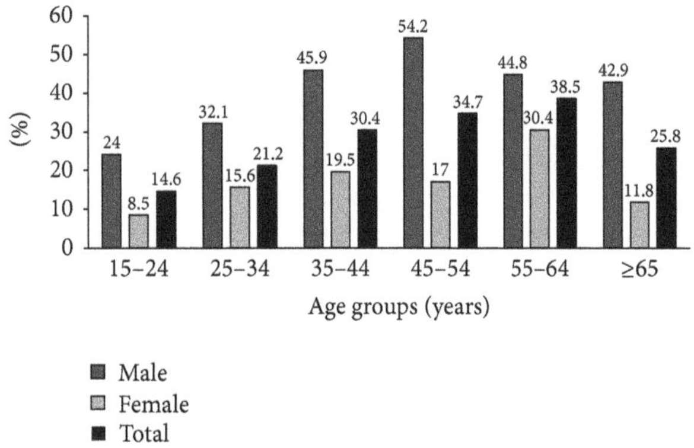

Figure 3: Prevalence (%) of current Smokeless tobacco in the study population according to the age group (n = 689). The categories are based on the WHO NCD risk factor steps survey manual [20]. Smokeless tobacco included products such as *gutka*, *khaini*, and *surti*. Dark and light grey bars are for men and women respectively, while the black bars represent both sexes.

of Myanmar (22.0%) [22] and the Chennai (20.2%) [23] and Patna (12.54%) [24] slums of India but lower than that in the Mumbai slum (66.7%) [18]. But compared to the urban poor from Kerala, India, there is not a large difference (37.3%) [25].

By gender-wise stratification also, more men and women in our study smoke compared to the of the Nepal's national data (31.2% and 15.5%) [19], the urban population of Myanmar (44.8 and 7.8%) [22], and the urban slum of Patna (21.15% and 5.91%) [24]. Comparatively, fewer women (12.2%) and more men (62.6%) in the Kerala slum smoked [25].

Regarding smokeless tobacco, the overall consumption rate in our study is 24.8% (men: 38.5%, women: 15.3%). Age-sex distribution of smokeless tobacco is shown in Figure 3. Compared to the national figures (18.6% for both sexes, 31.2% for men, and 4.6% for women), prevalence of consumption of smokeless tobacco is also higher in the study population [19]. The figures are however less compared to data from India and Myanmar. There are twice more consumers (55.4%) in the Mumbai slum [18] than in our study. Similarly, the prevalence in the urban Myanmar is also higher with 51.4% of the males and 16.1% of females consuming smokeless tobacco [22].

It is already an established fact that tobacco consumption is now universally more common among lower socioeconomic groups. For example, prevalence of tobacco chewing among women labourers in Dharan, Nepal (22%), was twice as much as among service class women (10%) [26].

3.2.2. Alcohol Consumption. Alcohol consumption in the slum is very high with 38.5% of the study population (58% of men and 24.9% of women) being current drinkers, that is, who had alcohol containing drink in the last 30 days. Among the current drinkers, one third consumes it daily (men: 34.6%, women: 31.1%). Comparatively, less people (31.2%) in the Mumbai slum drank [18]. Age-sex distribution of current drinkers is shown in Figure 4. Prevalences of alcohol consumption in the males and females of the study area were higher than the national averages for men (39.3%) and women (16.5%) [19]. Among males, the current drinking rate is higher than that in their counterparts from Patna (16.65%) [24] and Kerala (45.4%) [25]. The highest prevalence of current drinking was seen in the 35–44 years age group (72.1%). Similarly, more females in the Sinamangal slum drink more than the women of Patna slum (3.35%) [24] and in Kerala slum (1.0%) [25].

3.2.3. Fruits and Vegetable Consumption. The mean fruit consumption was less than two days per week with about 20% taking fruits less than once a week (Table 2). Comparatively, vegetable consumption was better with average six days per week. A higher level of fruit and vegetable intake has been observed among the urban slum dwellers in Chennai where more than half population consumed vegetables 5 days and fruits 3 days per week [27]. The mean number of servings of fruit and/or vegetables per day in the present study was low—one serving per day for fruits and two servings per day for vegetables (Table 2). Myanmar urban slum population had better fruit and vegetable consumption [22].

More than five servings of fruit and vegetables are recommended for healthy living, but 90.5% men and 93.3%

TABLE 2: Fruit and vegetable consumption in the study population (N = 689). One serving of fruit means one medium-sized piece of fruit (banana, apple, etc.) or half cup of raw, cooked or canned fruit, or a half cup of juice from a fruit (not artificially flavoured). One serving of vegetable is one cup of raw, leafy green vegetables, (spinach, salad, etc.), one half cup of other vegetables, cooked or raw (tomatoes, pumpkin, beans, etc.), or half cup of vegetable juice.

	Male		Female		Total	
	N	%	N	%	N	%
Fruit consumption						
Days/week						
0	60	21.2	79	19.5	139	20.2
1–3	181	64.0	272	67.0	453	65.7
4–6	29	10.2	42	10.3	71	10.3
7	13	4.6	13	3.2	26	3.8
Mean (SD)	**1.96 (1.76)**		**1.94 (1.66)**		**1.95 (1.70)**	
Servings/day						
0	60	21.2	79	19.5	139	20.2
1-2	204	72.1	312	76.8	516	74.9
≥3	19	6.7	15	3.7	34	4.9
Mean (SD)	**1.08 (0.81)**		**1.03 (0.72)**		**1.05 (0.76)**	
Vegetable consumption						
Days/week						
0	4	1.4	9	2.2	13	1.9
1–3	26	9.2	38	9.4	64	9.3
4–6	82	29.0	104	25.4	186	27.0
7	171	60.4	255	62.8	426	61.8
Mean (SD)	**6.01 (1.59)**		**5.95 (1.72)**		**5.98 (1.67)**	
Servings/day						
0	4	1.4	9	2.2	13	1.9
1-2	250	88.3	354	87.2	604	87.7
≥3	29	10.2	43	10.6	72	10.4
Mean (SD)	**1.80 (0.84)**		**1.73 (0.97)**		**1.76 (0.92)**	
Combined fruit and vegetable						
Servings						
<5	256	90.5	379	93.3	635	92.2
≥5	27	9.5	27	6.7	54	7.8
Mean (SD)	**2.88 (1.32)**		**2.76 (1.33)**		**2.81 (1.33)**	

SD: standard deviation.

women consume less than the recommended five servings of fruit and vegetables daily in the study area. The situation in the slum is worse compared to the average Nepalese data according to which 60.5% of men and 63.5% of women have inadequate fruit and vegetable consumption [19]. Our study population fared worse in comparison to other studies in the similar settings as well [22, 25, 27]. Low consumption of fruits and vegetables in the urban poor can be due to lack of health knowledge, poor economic status of urban poor, and preference for junk food that put them at high risk of developing NCDs.

3.2.4. High Salt Containing Food Consumption. About 14% of the respondents are taking high salt containing food such as chips, instant noodles, and pickles every day. While a quarter of the respondents are taking such food less than once a week or 1-2 times in a week, about 17% almost never had them.

3.2.5. Level of Physical Inactivity. One third of the study population in the slum have low physical activity. This contrasts with the lower prevalence of physical inactivity across Nepal (5.9%) [19] or the Kerala slum (4.5%) [25] but may be considered less compared to the very high physical inactivity Chennai figure of 95% [23]. The data is however similar to the one from the Patna slum (33.64%) [24].

Prevalence of low physical activity in the Sinamangal slum is higher in the females (39.4%) than in the males (21.9%). In fact, the women here are more inactive than those from Patna and Kerala slum settlements (37.65% and 4.9%, resp.) [24, 25]. At the same time, fewer males in the present study were physically inactive in contrast with 30.55% of males in the Patna slum [24]. Furthermore, low physical activity increased drastically from the average of 20% in the younger age group to around 60% in those aged 65 or more (Table 3). Those employed either in the government

Table 3: Prevalence (%) of low physical activity in the study population according to demographic variables ($N = 689$). The physical activity section included questions on number of days and time spent on vigorous and/or moderate activities at work, travel to and from places, and recreational activities. The responses were then converted to MET minutes/week. The respondents were labelled as having vigorous activity or moderate activity if they achieved certain MET minutes as given in the WHO steps manual [20]. Someone was termed as having low physical activity (LBA) if s/he did not fulfil the criteria of having vigorous or moderate activity.

	Male		Female		Total	
	N	%	*N*	%	*N*	%
Age (years)						
15–24	15	20.0	47	40.2	62	32.3
25–34	12	21.4	41	37.6	53	32.1
35–44	12	19.7	28	32.3	40	27.0
45–54	9	18.8	18	34.0	27	26.7
55–64	6	20.7	15	65.2	21	40.2
≥65	8	57.1	11	64.7	19	61.3
Ethnicity						
Hill Dalit	6	18.2	25	37.9	31	31.3
Disadvantaged Janajatis (Hill)	29	25.7	78	42.2	107	35.9
Relatively advantaged Janajatis	5	14.7	9	30.0	14	21.9
Upper caste groups	18	20.2	45	40.2	63	31.3
Others	4	28.6	3	23.1	7	25.9
Highest education						
No formal education	22	31.0	83	39.7	105	37.5
Less than primary	4	14.8	4	21.1	8	17.4
Primary completed	20	18.3	50	47.2	70	32.6
Secondary completed	13	22.4	16	29.1	29	25.7
High school or more	3	16.7	7	41.2	10	28.6
Occupation						
Employed (government/nongovernment)	3	5.2	6	18.8	9	10.0
Self-employed	26	19.0	36	33.0	62	25.2
Student	5	23.8	12	31.6	17	28.8
Housewife	—	—	64	40.3	64	40.3
Unemployed (able to work)	15	34.1	27	60.0	42	47.2
Others	13	68.4	15	65.2	28	66.7
Income status (NRs) ($n = 391$)						
1st quartile (≤5000)	13	23.6	20	22.0	33	22.6
2nd quartile (5001–7000)	4	12.5	12	34.3	16	23.9
3rd quartile (7001–10000)	6	11.8	19	45.2	25	26.9
4th quartile (≥10000)	7	11.9	11	42.3	18	21.2
Total	62	21.9	160	39.4	222	32.2

NRs: Nepalese rupees.

or nongovernmental organizations had less prevalence of low physical activity (10%). Whereas both men and women belonging to the lowest income group had similar prevalence of low physical activity, the women with high income tended to become less physically active compared to men of the same income group.

3.2.6. Blood Pressure Status. A respondent who was either a known hypertensive or was found to have high blood pressure during the survey was called having "hypertension." Twenty-eight percent of the respondents are thus found to have hypertension (Table 4). This prevalence is higher than the national average (21.5%) [19]. It is also high compared to the Indian slums of Chennai (22.8%) [23] and Patna (16.36%) [24]. On the other hand, the Kerala slum has a slightly higher (31%) prevalence of high blood pressure [25].

Prevalence of hypertension according to various demographic variables is given in Table 4. The males have a higher prevalence of hypertension (35.0%) than the females (23.2%). In fact, hypertension prevalence in the males of the slum is higher than the national average of 24.5% [19] and the urban males of Dharan town in the Eastern Nepal (22.7%) [28]. Furthermore, the prevalence rates are even higher than some of the slums of India such as Patna (18.79%) [24] and Kerala (31.0%) [25] but lower than the very high figure of Mumbai (71.2%) [18]. Though women in the slum had

TABLE 4: Prevalence of hypertension in the study population according to demographic variables (N = 689). Hypertensives included those who self-reported as having hypertension or those who had high blood pressure according to JNC-VII classification [21] during the time of survey.

	Male		Female		Total	
	N	%	N	%	N	%
Age (years)						
15–24	11	14.7	7	6.0	18	9.4
25–34	12	21.4	17	15.6	29	17.6
35–44	26	42.6	34	39.1	60	40.5
45–54	24	50.0	18	34.0	42	41.6
55–64	18	62.1	11	47.8	29	55.8
≥65	8	57.1	7	41.2	15	48.4
Ethnicity						
Hill Dalit	14	42.4	12	18.2	26	26.3
Disadvantaged Janajatis (Hill)	39	34.5	47	25.4	86	28.9
Relatively advantaged Janajatis	13	38.2	12	40.0	25	39.1
Upper caste groups	30	33.7	20	17.9	50	24.9
Others	3	21.4	3	23.1	6	22.2
Highest education						
No formal education	34	47.9	61	29.2	95	33.9
Less than primary	7	25.9	2	10.5	9	19.6
Primary completed	34	31.2	20	18.9	54	25.1
Secondary completed	16	27.6	8	14.5	24	21.2
High school or more	8	44.4	3	17.6	11	31.4
Occupation						
Employed (government/nongovernment)	20	34.5	3	9.4	23	25.6
Self-employed	49	35.8	30	27.5	79	32.1
Student	3	14.3	3	7.9	6	10.2
Housewife	—	—	37	23.3	37	23.3
Unemployed (able to work)	16	36.4	12	26.7	28	31.5
Others	11	57.9	9	39.1	20	47.6
Migration (years)						
<1	5	17.9	4	10.5	9	13.6
1–5	20	46.5	16	19.5	36	28.8
5–10	32	32.7	31	22.5	63	26.6
>10	42	36.8	43	29.3	85	32.6
Income status (NRs) (n = 391)						
1st quartile (≤5000)	15	27.3	18	19.8	33	22.6
2nd quartile (5001–7000)	13	40.6	10	28.6	23	34.3
3rd quartile (7001–10000)	21	41.2	10	23.8	31	33.3
4th quartile (≥10000)	21	35.6	8	30.8	29	34.1
Total	99	35.0	94	23.2	193	28.0

NRs: Nepalese rupees.

less hypertension compared to men, it was still high in comparison to the Nepalese average (18.1%) [19] and the Patna slum (14.48%) [24].

Blood pressure status of the population according to extent of awareness, treatment, and control is presented in Figure 5. About 63% of the study population had their blood pressure measured in the previous 12 months while 34.7% of the males and 29.8% of the females never had their blood pressure checked. Among the latter group, 49% of the males (i.e., 17% of the total male respondents) and 24.8% of the females (i.e., 7.4% of the total female respondents) were found to have high blood pressure during the survey—that is, undiagnosed hypertension. This prevalence of undiagnosed hypertension among both sexes in our study was about 20% which is higher than that in the Chennai slum study (15.4%) [23]. Likewise, our male population also had slightly higher prevalence of undiagnosed hypertension compared to the Dharan study (17% versus 14.4%) [28].

In our study, 17.6% males and 15.8% females were known hypertensives—among whom 50% males (i.e., 8.8%

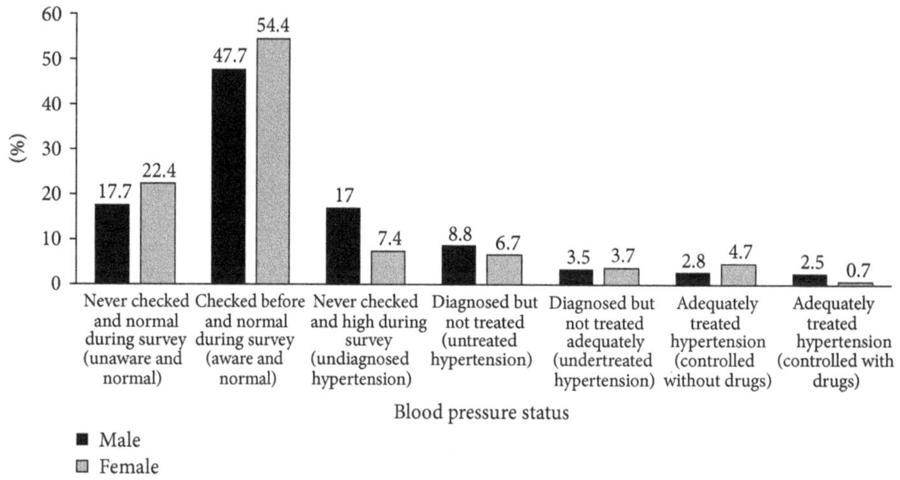

FIGURE 5: Blood pressure status of the study population according to different sub-categories of awareness, treatment and control (N = 689). Hypertensives included those who self-reported as having hypertension or those who had high blood pressure according to JNC-VII classification [21] during the time of survey. Black bars are for men and grey bars are for women respectively.

of total male respondents) and 42.4% (i.e., 6.7% of total female respondents) were untreated—that is, diagnosed but untreated hypertension. Among the hypertensive population who were receiving treatment, 39.8% of the males and 40.7% of the females still had high blood pressure during the survey—that is, 3.5% of the total male respondents and 3.7% of the total female respondents had undertreated hypertension. The remaining hypertensives had their blood pressure under control—that is, 5.3% of the total male respondents or 30.1% of the male hypertensives, and 5.4% of the total female respondents or 34.2% of the female hypertensives had their blood pressure under control with or without drugs. The control rate among the known male hypertensive population was less in our study compared to the study in the Dharan (30.1% versus 58.5%) [28].

3.2.7. General and Abdominal Obesity. According to their body mass index, almost one quarter of the respondents (26.0% of males and 23.9% of females) were overweight, while 5.8% were obese (Table 5). In the males, prevalence of overweight was the highest in the 35–44 years group (37.7%) while females had the highest percent (28.4%) of overweight in the 25–34 years group (Table 5). Ethnicity-wise, relatively advantaged Janajatis had the highest prevalence of overweight and obesity, while the prevalence was less in those who had studied more than secondary education and who were currently students. In terms of abdominal obesity, females had higher waist circumference across all demographic parameters than males (Table 5).

Unlike the other slum studies from India, the problem of high BMI is found to be more in males than in females in our study population. For example, the prevalence of overweight women was higher than men in the urban Myanmar (13.5% males and 22% females) [22] and in Kerala slums (men—29.7%, women—41%) [25]. Even in the Mumbai slum settlement, though 42.1% males were overweight compared to 11.7% females, 20% of women were obese in contrast to 0.8% males [18].

3.2.8. Combination of Risk Factors. About forty percent of the males and thirty percent of the females had 3–5 risk factors (Table 6). This is much higher than the 12.5% and 5.8% in the national representative data of Nepal [19]. In our study, the upper caste groups had the least occurrence of "3–5 risk factors" in both males and females. Those who were self-employed or were unemployed despite being able to work and those without formal education had more risk factors. Similarly, those who had lived for a longer time in the slum area were found to have more risk factors compared to those who had recently migrated. There was no definite relationship between income and number of risk factors.

3.3. Strengths and Limitations of the Study. Our study explored NCD risk factors in an urban slum for the first time in Nepal. Through this study, we intended to measure the status of NCD risk factors in this population group, so that appropriate recommendations could be made to improve any prevalent risk factors. We followed the WHO STEPwise approach to surveillance which is a standardized method for collecting, analysing, and disseminating data in WHO member countries. Data collection was done by trained medical students under continuous supervision of medical faculty. During the course of data collection, any needy respondent was referred to the hospital for further management ensuring that the study incorporated socio-ethical values.

Our study had certain limitations and weaknesses. There were disproportionately more women respondents (60%) in our study. Although there is no actual demographic data to compare if the male : female ratio is different in the population, unintentional oversampling of women is possible as the data collection was done during daytime when many

TABLE 5: Prevalence (%) of overweight and obesity, increased waist circumference, and increased waist hip ratio according to demographic variables ($n = 689$). Increased waist circumference is waist measurements of ≥80 cm for females and ≥90 cm for males; increased waist hip ratio is ≥0.85 for females and ≥0.90 for males. Income status data is only for 391 persons who disclosed their financial information.

	Body mass index				Increased waist circumference		Increased waist hip ratio	
	Overweight (25–29.9 kg/m^2)		Obesity (≥30 kg/m^2)					
	Male	Female	Male	Female	Male	Female	Male	Female
Age (years)								
15–24	8.0	9.4	5.3	0.9	10.7	17.1	49.3	54.7
25–34	28.6	28.4	0.0	3.7	14.3	45.9	50.0	59.6
35–44	37.7	25.3	11.5	8.0	32.8	51.7	63.9	71.3
45–54	31.2	24.5	8.3	9.4	27.1	56.6	60.4	69.8
55–64	17.2	26.1	3.4	4.3	37.9	43.5	58.6	34.8
≥65	28.6	17.6	7.1	5.9	35.7	52.9	71.4	52.9
Ethnicity								
Hill Dalit	21.2	16.9	6.1	3.0	18.2	40.9	39.4	48.5
Disadvantaged Janajatis (Hill)	26.5	23.6	6.2	4.3	21.2	43.2	58.4	65.9
Relatively advantaged Janajatis	32.4	30.8	8.8	13.3	29.4	43.3	70.6	60.0
Upper caste groups	20.2	25.3	4.5	4.5	23.6	34.8	53.9	58.9
Others	21.4	36.4	7.1	0	28.6	38.5	64.3	53.8
Highest education								
No formal education	21.1	25.8	9.9	6.2	26.8	49.8	59.2	60.8
Less than primary	37.0	21.1	7.4	0	18.5	47.4	59.3	57.9
Primary completed	22.0	27.7	4.6	5.7	16.5	31.1	54.1	62.3
Secondary completed	15.5	12.5	3.4	0	22.4	29.1	56.9	56.4
High school or more	61.1	17.6	5.6	0	55.6	11.8	55.6	58.8
Occupation								
Employed (government/nongovernment)	29.3	25.9	5.2	6.2	27.6	34.4	53.4	59.4
Self-employed	28.5	21.6	8.0	7.3	23.4	38.5	60.6	56.9
Student	—	6.1	0	0	9.5	10.5	33.3	50.0
Housewife	—	29.5	—	3.1	—	50.9	—	68.6
Unemployed (able to work)	22.7	23.1	6.8	6.7	29.5	37.8	59.1	53.3
Others	15.8	22.2	0	4.3	10.5	39.1	52.6	52.2
Migration								
<1	14.3	17.1	3.6	0	17.9	26.3	25.0	50.0
1–5	25.6	25.6	9.3	8.5	23.3	41.5	72.1	61.0
5–10	28.6	21.4	5.1	5.7	21.4	38.8	58.2	63.3
>10	22.8	25.4	6.1	3.2	25.4	44.9	57.0	59.9
Income status (NRs)								
1st quartile (≤5000)	31.3	19.0	2.1	6.3	20.8	43.0	68.8	60.8
2nd quartile (5001–7000)	29.0	33.3	6.5	13.3	27.6	39.4	65.5	66.7
3rd quartile (7001–10000)	38.8	26.3	10.2	0.0	28.9	53.8	62.2	76.9
4th quartile (≥10000)	32.8	33.3	8.6	8.3	29.3	43.5	60.3	65.2
Total	26.0	23.9	6.4	5.3	25.8	45.1	63.5	67.3

NRs: Nepalese rupees.

men may have gone for work. We tried to minimize this by visiting the households in the morning time before the men left for work. Also, we did stratified analysis for men and women to eliminate this selection bias.

Certain biological risk factors such as blood glucose and cholesterol were not included in the study due to logistic limitations. Because the sample size is moderate, only one slum area was studied and nonprobability sampling was

Table 6: Summary of combined risk factors in the study population, shown in percentage ($N = 689$). The following risk factors were considered while counting the number of risk factors present: current daily smoker, less than 5 servings of fruits and vegetables per day, low physical activity (<600 MET-minutes), overweight or obese (BMI ≥ 25 kg/m^2), raised BP (SBP ≥ 140 and/or DBP ≥ 90 mmHg, or currently on medication fro raised BP [20].

	Male			Female			Total		
	Number of risk factors			Number of risk factors			Number of risk factors		
	0	1-2	3–5	0	1-2	3–5	0	1-2	3–5
Age (years)									
15–24	2.7	81.3	16.0	6.0	82.9	11.1	4.7	82.3	13.0
25–34	1.8	57.1	41.1	2.8	67.0	30.3	2.4	63.6	33.9
35–44	0.0	49.2	50.8	1.1	58.6	40.2	0.7	54.7	44.6
45–54	0.0	43.8	56.3	0.0	62.3	37.7	0.0	53.5	46.5
55–64	0.0	55.2	44.8	0.0	39.1	60.9	0.0	48.1	51.9
≥65	0.0	28.6	71.4	0.0	47.1	52.9	0.0	38.7	61.3
Ethnicity									
Hill Dalit	0.0	54.5	45.5	1.5	65.2	33.3	1.0	61.6	37.4
Disadvantaged Janajatis (Hill)	0.0	57.1	42.9	2.7	63.2	34.1	1.7	60.4	37.9
Relatively advantaged Janajatis	5.9	50.0	44.1	3.3	56.7	40.0	4.7	53.1	42.2
Upper caste groups	1.1	65.2	33.7	2.7	75.9	21.4	2.0	71.1	26.9
Others	0.0	57.1	42.9	7.7	69.2	23.1	3.7	63.0	33.3
Highest education									
No formal education	0.0	49.3	50.7	2.4	57.9	39.7	1.8	55.7	42.5
Less than primary	0.0	55.6	44.4	5.3	73.7	21.1	2.2	63.0	34.8
Primary completed	0.9	63.3	35.8	1.9	72.6	25.5	1.4	67.9	30.7
Secondary completed	3.4	58.6	37.9	5.5	81.8	12.7	4.4	69.9	25.7
High school or more	0.0	61.1	38.9	0.0	82.4	17.6	0.0	71.4	28.6
Occupation									
Employed (gov/nongov)	0.0	70.7	29.3	9.4	71.9	18.8	3.3	71.1	25.6
Self-employed	0.0	53.3	46.7	0.9	63.3	35.8	0.4	57.7	41.9
Student	9.5	76.2	14.3	10.5	81.6	7.9	10.2	79.7	10.2
Housewife	—	—	—	1.9	71.7	26.4	1.9	71.7	26.4
Unemployed (able to work)	0.0	52.3	47.7	0.0	53.3	46.7	0.0	52.8	47.2
Others	0.0	42.1	57.9	0.0	43.5	56.5	0.0	42.9	57.1
Migration (years)									
<1	3.6	78.6	17.9	0.0	73.7	26.3	1.5	75.8	22.7
1–5	2.3	44.2	53.5	3.7	73.2	23.2	3.2	63.2	33.6
5–10	1.0	57.1	41.8	3.6	65.5	30.9	2.5	62.0	35.4
>10	0.0	58.8	41.2	2.0	62.6	35.4	1.1	60.9	37.9
Income status (NRs) ($n = 391$)									
1st quartile (≤5000)	0.0	60.0	40.0	4.4	67.0	28.6	2.7	64.4	32.9
2ndquartile (5001–7000)	0.0	43.8	56.3	2.9	62.9	34.3	1.5	53.7	44.8
3rd quartile (7001–10000)	0.0	56.9	43.1	0.0	73.8	26.2	0.0	64.5	35.5
4th quartile (≥10000)	0.0	57.6	42.4	3.8	53.8	42.3	1.2	56.5	42.4
Total	1.1	58.0	41.0	2.7	66.7	30.5	2.0	63.1	34.8

NRs: Nepalese rupees.

opted, the results may not be generalized to other slum populations.

4. Conclusions

NCDs are emerging as a public health problem in Nepal. Hence, surveillance of its risk factors in different population subgroups, including the urban poor, is essential for future policy making and planning by the government and other stakeholders. Our study has shown that the behavioural risk factors of NCDs are very common in the urban poor population of Kathmandu. In fact, most of the risk factors are present in at least a quarter of the slum population: smokeless tobacco, high BMI and waist hip ratio, and hypertension. Other risk factors such as tobacco smoking, current alcohol drinking, and low physical activity are found in one third of them. Fruit and vegetable consumption is very low with 92.2% of the population not consuming 5 or more servings. One third of the population have 3–5 risk factors.

Health system of Nepal is based on primary health care with focus on rural health and with emphasis on communicable diseases, maternal, and child health issues including nutrition. Thus, as both urban poor population and NCDs have remained neglected by the government and other stakeholders, the urban poor are having a double jeopardy when it comes to NCDs. With such a huge burden of risk factors, even the burden of NCDs can be expected to be high among the urban poor. Tragically, though the facilities are often nearby, they cannot afford the costly diagnostic and treatment modalities that are accessible only to the higher socioeconomic stratum. Thus, in lack of access to proper promotive, preventive and curative services, and in absence of a civic system that acknowledges their existence, the slum people may therefore be suffering and dying from NCDs unnoticed and unaccounted.

Despite all this, it is indeed very heartening to note that the government has recently finalized the final draft of the National Urban Health Policy. Under this, free primary health care will be given to urban dwellers with low economic status, targeting mainly the poor living in the slum areas. We recommend that, because the slum people are probably the most severely hit population in terms of double burden of disease, the policy should give equal emphasis, if not more, to the NCDs and the underlying risk factors.

Conflict of Interests

The authors declared that there is no conflict of interests.

Authors' Contribution

The study concept was conceived by Natalia Oli. Tool preparation, training, and data collection supervision were carried out by Natalia Oli, and Abhinav Vaidya. Data entry was done by Gobardhan Thapa, Natalia Oli and Abhinav Vaidya. Data analysis was done by Abhinav Vaidya and Natalia Oli. The paper was written by Natalia Oli, Abhinav Vaidya, and Gobardhan Thapa.

Acknowledgments

The authors are highly obliged to all the participants of the study and the local leaders who facilitated conduction of the study. They are thankful to the medical students of the 13th batch of the Kathmandu Medical College for their contribution in data collection. They would also like to thank the post-graduate students, faculty members, and staff of Department of Community Medicine for their cooperation and support.

References

[1] World Health Organization, *Non-Communicable Diseases in the South-East Asia Region: Situation and Response 2011*, World Health Organization, New Delhi, India, 2011.

[2] D. Yach and C. Hawkes, "Chronic diseases and risks," in *International Public Health*, M. Merson, R. E. Black, and A. J. Mills, Eds., pp. 273–313, Jones & Bartlett Publishers, Burlington, Mass, USA, 2006.

[3] S. Mendis, P. Puska, and B. Norrving, *Global Atlas on Cardiovascular Disease Prevention and Control*, World Health Organization, Geneva, Switzerland, 2011.

[4] M. M. Engelgau, S. El-Saharty, P. Kudesia, V. Rajan, and S. Rosenhouse, *Capitalizing on the Demographic Transition: Tackling Noncommunicable Diseases in South Asia*, World Bank Publications, 2011.

[5] A. Vaidya, S. Shakya, and A. Krettek, "Obesity prevalence in nepal: public health challenges in a low-income nation during an alarming worldwide trend," *International Journal of Environmental Research and Public Health*, vol. 7, no. 6, pp. 2726–2744, 2010.

[6] K. Anand, B. Shah, K. Yadav et al., "Are the urban poor vulnerable to non-communicable diseases? A survey of risk factors for non-communicable diseases in urban slums of Faridabad," *National Medical Journal of India*, vol. 20, no. 3, pp. 115–120, 2007.

[7] Linking Population, poverty and development, http://www.unfpa.org/pds/urbanization.htm.

[8] M. R. Montgomery and A. C. Ezeh, "The health of urban populations in developing countries," in *Handbook of Urban Health*, pp. 201–222, Springer, New York, NY, USA, 2005.

[9] Central Bureau of Statistics, *National Population and Housing Census 2011*, National Planning Commission Secretariat, 2012.

[10] CARE Nepal, *Health Problems among Urban Poor in Selected Slums along Bishunumati River in Kathmandu*, CARE Nepal Publications, 2008.

[11] A. Vaidya, "Tackling cardiovascular health and disease in Nepal: epidemiology, strategies and implementation," *Heart Asia*, vol. 3, no. 1, pp. 87–91, 2011.

[12] Nepal Health Research Council, *Prevalence of Non-Communicable Disease in Nepal: Hospital-Based Study*, Nepal Health Research Council, 2010.

[13] World Health Organization, *2008–2013 Action Plan for the Global Strategy for the Prevention and Control of Non-Communicable Diseases*, World Health Organization, Geneva, Switzerland, 2010.

[14] "300 families screened in slums," http://www.hollows.org.au/news-media/300-families-screened-slums.

[15] "Nepal—city slum dwellers' health condition appalling," http://urbanhealthupdates.wordpress.com/2011/04/01/nepal-city-slum-dwellers-health-condition-appalling/.

[16] "Mobile health clinics to target city slums," http://www.myrepublica.com/portal/index.php?action=news_details&news_id=34541.

[17] L. W. Riley, A. I. Ko, A. Unger, and M. G. Reis, "Slum health: diseases of neglected populations," *BMC International Health and Human Rights*, vol. 7, article 2, 2007.

[18] P. Waingankar and D. Pandit, "A cross sectional study of coronary heart disease in Urban slum population of Mumbai," *International Journal of Medical and Clinical Research*, vol. 3, no. 5, pp. 180–189, 2012.

[19] Ministry of Health and Population, *Nepal Non-Communicable Diseases Risk Factors Survey 2007*, Ministry of Health and Population, Kathmandu, Nepal, 2008.

[20] World Health Organization, *WHO Steps Instrument Question-by-Question Guide (Core and Expanded)*, World Health Organization, Geneva, Switzerland, 2008.

[21] A. V. Chobanian, G. L. Bakris, H. R. Black et al., "Seventh report of the joint national committee on prevention, detection, evaluation, and treatment of high blood pressure," *Hypertension*, vol. 42, no. 6, pp. 1206–1252, 2003.

[22] World Health Organization, *Non-Communicable Disease Risk Factor Survey Myanmar 2009*, World Health Organization, 2011.

[23] World Health Organization and Indian Council of Medical Research, *Report of the Surveillance of Risk Factors of Non-Communicable Diseases (STEP 1 and 2) from Chennai*, World Health Organization and Indian Council of Medical Research, 2002.

[24] R. Singh, M. Mukherjee, R. Kumar, and R. Pal, "Study of risk factors of coronary heart disease in Urban slums of patna," *Nepal Journal of Epidemiology*, vol. 2, no. 3, pp. 205–212, 2012.

[25] K. R. Thankappan, B. Shah, P. Mathur et al., "Risk factor profile for chronic non-communicable diseases: results of a community-based study in Kerala, India," *Indian Journal of Medical Research*, vol. 131, no. 1, pp. 53–63, 2010.

[26] S. R. Niraula, "Tobacco use among women in Dharan, Eastern Nepal," *Journal of Health, Population and Nutrition*, vol. 22, no. 1, pp. 68–74, 2004.

[27] A. Nath, S. Garg, S. Deb, A. Ray, and R. Kaur, "A study of the profile of behavioral risk factors of non communicable diseases in an urban setting using the WHO steps 1 approach," *Annals of Tropical Medicine and Public Health*, vol. 2, no. 1, pp. 15–19, 2009.

[28] A. Vaidya, P. K. Pokharel, P. Karki, and S. Nagesh, "Exploring the iceberg of hypertension: a community based study in an eastern Nepal town," *Kathmandu University Medical Journal*, vol. 5, no. 19, pp. 349–359, 2007.

Permissions

The contributors of this book come from diverse backgrounds, making this book a truly international effort. This book will bring forth new frontiers with its revolutionizing research information and detailed analysis of the nascent developments around the world.

We would like to thank all the contributing authors for lending their expertise to make the book truly unique. They have played a crucial role in the development of this book. Without their invaluable contributions this book wouldn't have been possible. They have made vital efforts to compile up to date information on the varied aspects of this subject to make this book a valuable addition to the collection of many professionals and students.

This book was conceptualized with the vision of imparting up-to-date information and advanced data in this field. To ensure the same, a matchless editorial board was set up. Every individual on the board went through rigorous rounds of assessment to prove their worth. After which they invested a large part of their time researching and compiling the most relevant data for our readers. Conferences and sessions were held from time to time between the editorial board and the contributing authors to present the data in the most comprehensible form. The editorial team has worked tirelessly to provide valuable and valid information to help people across the globe.

Every chapter published in this book has been scrutinized by our experts. Their significance has been extensively debated. The topics covered herein carry significant findings which will fuel the growth of the discipline. They may even be implemented as practical applications or may be referred to as a beginning point for another development. Chapters in this book were first published by Hindawi Publishing Corporation; hereby published with permission under the Creative Commons Attribution License or equivalent.

The editorial board has been involved in producing this book since its inception. They have spent rigorous hours researching and exploring the diverse topics which have resulted in the successful publishing of this book. They have passed on their knowledge of decades through this book. To expedite this challenging task, the publisher supported the team at every step. A small team of assistant editors was also appointed to further simplify the editing procedure and attain best results for the readers.

Our editorial team has been hand-picked from every corner of the world. Their multi-ethnicity adds dynamic inputs to the discussions which result in innovative outcomes. These outcomes are then further discussed with the researchers and contributors who give their valuable feedback and opinion regarding the same. The feedback is then collaborated with the researches and they are edited in a comprehensive manner to aid the understanding of the subject.

Apart from the editorial board, the designing team has also invested a significant amount of their time in understanding the subject and creating the most relevant covers. They scrutinized every image to scout for the most suitable representation of the subject and create an appropriate cover for the book.

The publishing team has been involved in this book since its early stages. They were actively engaged in every process, be it collecting the data, connecting with the contributors or procuring relevant information. The team has been an ardent support to the editorial, designing and production team. Their endless efforts to recruit the best for this project, has resulted in the accomplishment of this book. They are a veteran in the field of academics and their pool of knowledge is as vast as their experience in printing. Their expertise and guidance has proved useful at every step. Their uncompromising quality standards have made this book an exceptional effort. Their encouragement from time to time has been an inspiration for everyone.

The publisher and the editorial board hope that this book will prove to be a valuable piece of knowledge for researchers, students, practitioners and scholars across the globe.

List of Contributors

Abdullah Balkhair, Zakariya Al-Muharrmi, Raiya Al-Rashdi, Mansoor Al-Jabri and Fatma Neilson
Department of Infection Control, Sultan Qaboos University Hospital, Sultan Qaboos University, Muscat, Oman

Yahya M. Al-Farsi and Marah El-Beeli
Department of Family Medicine and Public Health, College of Medicine and Health Sciences, Sultan Qaboos University, P.O. Box 35, P.C. 123 Al-Khoud, Muscat, Oman

Sara S. Al-Adawi
Oman Medical College, Sohar Campus, Al Tareef, Sohar, Oman

Samir Al-Adawi
Department of Behavioral Medicine, College of Medicine and Health Sciences, Sultan Qaboos University, Muscat, Oman

Sandra C. Fuchs
Postgraduate Studies Program in Cardiology, School of Medicine, Clinical Research Center, No. 5 Andar, Hospital de Clinicas de Porto Alegre, Universidade Federal do Rio Grande do Sul, Rua Ramiro Barcelos 2350, 90035-903 Porto Alegre, RS, Brazil
Postgraduate Studies Program in Epidemiology, School of Medicine, Universidade Federal do Rio Grande do Sul, 90035-003 Porto Alegre, RS, Brazil
National Institute for Health Technology Assessment (IATS/CNPq), Hospital de Clinicas de Porto Alegre, 90035-903 Porto Alegre, RS, Brazil

Maria Letícia R. Ikeda
Postgraduate Studies Program in Cardiology, School of Medicine, Clinical Research Center, No. 5 Andar, Hospital de Clinicas de Porto Alegre, Universidade Federal do Rio Grande do Sul, Rua Ramiro Barcelos 2350, 90035-903 Porto Alegre, RS, Brazil

Ajácio B. M. Brandão and Paulo R. Alencastro
National Institute for Health Technology Assessment (IATS/CNPq), Hospital de Clinicas de Porto Alegre, 90035-903 Porto Alegre, RS, Brazil

Ricardo A. A. Ximenes
National Institute for Health Technology Assessment (IATS/CNPq), Hospital de Clinicas de Porto Alegre, 90035-903 Porto Alegre, RS, Brazil
Department of Clinical Medicine, Universidade de Pernambuco, 50670-901 Recife, PE, Brazil

Heloísa Ramos Lacerda
Department of Tropical Medicine, Universidade Federal de Pernambuco, 50610-110 Recife, PE, Brazil

Maria de Fátima P. M. de Albuquerque
Research Center Aggeu Magalhaes, Fundacao Oswaldo Cruz, 50.670-420 Recife, PE, Brazil

Ulisses Ramos Montarroyos
Institute of Biological Sciences, Universidade de Pernambuco, 50670-901 Recife, PE, Brazil

Max W. Nery
Institute of Tropical Pathology and Public Health, Universidade Federal de Goias, 74605050 Goiania, GO, Brazil

Nêmora T. Barcellos and Fernando H. Wolff
Postgraduate Studies Program in Cardiology, School of Medicine, Clinical Research Center, No. 5 Andar, Hospital de Clinicas de Porto Alegre, Universidade Federal do Rio Grande do Sul, Rua Ramiro Barcelos 2350, 90035-903 Porto Alegre, RS, Brazil
National Institute for Health Technology Assessment (IATS/CNPq), Hospital de Clinicas de Porto Alegre, 90035-903 Porto Alegre, RS, Brazil

Demócrito de B. Miranda-Filho
National Institute for Health Technology Assessment (IATS/CNPq), Hospital de Clinicas de Porto Alegre, 90035-903 Porto Alegre, RS, Brazil
Department of Clinical Medicine, Universidade de Pernambuco, 50670-901 Recife, PE, Brazil
Department of Tropical Medicine, Universidade Federal de Pernambuco, 50610-110 Recife, PE, Brazil

Marilia D. Turchi
National Institute for Health Technology Assessment (IATS/CNPq), Hospital de Clinicas de Porto Alegre, 90035-903 Porto Alegre, RS, Brazil
Institute of Tropical Pathology and Public Health, Universidade Federal de Goi´as, 74605050 Goiania, GO, Brazil

Flávio D. Fuchs
Postgraduate Program in Cardiology, School of Medicine, Universidade Federal do Rio Grande do Sul, R. Ramiro Barcelos 2600, 90035-003 Porto Alegre, RS, Brazil
National Institute for Health Technology Assessment (IATS/CNPq), Clinical Research Center, Hospital de Clinicas de Porto Alegre, R. Ramiro Barcelos 2350, 90035-003 Porto Alegre, RS, Brazil

Rosmeri K. Lazzaretti and Regina Kuhmmer
Servico de Cardiologia, Hospital de Clınicas de Porto Alegre, Universidade Federal do Rio Grande do Sul, 90035-903 Porto Alegre, RS, Brazil

Aline S. Gasparotto, Marina G. de M. Sassi and Vanessa S. Mattevi
Universidade Federal de Ciencias da Saude de Porto Alegre, Rua Sarmento Leite 245, Sala 309, 90050-170 Porto Alegre, RS, Brazil

Jussara M. Silveira
Hospital Universitario Dr. Miguel Riet Correa Jr., 96200-000 Rio Grande, RS, Brazil

Mariângela F. Silveira and Cezar A. T. Pinheiro
Servico de Assistencia Especializada em HIV/AIDS, Universidade Federal de Pelotas, 96030-001 Pelotas, RS, Brazil

Eduardo Sprinz
Servico de Medicina Interna, Hospital de Clınicas de Porto Alegre, Universidade Federal do Rio Grande do Sul, 90035-903 Porto Alegre, RS, Brazil

Carísi A. Polanczyk
Servico de Cardiologia, Hospital de Cınicas de Porto Alegre, Universidade Federal do Rio Grande do Sul, 90035-903 Porto Alegre, RS, Brazil
Servico de Cardiologia, Hospital de Clınicas de Porto Alegre, Universidade Federal do Rio Grande do Sul, Instituto de Avaliac¸˜ao de Tecnologias em Sa´ude, 90035-903 Porto Alegre, RS, Brazil

Rossana P. Basso
Hospital Universitario Dr. Miguel Riet Correa Jr., 96200-000 Rio Grande, RS, Brazil
Servico de Assistencia Especializada em HIV/AIDS, Universidade Federal de Pelotas, 96030-001 Pelotas, RS, Brazil

Denizar Vianna Araújo and Luciana Bahia
Department of Internal Medicine, State University of Rio de Janeiro, Boulevard 28 de Setembro, No. 77, Room 329, 20551-030 Rio de Janeiro, RJ, Brazil
National Institute of Science and Technology for Health Technology Assessment (IATS), CNPq, Rua Ramiro Barcelos, No. 2359, 90035-903 Porto Alegre, RS, Brazil

Steffan Frosi Stella
National Institute of Science and Technology for Health Technology Assessment (IATS), CNPq, Rua Ramiro Barcelos, No. 2359, 90035-903 Porto Alegre, RS, Brazil

Max Weyler Nery
Postgraduate Studies Program, Institute of Tropical Pathology and Public Health, Federal University of Goias, Brazil
Department of Medicine, Catholic University of Goias, Brazil

Luis Carlos Silva e Souza
Institute of Tropical Pathology and Public Health, Federal University of Goias, Brazil

Aline de Cássia Oliveira de Castro and Marianne de Oliveira Falco
Postgraduate Studies Program in Health Sciences, School of Medicine, Federal University of Goias, Brazil

Clarissa Alencar de Sousa and Jorge Tannus Esper
Postgraduate Studies Program, Institute of Tropical Pathology and Public Health, Federal University of Goias, Brazil

Erika Aparecida Silveira
School of Nutrition, Federal University of Goias, Brazil
Postgraduate Studies Program in Health Sciences, School of Medicine, Federal University of Goias, Brazil

Celina Maria Turchi Martelli
Postgraduate Studies Program, Institute of Tropical Pathology and Public Health, Federal University of Goias, Brazil
Institute of Tropical Pathology and Public Health, Federal University of Goias, Brazil
National Institute for Health Technology Assessement, Brazil

Erika Aparecida Silveira
School of Nutrition, Federal University of Goias, Brazil
Postgraduate Studies Program in Health Sciences, School of Medicine, Federal University of Goias, Brazil

Marília Dalva Turchi
Postgraduate Studies Program, Institute of Tropical Pathology and Public Health, Federal University of Goias, Brazil
Institute of Tropical Pathology and Public Health, Federal University of Goias, Brazil
National Institute for Health Technology Assessement, Brazil
Postgraduate Studies Program in Health Sciences, School of Medicine, Federal University of Goias, Brazil

Adrian Zaragoza Bastida, Lilia P. Bustamante Montes and Ninfa Ramırez Duran
Facultad de Medicina, Universidad Aut´onoma del Estado de M´exico, 50180, Toluca, MEX, Mexico

Marivel Hernandez Tellez
Centro Interamericano de Recursos del Agua, Universidad Aut´onoma del Estado de M´exico, 50200, Toluca, MEX, Mexico

Imelda Medina Torres and Jaime Nicolas Jaramillo Paniagua
Facultad de Medicina Veterinaria Zootecnia, Universidad Autonoma del Estado de Mexico, 50200, Toluca, MEX, Mexico

German David Mendoza Martınez
Departamento de Produccion Agrıcola y Animal, Universidad Autonoma Metropolitana, 04960, Mexico, DF, Mexico

Ali Reza Rezaee
Department of Animal Science, Faculty of Agriculture, Ferdowsi University of Mashhad, Mashhad, Iran

Mohammad Mehdi Banoei and Massoud Houshmand
Department of Medical Genetics, National Institute of Genetic Engineering and Biotechnology, Tehran 14155-6343, Iran

Elham Khalili
Department of Genetics, Special Medical Center, Tehran, Iran

Mohamed A. Daw
Department of Medical Microbiology & Immunology, Tripoli Medical Centre, Faculty of Medicine Tripoli,
P.O. Box 82668, Tripoli, Libya

Aghnaya A. Dau
Department of Vascular Surgery, Tripoli Medical Centre, Faculty of Medicine Tripoli,
P.O. Box 82664, Tripoli, Libya

Feng-Jiao Li, Hong-Fang Ji and Liang Shen
Shandong Provincial Research Center for Bio informatic Engineering and Technique, Shandong University of Technology, Zibo 255049, China

Vjekoslav Bakašun and Yana Pahor
Public Health Institute, 51000 Rijeka, Croatia

Angela Andréia Franca Gravena, William Augusto de Mello, Deise Helena Pelloso Borghesan, Sheila Cristina Rocha Brischiliari and Maria Dalva de Barros Carvalho
Postgraduate Health Sciences Program, Maringa State University, Colombo Avenue 5790, 87020-900 Maringa, PR, Brazil

Catia Milene Dell Agnolo, Tiara Cristina Romeiro Lopes and Marcela de Oliveira Demitto
Department of Nursing, Postgraduate Nursing Program, Maringa State University, Nossa Senhora da Gloria Street, 56-A Jardim, Sao Jorge, 87080-620 Maringa, PR, Brazil

Sandra Marisa Pelloso
Postgraduate Health Sciences Program, Maringa State University, Colombo Avenue 5790, 87020-900 Maringa, PR, Brazil
Department of Nursing, Postgraduate Nursing Program, Maringa State University, Nossa Senhora da Gloria Street, 56-A Jardim, Sao Jorge, 87080-620 Maringa, PR, Brazil

Alexandra-Cristina Paunescu, Sylvie Dodin, Éric Dewailly and Suzanne Côté
Axe Sante des Populations et Pratiques Optimales en Sante, Centre de Recherche du CHU de Quebec, Quebec, QC, Canada G1V 2M2

Pierre Ayotte
Axe Sante des Populations et Pratiques Optimales en Sante, Centre de Recherche du CHU de Quebec, Quebec, QC, Canada G1V 2M2
Laboratoire de Toxicologie, Institut National de Sante Publique du Quebec, 945 AvenueWolfe, Quebec, QC, Canada G1V 5B3

Gert Mulvad
Center of Primary Health Care, Queen Ingrid's Hospital and Greenland Center for Health Research, University of Greenland, Nuuk 3900, Greenland

Henning S. Pedersen
Medical Centre, Dronning Ingrids Hospital, Nuuk 3900, Greenland

Alison Reid, Susan Peters and Lin Fritschi
Harry Perkins Institute of Medical Research, The University of Western Australia, Perth, WA 6009, Australia

Alison Reid, Susan Peters and Lin Fritschi
Harry Perkins Institute of Medical Research, The University of Western Australia, Perth, WA 6009, Australia

Renee N. Carey
Harry Perkins Institute of Medical Research, The University of Western Australia, Perth, WA 6009, Australia
Sir Charles Gairdner Hospital, B Block, Hospital Avenue, Nedlands, WA 6009, Australia

A. M. Qasim
Department of Community Health, University of Benin, Benin City, Nigeria
National Veterinary Research Institute, Livestock Investigation Department, Poultry Division, Vom, Nigeria

V. Y. Adam
Department of Community Health, University of Benin, Benin City, Nigeria

M. O. Kazeem
Department of Microbiology, University of Ilorin, Ilorin, Nigeria

Vanessa L. Short
Mississippi State Department of Health, 570 East Woodrow Wilson, Osborne-429B, Jackson, MS 39215, USA

Tameka Ivory-Walls
Office of Preventive Health, Mississippi State Department of Health, 522West Park Avenue, Suite P, Greenwood, MS 38930, USA

Larry Smith
Office of Preventive Health, Mississippi State Department of Health, 570 East Woodrow Wilson, Osborne-429B, Jackson, MS 39215, USA

Fleetwood Loustalot
Division for Heart Disease and Stroke Prevention, Centers for Disease Control and Prevention, 1600 Clifton Road, Atlanta, GA 30333, USA

R. V. Sudershan, R. Naveen Kumar, L. Kashinath and K. Polasa
Food and Drug Toxicology Research Center, National Institute of Nutrition, Indian Council of Medical Research (ICMR), Jamai-Osmania, Tarnaka, Hyderabad 500007, India

V. Bhaskar
Statistical Division, National Institute of Nutrition, Indian Council of Medical Research (ICMR), Hyderabad 500007, India

Waqar Al-Kubaisy and Nik Nairan Abdullah
Population Health & Preventive Medicine, Faculty of Medicine, Universiti Teknologi MARA (UiTM), Sungai Buloh Campus, Jalan Hospital, 47000 Sungai Buloh, Selangor, Malaysia

Sabzali Musa Kahn
Cultural Centre, University of Malaya, Lembah Pantai, 50603 Kuala Lumpur, Malaysia

Maram Zia
Faculty of Medicine, Syrian International University for Science and Technology (SIUST), Dara'a, Damascus, Syria

Adesola O. Sangowawa, Olukemi K. Amodu, Subulade A. Olaniyan, Folakemi A. Amodu, Peter E. Olumese and Olayemi O. Omotade
Institute of Child Health, College of Medicine, University of Ibadan, Ibadan 200001, Nigeria

Takashi Yamashita
Department of Sociology, University of Nevada, Las Vegas, Las Vegas, NV 89154, USA

Douglas A. Noe
Department of Statistics, Miami University, Oxford, OH 45056, USA

A. John Bailer
Department of Statistics, Miami University, Oxford, OH 45056, USA
Scripps Gerontology Center, Miami University, Oxford, OH 45056, USA

Adam J. Branscum
Biostatistics Program, College of Public Health and Human Sciences, Oregon State University, Corvallis, OR 97331, USA

Wesley O. Johnson
Department of Statistics, University of California, Irvine, CA 92697, USA

Andre T. Baron
Tumor Biology Investment Group, Inc., Richmond, KY 40475, USA

Natalia Oli and Abhinav Vaidya
Department of Community Medicine, Kathmandu Medical College, Sinamangal, Kathmandu, Nepal

Gobardhan Thapa
Kathmandu Medical College, Sinamangal, Kathmandu, Nepal